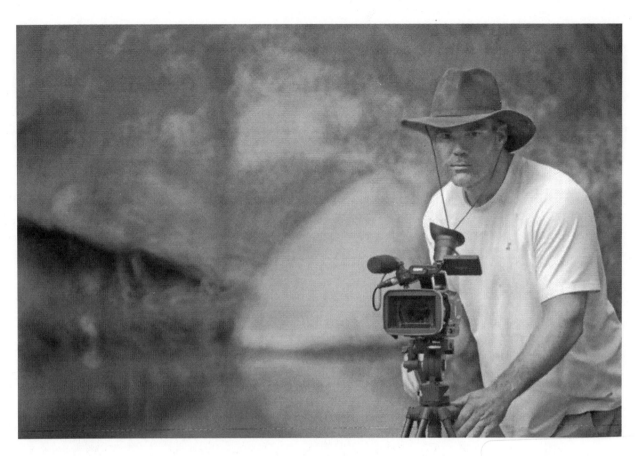

iCureCancer.com: The Book

By Ian Jacklin

www.archangelstudios.org

www.icurecancer.com

I Cure Cancer – The Book

Written and Published by

Ian Jacklin

1st Edition

May 2019

Ordering Information:

Quantity sales. Special discounts are available on quantity purchases by corporations, associations, and others. For details, contact the publisher at the address above.

Orders by U.S. trade bookstores and wholesalers. Please contact Big Distribution:

www.archangelstudios.org

email: gijacklin@yahoo.com

Printed in the United States of America

DISCLAIMERS

DEDICATIONS

I dedicate this book to my mom and dad, Gord and Carol Jacklin, who adopted me Aug. 22, 1968, and to my sister Mary; all of whom I worried could get cancer, so I wanted to be prepared. Also, to the two crazy, young kids Johnny and Mariah, my biological parents, for having me. Oh, and my nephews Breven and Tayvin for keeping me young.

Hope I don't forget anyone here, but I am who I am, to write this book now, thanks to these other folks too: Big Ian. I don't know his last name. He was probably 16 or so when I was 3. His name was Ian as well was known on the street as "Big Ian" and I was Little Ian. The point is, I knew someday I'd be Big Ian, and couldn't wait.

To Mrs. Ferguson, my Tecumseh public school 1st-grade teacher - She thought I could write well and told me to never stop! That was good for me to hear then and I didn't. I just wish they had spell check sooner! Mr. Doug Dyer and Mrs. Walmsly who also helped me in public school. I'll never forget them including Mr. Green at H. B. Beal Secondary School.

My childhood friends, Lorne Albert and Howie Perkins from the Grey St. / Simcoe St. in London, Ontario, Canada. I learned the street from these guys. Even though my adopted parents lived in the middle-class area in South London I, for some reason, felt drawn to the north of the bridge, "The Hood" right before downtown. Although I was born in Chatham, Ontario, Canada I was later to find out my biological mom was indeed from and back in London. Turns out it was just 4 blocks away from Lorne's house. John Paul Clancy, Chris Clancy, and Rob Walker, spiritual brothers forever. My cousin Duaigne Little for the hunting daze. Frogs and women when we were older. Oh, and Joel Croncrieght, who got beat up in front of me in grade nine which made me join karate. That was huge.

Ken from London's Boys and Girls Club - Boxing. Terry Albert. Ralph Chinnick RIP who was my karate master in Kenpo Karate at Professional Self Defense Studios. His black belt Rene... and for the life of me, I can't remember his last name, sorry. Probably becasue he kicked me in the head too many times. Great kicker that Rene! He and Paul Roemelle were my first sparring partners and really set me in the right direction for the fight game. Leo Loucks. Martin Freetolay. Peter Free and all the Kitchen Kicks guys. Ernie Bheem.

Mike Bernardo's Karate. N'Amerind Boxing. East Side Boxing, Rob Caron, Frank Rodriguez, Jim Reed, Jim Fields, Ron Day, John Davenport, Harold "The Shadow" Knight, Antoine Tarver, and Lennox Lewis.

Mr. Rodriguez from Elmonte Kickboxing. Ruben Urquidez, Javier Mendez of AKA and all the fighters that got in the ring with me. Don "The Dragon" Wilson for everything! David Huey for Expert Weapon.

Reuben Urkquidez, Efren Contreas, Hector Pena, Benny "The Jet" Urquidez for the Jet Center and choreography for Death Match. Joanne Baron DW Brown Acting Studios, Tom and Mary. The Roxbury. My theatrical agent Joe Kolkowitz of Players Talent. Jay Davis. Oleg Zatsepin for the comedy relief! Sha Ali for always being there. Max Davidson too. The Irish Times. Hilary for all the great photo shoots in LA! David Paul the Barbarian / Photographer. Todd Stewart. Bobnoxious, Joe Mitchell for "The Jackal" mini-doc.

Rob Walker, Lynn Dwight, Jack and Les Sickles, London's favorite Chiropractor, Dr. Hardick – love my Cancer Killer Shirt! Adrenaline MMA, Turners Drug Store for also having holistic medicine! London Free Press for all the articles and CFPL channel 10. Rogers cable 13. CJBK FM 96 CKSL and what the heck, everyone in Canada!

Bobby Williams and Mariel Hemingway for everything. J. Cynthia Brooks for inspiring the movie which led to this, book. Rev Lynne Deverges, she is an Essene master. Dr. Bernardo for his warriorship, love, and light he had for the human race. The Cancer Control Society & Frank & Lorraine! Emily Woods for teaching me how to be a boss. Brent Beaty and Debora Berg my American mom and lil' bro. Dan James for the numerology! Raul Rodriguez my big brother from another mother... Everyone in the movie and this book. Rose Bud, Charles Foster Cane.

Ian Jacklin

FOREWARD

Ian Jacklin is an amazing and unique addition to the alternative cancer solution scene. Alternative simply means natural approaches that work without harmful side effects compared to the accepted cancer treatments that have created the multi-billion dollar "cancer industry" with its dismal cure rate. Ian grew up in Canada and became a North America kick-boxing champion who was ranked number two in the world at one time. During that time, he moved to Los Angeles where he achieved his North American kickboxing championship and got involved as an actor in several martial arts movies that were popular during the 1990s. During that time, he got personally involved with another young actress who had survived terminal cervical cancer without submitting to the accepted orthodox cancer industry of cut, burn, and poison (surgery, radiation therapy, and chemotherapy). She opened his eyes to the fact that cancer victims don't have to be chemo or radiation victims to survive cancer with good health. The same attitude that inspired him to become the best fighter he could be after helplessly watching his ninth-grade school buddy get beat up became an inspiration to spread the word of how a bully cancer industry creates cowed victims who succumb to harmful treatments. The adverse effects that cause many deaths are attributed to cancer and swept under the rug. So, he began filming documentaries and interviews of cancer survivors and medical practitioners who use natural means for re-establishing health as the solution over cancers of all kinds. Unlike most writers, myself included, who are not health practitioners or cancer survivors, Ian did not get his material for this book from other published sources. His thirst for knowledge and his unbridled pursuit of cancer health truth has led to recording direct communication with several in the field of alternative cancer solutions, both preventative and curative. From Ian's relentless pursuit of picking the finest brains within the alternative cancer therapy field, a lot of information has been amassed to offer several options for preventing and curing cancer. This wide variety of options inspires a great deal of hope and confidence that will encourage anyone, with or without cancer, to understand what he or she can do to both prevent and cure cancer without the rigors and expense of what the cancer industry insists is the only solution. It also allows the reader to cherry pick healing options that resonate. And as you may assume from Ian's background as a fighter, actor, and documentary filmmaker, this book is not written in a dry academic style. He doesn't pull punches and kicks. It's packed with passion and the enthusiasm of one who is discovering the suppressed health information that the arrogant cancer establishment manages to maintain despite continually losing its half-century trillion dollars wasted "war on cancer." **- Paul Fossa, Holistic Author**

Dr. Bernardo C. Majalca was a giant in a league of a handful of cancer specialists worldwide. He would try every new modality to help his (typically) late-stage cancer patients; the majority considered terminal. It was rare that he would find something that clinically worked for his patients. Many times, I would read in the medical journals something that appears as it should work theoretically, but time and time again he would tell me it doesn't work clinically, in patients. Medicine is typically very collegial and friendly among practitioners — everyone is considered 'right' to some degree. But Dr. B. would be brutally frank and would never equivocate — it either works or it doesn't, period. I respected that quality. His unprecedented number of successes speak for themselves. Ian's film depicts Dr. B. brilliantly.

Dr. Bernardo was remarkable, to say the least. In 1986 he began Preventive Medical Research. For more than 20 years, his objective was to research the published medical literature and look for the missing links for a cure for cancer with alternative therapies. He embraced my work on Essential Oils (EFA's) as a 'missing link' and added it to his protocol, improving patient results. Dr. B Bernardo never stopped working and researching. His passion for helping his patients, regardless of personal financial gain, was always his priority. He was the rarest of gems. - **Prof. Brian Peskin, Author**

Clinical Results with the Peskin Protocol Physicians utilizing the Peskin Protocol report significant improvements in patient outcomes across a broad spectrum of conditions. "The Hidden Story of Cancer" has provided a great breakthrough in the treatment of our cancer patients. The addition of 5-725 mg Peskin Protocol EFA capsules t.i.d. along with our protocol has brought a dramatic difference, unbelievable and rapid improvement.

Patient 1: 80-lb female with stage III lung cancer was in full remission in 90 days.

Patient 2: Two inoperable brain tumors (1 cm), unable to speak or navigate had 40% reduction of both tumors in 60 days. Patient is able to walk and speak almost normally.

Patient 3: 8cm x 3 cm liver tumor told by his physician he had 30 days survival time. In 60 days of therapy, patient gained 30 pounds, 80% of tumor had calcified. Patient felt strong enough to return to work.

Patient 4: P.A.D. unable to walk more than 30 feet; with seven days of Peskin Protocol EFAs, she could walk four blocks. In ten days' time one can see a physical improvement in patient condition. We believe Peskin Protocol EFAs are the 'missing link' in cancer therapy.

The cost of treating our patients has dropped from $20,000 (USD) per month to $1,500 per month by eliminating the use of eight IVs daily. We saw no side effects. Within two weeks, patients typically see a great physical and mental improvement.

Bernardo C. Majalca, ND
Stage 4 Cancer Researcher and Consultant
San Diego, California

PREFACE

Hi, everybody! This is Ian Jacklin. Although much of this book is transcribed interviews, I do write some throughout the book and this preface is a good intro to what I do and what this book will do for you. We are talking about cancer. If you want to cure yourself, follow Dr. Bernardo's protocol in Chapter 7. Don't falter. Don't fall. This isn't a Jenny Craig diet. You screw this diet up, you not only don't lose weight, but you also stay acidic and die. So, listen up!

Okay, well here's the gist:

I found out in 1997 cancer is curable if you stay away from your oncologist. Turns out "Rockefeller Medicine" via the Rothschild's aka Western Medicine has the sole purpose of feeding the Archons aka Evil Spirits. Satan. The Boogeyman...with death and suffering. And making their minions - the Illuminati - rich and powerful. Yada, yadda. Rockefeller, the monopolist, had to figure out a way to get rid of his biggest competition. So, he used the classic strategy of "problem-reaction-solution." That is, create a problem and scare people, and then offer a (pre-planned) solution. (Similar to our terrorism scare, followed by the "Patriot Act"). He went to his buddy, Andrew Carnegie – another plutocrat who made his money from monopolizing the steel industry – who devised a scheme. From the prestigious Carnegie Foundation, they sent Abraham Flexner to travel around the country and report on the status of medical colleges and hospitals. This led to the Flexner Report, which gave birth to modern medicine as we know it. Needless to say, the report talked about the need for revamping and centralizing our medical institutions.

Based on this report, more than half of all medical colleges were soon closed. Homeopathy and natural medicines were mocked and demonized, and doctors were even jailed. http://woked.co/rockefeller-natural-cures-big-pharma . The point is, chemo and radiation work, sometimes, but with a whole load of side effects. In the meantime, Big Pharma makes a killing. Oh, and it usually kills you quicker and in a worse way than the actual disease.

This is why I made the film "iCureCancer.com" in 2006, it is free on YouTube now, to show the world there is a whole new paradigm out there called Holistic Medicine. Dr. Bernardo Maljaca's protocol was best then and it is still best now, so it's starring in my book about curing cancer. No one did it better than Dr. Bernardo and may he rest in peace. This is why I teach his protocol in this book. I pieced it together with his patients over the years and give it out to new ones. It's also on my I Cure Cancer FaceBook group, because it's what I'd do if I had cancer.

Remember, always say the words daily to yourself, "I Cure Cancer," because you do. After Dr. B's protocol, there are a number of interviews I did with prominent people in the cancer curing area. That's what I was studying here - how to cure cancer. I hope you like it.

Thanks, Lisa Smith, Carol Lirette, Jen Smith, and Dr. Ken W. Anderson for transcribing the interviews and making this become a reality in paper and ebook. Much appreciated.

Listen to everyone's heart and follow your own. Godspeed. **- Ian Jacklin**

TABLE OF CONTENTS

Chapter 1: Chris Wark Interview

Chapter 2: Background on Yours Truly

Chapter 3: What I Would Do If I Were You

Chapter 4: If I Had Money for A Holistic Treatment Center

Chapter 5: Too Broke for A Treatment Center?

Chapter 6: Dr. Bernardo's - (Excerpt from I Cure Cancer.Com)

Chapter 7: Dr. Bernardo's Protocols with Supplements

Chapter 8: Interview with Rhonda Majalca And Constantine Kotsanis MD

Chapter 9: Interview with Professor Brian Peskin, Essential Fatty Acid for Cancer

Chapter 10: Ian Jacklin interview with Burton Goldberg

Chapter 11: Ronnie Smith on Cannabis Hemp Oil

Chapter 12: Ian with Rick Simpson

Chapter 13: Dr. Vickers on the Improved Gerson Therapy

Chapter 14: Testimonial with Cynthia Brooks

Chapter 15: Dr. Nick Gonzalez - I Cure Cancer II Excerpt

Chapter 16: Rev. Lynne Herod-DeVerges – Spiritual Chapter

Chapter 17: Skin Cancer Cured Naturally – Gerson Therapy

Chapter 18: American Bio-Dental Center (Tijuana)

Chapter 19: Vandana Shiva – Venice Beach

Chapter 20: Robert Scott Bell of Natural News

Chapter 21: Interview Ian Jacklin with Dr. Matthew Loop

Chapter 22: Ian Jacklin Interview with Ty Bollinger

Chapter 23: Ian Jacklin interviewing Dr. Kelly Raber

Chapter 24: Richard Gordon - Quantum Touch

Chapter 25: Bob Williams and Mariel Hemingway

Chapter 26: Dr. Wallach (Dead Doctors Don't Lie) clip from icurecancer.com

Chapter 27: Extras

CHAPTER 1

CHRIS WARK INTERVIEW

Chris: Hey what's up, it's Chris from http://www.ChrisBeatCancer.com/ and today I have the pleasure of talking with and interviewing Ian Jacklin. Ian is a documentary filmmaker and kickboxing champion and he made a really, really, amazing documentary about people who've cured themselves of cancer, you know after their doctor's wanna... basically unable to help them and that movie is called icurecancer.com and when I saw it I was like man, I gotta interview Ian, clearly is an awesome dude. So, I wanna help share his story and what he is doing now.

Chris: So anyway, Ian, thanks for talking with me.

Ian: Hey, my pleasure. It's funny, I had already been following some of your posts and I thought, man, this is a young guy and he has really got his act together, he knows what he's talking about and he's taking steps to try and help others and that's the key. You know, a lot of people might discover that cancer is curable, do it on their own and then go back into the woodwork. You're standing up and shooting at the top of your lungs, 'LOOK FOLKS YOU DON'T HAVE TO DIE, you've been misled" and I really respect that. So, it's a pleasure for me to be here with you, brother.

Chris: Man, thanks so much. And you know, it's funny that you said that too because I was almost one of those people.

Ian: Really?

Chris: Yeah, I did, I went back into the woodwork. You know, I had cancer in 2003 and I had surgery then I used nutrition and natural therapies instead of chemotherapy to heal myself and restore my health. Of course, all of that is on my site. ChrisBeatCancer.com. But you know, basically, I just went back to work. And after about 7 years, you know, 7 years later I was like, people kept hearing about what I did and asking me and you know, kind of word got around and I kind of thought, "Alright, well it's been 7 years, may I should, you know, try to share my story publicly, maybe I can help more people." And that's when I started my blog or whatever. So... but yeah, I mean, you're right, there are so many people out there, you don't even hear about them that have healed themselves of cancer and they just, you know, get on with their life. And so that's part of my mission to like you is to share as many of those stories as possible because I really believe we can learn from the experience of others.

Ian: Yeah, back the late '90s, when I first learned about this... and this is cool, cause, it will explain my story real quick in a nutshell. I was dating this girl, J. Cynthia Brooks, we're were doing a play together, a beautiful actress, I always had a crush on her, as the story goes and we're still good friends to this day. She had just cured herself of terminal cervical cancer and it just blew my mind. So, I have never had cancer. A lot of people think I have and that's why I do what I do. No, she tossed me the ball and I was like, "Alright, I'm going for a touchdown with this because this is going to help other people and if I ever did get cancer, I'd also know what to do or my family. So, basically, I just learned that and figured that you know, if this story was on the nightly news... these stories... everybody was seeing, "Oh, they just cured themselves of terminal lung cancer." You know, then it would get in their psyche that that is possible. Right now, there is nothing like that. As you know, it's the medical mafia runs our medical system right now. So, you're never gonna hear the truth unless you get on the internet like this. And thank God for the internet, cause if it wasn't for this, we'd still all be in the dark ages, you know.

Chris: Yeah, absolutely. Absolutely. Yeah, as long as the internet is still uncensored which (chuckling)...

Ian: Yeah.

Chris: I don't know how much longer that'll go.

Ian: If they take that away, they may get the revolution they've been looking for (chuckling).

Chris: Yeah. Yeah, there'd be some trouble. So, ok, so, your girlfriend had it, and I mean it just kind of blew up in your mind and you're just like, this is amazing I gotta do something with this. I gotta make a documentary about it? I mean, how did that all come together.

Ian: Yeah, basically... cause, I didn't even believe her at first (chuckling)... at first, I was thinking, maybe she's just saying this to be cool, you know, to try and impress me or something, which is silly. But it was just so hard to believe, you know, that my doctor... and again, I only liken anything to my mother or my family, my loved ones, like if they went to the doctor, sent to an oncologist, would be sent to get radiation, chemotherapy, surgery, end of story. And I did not understand that. So, I just... it was good. I was a skeptic, 'cause there are so many skeptics out there still that I have to confront, or they confront me all the time, who I can always disarm in a matter of moments cause, I've got enough up here now in my brain. But that's because I played the skeptic, I played... when I was making, I said, "Okay, the best way to get to people, is documentaries, you know."

I was just an actor at the time, I didn't even know how to shoot or edit or anything. So, I taught myself. I was looking for money all along to fund it. I had friends, that had millions of dollars, you know, like $50,000, or $100,000, would have been a drop in the bucket to them. Either they didn't believe it, or they just... you know, rich people that don't like to part with their money even for good causes. So, I said, "The Hell with it." And I taught myself how to shoot and how to edit with a couple of rockumentaries I made. One in New York City, one in upstate New York. And then as soon as I thought I was good enough, I just started shooting cancer patients that had cured themselves of cancer cause as a fighter, I don't know if we've mentioned this yet, but I used to be a kickboxing champion and I also boxed with Lennox Lewis. So, I always went with the best of the best and who were the champions, I wanted to be champion, who's the champion, Lennox Lewis. I got to train with him. And some of the best kick boxers in the world. So, the same thing with anything else. I just started putting the camera in front of people... as far as I'm concerned, of people like yourself, you're the heavyweight champ or the world, for cancer curing, cause, you did it all on your own with no side effects and it's probably not gonna come back. You know, so that's what I started to do was study the champions basically and put it on tape for others to see, cause, the eyes don't lie. You know, we're looking at your soul when we're doing this whether it's on video or not. So, you can tell if someone is giving you the gears or not, more or less. I mean, the odd shyster might slip through, but in general, you know, and especially if I'm the one doing the interviews. I'm talking to them off camera, beforehand to people they know, and I can read energy pretty well and tell if someone is giving me the gears or not. And they never are. Why would anybody go out of their way, you know what I mean, to mislead someone? They're like you, you cured yourself, holy crap this works, you know. And you're very smart at colon cancer that you had cause Dr. Bernardo, who's you know the star of my first film, one of the stars, remember him screaming at the camera, "IF YOU HAVE COLON CANCER, IT WILL ALWAYS, ALWAYS, COME BACK... WHY... YOU DIDN'T ADDRESS THE PROBLEM... THE PROBLEM IS ACIDOSIS. YOU DIE OF ACIDOSIS YOU DON'T DIE OF CANCER USUALLY." And that's the thing if they were to cut out your tumor, fine, and then they think, "Oh, chemo and radiation, just in case there are any rogue cells." Oh, ya think? They just cut into it. They cut it out, they're flowing all through your body now, you know. So basically, those who've done the alkaline diet, which I'm sure you did, raise your pH, correct? Is that how you did it?

Chris: Yup. Yup, a big part of it.

Ian: That's the way to do it, the only way to do it. They just did a story on, I don't know if you caught that... well, it wasn't on me, it was on Jeff Speakman the martial art guy from back in the '90s, he had a big movie out called, The Perfect Weapon, he was like a hero for all us young guys coming up. Now he's got throat cancer, so one guy that has interviewed me before because of my kickboxing years, he also knows I'm now fighting the whole cancer industry, so he asked my opinion. So, half the article is about poor Jeff Speakman getting this cancer and I didn't know he was gonna write all of this in, but he said, "Yeah, Jeff said, the doctor said I got a 90 percent..." he's got stage 4 throat cancer, which means it's spread everywhere and it's really bad and he can't get surgery because of the vocal cords and it's a 90 percent chance that the doctors at this hospital are gonna help him. Now I hope and pray that's true. But from what I know, nobody has a 90 percent success rate in stage 4 cancers other than Dr. Kelly who had the enzyme protocols who Dr. Gonzalez in New York City is now doing that program. So, he may have a 90 percent success rate with pancreatic cancer and probably most cancers, but no western medicine has that.

I don't know if Jeff was trying to be kind to his fans and didn't wanna worry them, but if you got stage 4. and so I go on... basically, he asked me what I would do if I was in his situation. I said, "Well if it's a tumor, 3 percent success rate with chemo, that's a known fact across the board, you can look it up in different countries, different studies, 3 percent. The placebo effect is upwards of 20 percent in some cases so you're better off doing nothing than you are getting chemo. And I basically went on the say if you did what you did, alkaline diet, detox the system, pump up the immune system, he has a good chance of not only getting rid of it but if never coming back. But he's going for full-on radiation and chemo. And I just feel so bad. I mean, I don't know, maybe I'm wrong, maybe he's gonna make it. I really hope he does. It's just that everybody... Patrick Swayze, came along and I was trying to get a hold of him. Because, again, he had pancreatic cancer, Dr. Kelly which you can get via Dr. Gonzalez, 90 percent success rate with that, western medicine can't touch that figure. There's every star you can think of for the last... ever since I've been doing this, 15 years or so, I wanted to get a hold of them and say, "Look, just have an open mind and look at this." And not just stars either, any human being that crosses my path I try and put them on the straight and narrow, which the unfortunate part is, they've been brainwashed, you know, as I was when I was making the film, I kept thinking, "I'm gonna prove these guys to be quacks and that my doctor, oncologist, whoever, is right. These guys are quacks. There's no way this kind of travesty could be going on in this day and age. But it is." It's sad.

Chris: It is. Well you know, it's really interesting that you said that and I'm glad you just said the bit about, you know, the celebrities. Because you know, I get that question I'd say kind of frequently where people... this is a common question, "Well what about Steve Jobs? What about Farrah Faucet? I mean, you know, they had all this money, how come they couldn't cure their cancer?" And you know, my answer to that question is, "It doesn't matter how much money you have, it's all about the decision you make to treat yourself," you know.

Ian: The other thing, there is no silver bullet, you know. That's the first thing I tell people, "Look, this isn't, you know, magic. You... I'll tell you the statistics are 3 percent success rate for most chemos, most cancers, up to 40 percent for some of the blood cancers, but even 40-50 percent, that's horrible when you look at cannabis oil is almost 100 percent skin cancer. That's the latest thing, anybody out there who has cancer right now, I don't care how you get it, get some cannabis oil, you'll be very pleased in a couple few months from what I hear."

Chris: You're talking about cannabis oil, right?

Ian: Yeah, cannabis oil from Rick Simpson. I've been investigating a lot of that lately and I've been on the radio with Rick Simpson himself a couple of times. And you just look on YouTube, Google, Rick Simpson oil and look at how many people are getting on their saying, "Look, I used to have skin cancer, right here, here are the pictures." And they'll show you the boom, boom, boom, boom, all the way along until it's gone. I mean the proof is in the pudding, so that's another great thing. But we're getting offline there, what were we originally talking about... oh, Steve Jobs, I have to say this, because I get that one all the time too. Steve Jobs, (chuckling) they think he was... you know, sometimes geniuses are so smart they're stupid. I know, cause a lot of my friends are geniuses, 200 IQ's, but they can't walk and chew gum at the same time sometimes, you know. And I think some of them may get arrogant, I don't know what his issue was, I never met him, but I know that people are trying to put alternative medicine as a bad thing because he tried it and it didn't work. He didn't. He was just a vegan. And being a vegan is not good for you. A lot of people are gonna be pissed at me for saying that, but it's true, 6 percent of the population can handle a vegan lifestyle, everybody else needs meat, it's just the way we're made. There's a book called Eat For Your Blood Type or something... you know, I'm type O, I'm definitely a meat eater.

Chris: So am I.

Ian: But for spiritual reasons and acidosis, I only eat it once a week nowadays, and then I'm not talking factory farming meat, I'm talking organic free-range. That kind of thing, nothing from the regular superstore, factory farming is so full of steroids and crap it's disgusting. But, anyway, the Steve Jobs story, "Well he tried alternative and it didn't work." "No, he didn't try an alternative, he was just a vegan his whole life which was bad for him and that's probably why he got cancer, you need to eat meat." And so that's it, you know. That was his story. And that's too bad, even if you go vegan say 3 months, it's ok, cause it helps to detox, so if he would have done it three months, but took enzymes, but took high dose vitamin C, took laetrile, took DMSO to put all that as a penetrator into the cells... I bet he would have made it, you know.

Chris: Yeah, you know the one thing they never said about Steve Jobs, they definitely used his story to try to demonize nutrition and natural therapies. But you notice they never said what he did. And I've looked and looked and looked... what did he do? I wanna know. What did he do?

Ian: I really had to dig to find it. And I found guys like you and I that are already in this who have been doing it longer, that's where I heard it, you know, word around the campfire. I had it on one of my Facebook posts at one time. Yeah, that's all he did was maintain the vegan thing and that was it. And that's not enough.

Chris: Yeah. No, it's... you know, it's funny that you said, three months... that's what I did. I did 3 months of raw vegan. That was like phase one. And then I was working with a naturopath and he added clean meat, just like we talked about, organic, grass-fed, free-range meat back into my diet because I was not able to maintain a healthy weight on a raw vegan diet. I mean literally, I was 6'2" 135 pounds.

Ian: Woooahhh...

Chris: So, yeah, like, skeleton man... (chuckling)

Ian: (Laughing)

Chris: And so again, it's a very powerful detoxification diet, cleansing diet, healing diet... but for a lot of people it's not sustainable long term. And that's the main thing, it's like I don't wanna get in fights with vegans about this, but a lot of people get really caught up in the dogma of veganism as the healthiest diet for all. And you really have to eat a diet that works best for your metabolic type, your blood type, and your body type. You know, we're different body types, we're the same blood type, you and I, but I'm an ectomorph, you know, I'm a skinny guy anyway. And I have a super high metabolism.

Ian: Right, and I'm right in the middle. So, that's different, yeah.

Chris: Yeah, so anyway... but you know, for anybody listening, it's really important that you look at your blood markers and your bio-markers and really see what impact your diet is having on your physiology.

Ian: Yeah, the smartest guy I've probably interviewed to date, his name is Dr. Nick Gonzalez, he's the...

Chris: Oh yeah.

Ian: He was in Suzanne Somer's book, he's the enzyme therapy guy. And who I was just talking about that has the 90 percent success rate... or at least Dr. Kelly's studies say 90 percent on pancreatic cancer. He told me... he goes, "You're a meat eater." I go, "Yeah, yeah, how'd you know?" He goes, "I can just tell you are kind of ... you're energetic, you're an action kind of guy, you're a leader." I mean just, "You don't need blood tests or anything like that to figure out if you're a meat eater or not, if you wake up dreaming of bacon, you're a meat eater." (Laughing)

Chris: (Chuckling)

Ian: I do that all the time, I love bacon... shit... I'd eat bacon ice cream if they had it. (Chuckling) So yeah, and it's very true. So he's got 10 different diets, I'm almost full vegan nowadays!

Chris: Yeah...

Ian: He also taught me something too, which I haven't researched enough yet, but he taught me that... cause I always thought anybody that had cancer it's cause they're acidic, their pH level is low down around 5 and if you get it up to 7.2 – 7.4 as you know, cancer can't live. Well apparently, with the blood cancers, he's telling me it's the opposite. That you're too alkaline. Have you heard this before?

Chris: Yeah. I absolutely have heard that.

Ian: One of my friends now, whom I'm following for my movie, iCureCancer.com Part II, which is focusing on the fact, that even though you did and I now know how to cure cancer, right... you especially because you did it. Let's say you have a child. And your child has brain cancer or some kind of cancer and you want to treat them holistically because you know how to do it, you know it's gonna work and you know chemo, radiation and surgery is gonna kill 'em. You can't do that. Legally they will take your child away from you, throw you in jail and force that child chemo. I am following two families going through this right now. And I hate to say it, I don't see happy endings, but I'm hoping for it, but they've got 'em.... the kids are being forced the chemo. There's nothing they can do about it, it's murder. It's pure murder. There's a great movie called Cut, Poison and Burn.

Chris: Yeah.

Ian: I follow a couple of other families that went through this and it's just... I don't know how... I mean I understand them maybe not having any feelings for us adults because we're just numbers to them, useless eaters as they call us. But children? You're gonna do this to children? So that's why... I wanted to call Part II Baby Killers... but people are kind of saying, "Well that's kind of negative."

Chris: (Laughing)

Ian: But that's what they are, you know... guys like Ty Bollinger, you know, of Natural News.com... he's saying, "No, call them that. That's what they are." Usually, he's energetic and a warrior like me, he's like, "Call it Baby Killers." But anyway, I haven't decided on that, but I'm following these two families and just hoping, well, there's really nothing you can do, once they get you, you're kind of screwed.

Chris: Yeah. Once you're on their radar and I have seen Cut, Poison, Burn. In fact, I saw the screening at the Cancer Control Society a couple of years ago.

Ian: Ahh...

Chris: When it first came out. But you know, it's a very powerful movie and a lot of people don't realize that if you try to pursue any kind of nutrition or natural therapies for your child instead of chemo and radiation that you will be in jeopardy of the government taking your child away from you. Child protective services taking your child away from you and forcing chemotherapy and radiation on your child, is terrifying. Even for somebody like me, that has all this information and I just packed my head full of knowledge. I mean, still, the thought of having to deal with that is extremely scary and I hope I never have to. So, let me make sure, cause for anybody watching this, they've got to watch your first movie. It's ICureCancer.Com. I don't know if we've plugged it yet, but I want to make sure I plug it. Because it's really, really awesome. I mean it's just... it's just... you wanna hear from more survivors and doctors that are treating cancer successfully, naturally... and survivors that have done it, here's a bunch of them, www.icurecancer.com and you can go there, buy a copy of the movie and also donate to help fund Ian's new project which is basically Part II, that's what he's talking about right now, which is really focused in on... well like you said, about what to do if your child has cancer, like kind of like the industry works, right?

Ian: Yeah. Yeah, absolutely, thanks for reminding me about that. Yeah, and again, nobody is funding me for this. Again, I thought after I proved myself by making the first one on my own, you know, somebody would come along and go, "You know what you're doing kid, and you got a good heart. Here's a $100,000, here's $50,000, whatever, go do it. Just keep doing what you're doing." Now I've got the people behind me that are doing that, they don't have the $100,000, or $50,000 to give me, so they'll buy a movie for $35. Sometimes somebody will send me 3 dollars because they really believe in what I'm doing but they can't afford it, which I totally understand. Month-to-month I live, you know, my rent is due in a couple of weeks, I've got, I think maybe $7 dollars to my name, and I have to come up with a thousand.

And I'm not working, I can't work cause of my kickboxing days, I got a bad hip, I think I need a hip replacement, like Chuck Norris, had both his hips replaced, a couple of the guys I study, I guess it's par for the course when you're a wicked kicker, like I was known for being one of the best kickers. I'm paying for it now. So, it's just kind of a nightmare, but I never got anything. I don't have Hollywood people to come behind me because again, I'm trashing big pharma; I'm trashing the Illuminati, if you look, not to get too deep and crazy. I'm always told by my friends, don't talk so much about the Illuminati.

Chris: (Laughing)

Ian: …because it will take away from your message. I'm like, "Yeah, but it's true. And I learned it from this cancer thing." You know, I found out that Rockefeller, who is Illuminati, right up there with the Rothschild's owned the pharmaceutical companies in the early 1900s and this is why our medical system is screwed today. He invested into the medical schools, got members on the board and next thing you know, big pharma controls what our doctors learn. So, our doctors giving us the chemo and radiation. A lot of them don't even know that what they're doing is wrong. They believe in it. They don't know. They are so smart, but these highly intelligent people don't know how to think outside of the box.

That's the first thing I did was go back to, "Well where did it all change?" And that's when I figured out, "Oh, so… but what is Illuminati?" I said, so I looked that up. And then I found out about 911. After researching that, there's no denying, you know, without getting into it, but they lied to us about that one. And again, so that's the major problem of the world is the elite, the one percent. And I am grateful for that one movement that got kind of started there, you know, the Occupy Wall Street stuff, because at least now it's in our consciousness, it's in our vocabulary. If I say, "One percent, the elite…" the masses now know what that means, before they didn't, you know. So that's good, instead of saying Illuminati or Zionists or this or that I just go, "The elite, the one percent, the banks, the bankers, the billionaires that run everything." That's why we are in the situation we are.

We have to be our own doctors. Like you are, we have to be self-educated and thank God for the internet, we can be. You can learn more. I think Bill Henderson said this, in six hours on the internet than any oncologist out there. Cause you just go to what works, whereas they are taught, you know, what big pharma wants them to learn.

So that's very important people out there, you want to cure your own cancer man, it's not that difficult. Again, no silver bullet, but we're looking at success, in all my time, I'd say low end 60 to 70 percent success rates in end-stage cases using a good holistic alternative program which must include getting your pH level up, especially if you have a tumor type cancer, you need to get your pH from 5, which it probably is if you have cancer, to 7.2 or so. A pH level of 7.2 – 7.4 and cancer can't live and that's the one main thread through all protocols. But I will say this, again, looking at all this cannabis oil, Rick Simpson told me himself, cause he's been helping cure people for years now, decades, with the oil, that a lot of his people, he'll tell them, "Get on an alkaline diet, take the supplements, do this..." and they're just like regular people, they don't care, you know. They don't care, they just take the oil and it still works. And most interesting, and I plan on getting this family on tape if I can. It was awesome, after him and I did a radio interview, he called me at home and we just thought they should have recorded that, because we went on for about two hours.

He told me about this one family, that their child is right now in the hospital getting chemo, so they started sneaking cannabis oil into her feeding tube and a few months later the kid is cured of cancer. Now, of course, the doctor is saying, "Well the chemo is working we gotta keep going with the chemo." They're like, "No, no, no we used oil behind your backs, scum bag." (Chuckling) And still, he won't allow it, "Nope, you gotta stay on the chemo." See, if that was my kid, and that's probably why I don't have a kid right now, 'cause I would probably kill people. I would want to, especially if I didn't have a wife, say, if it was just me, single dad, and they murdered my child, I'd be like that cop right now running around LA shooting everybody. But I wouldn't be shooting the cops, I'd be shooting freakin' you know, the Illuminati, the politicians, the oncologists. I'm just kidding! Just kidding!

Chris: (Laughing)

Ian: (Chuckling) Well, you know, what I'm saying, it would drive you insane to watch, if you know how to save your child and they won't even give you that option, and you've got to sit there and watch them murder it. You know, I take my hat off to a number of people that I know are going through this right now.

Chris: I can't even imagine what that's like, as a dad... I mean, I've got two little girls. I'm a dad. And my girls are 4 and 8, and yeah, I cannot even imagine watching them suffer and being powerless to do anything about it.

Ian: Yeah, I wish – I'm shooting this film, right, ICureCancer Part II and I'm following Jay Matthews and his family, we're not allowed to mention his daughter's name anymore because that got brought up in court. They actually said that, "Who's this Ian Jacklin guy said he would kill anybody that did that (chuckling) to their kids?" Well, you know what do you expect, you're trying to murder my child, you know. But anyway, I stayed at his house and was getting his story. And every morning, the poor little girl, I would hear the screams, the first morning it happened, I was scared. I thought somebody had broken into the home and it was a home invasion, and somebody was being tortured with drills and vice grips and tortures. It scared the Hell out of me. Then I remember he told they have to go through that every morning, cause one of the medications that aren't even the chemo does that to her. They have to hold her down and giver her this shot and she's screaming murder, could you imagine having to even hear that happen to your daughter, let alone having to do it. I mean it's… what they're doing to that man is just horrifying... horrifying.

Chris: Wow, yeah. Unbelievable. Well, let me plug your site again. ICureCancer.Com. Go there, buy a copy of the first movie, donate to help Ian, I am personally pledging to donate to help Ian fund this next deal because it is important. What he is doing... he is doing what I'm doing. We're doing the same thing (chuckling) we're on the same team, that's why I'm excited to be able to share his story. But we gotta take a quick commercial break. We'll be right back.

Chris: Ok. We're back. Alright, so Ian, we're talking about ICureCancer.Com your first movie and Part II the movie you're working on. And let me ask you, when people, you know I feel like I know the answer you're gonna say, but I really wanna hear it. But when people say like, "You know, what do you mean, you know, natural therapies? What do you mean alternative therapies? Man, that stuff doesn't work, if that worked, they'd be using it." What do you say to that when people say that to you?

Ian: Well, it's great because that's what I used to say. And you know what's funny, Patrick Swayze said that. I always liked Patrick Swayze and people always called me Patrick Swayze when I was younger and I really wanted to reach that guy. When I saw him on Barbara Walters and he said those exact same words only he was really arrogant about it too, "Ehh my doctor would know it... blah blah blah..." and it turned around and bit him in the ass. So, I just tell them, you've been brainwashed. I tell them the story about Rockefeller, you know, so they understand where it started. Back in the day, medicine was okay, it was coming along they used what worked, then Rockefeller ruined it by big pharma. Now your doctor probably doesn't even know what he is doing is gonna kill you. What's worse is some of them do and they still do it. I think 75 percent of oncologists said they would never do their treatments they give to others.

Now to me, that means, you're a murderer. You're just committing manslaughter if you're killing people not knowing it, but if you know, that you wouldn't even do that, to me you're a murderer and I don't know how you sleep at night. But I basically explain to them that they've been brainwashed and then I have to get into that whole thing; the elite, the one percent run the world and we're just numbers to them, we're just useless eating animals the way they treat us. So, once they kind of understand that they're on their own and hopefully, you know, if they're 18 and above then they can make their own decisions, that's the only thing we got going for us there. But again, the child thing, that's why I'm hoping this film will help. I don't know how I'm gonna change it cause every state is the same, it doesn't matter. I've talked to parents and they've gone to every state and it's the same there's a standard of care, the standard of protocol that every oncologist has to follow with a child and its chemo, radiation, and surgery and none of them work. Not like the natural stuff does.

Chris: You know, something I want to inject is just right along with what we're talking about is, you know, there are studies that are published every year, hundreds of studies are published every year on natural compounds that can slow the growth of cancer, reverse the growth of cancer and kill cancer cells, published peer-reviewed studies. They come out every week practically. And so, the proof is already out there, it exists, and you can find it on pub-med. I mean, heck, you can get on pub-med and search for garlic and cancer, green tea extract and cancer, turmeric and cancer, you'll find all this amazing research.

But the problem is, you know, that argument that "Oh, if there was something better, we'd be using it, or we'd know about it." But the thing is, it costs $4 billion dollars, $4 billion, on average, to get a drug approved by the FDA. So even though there's research that shows these amazing anti-cancer compounds from nature, they can't be patented and there's no way they're gonna make their 4 billion dollars back.

Ian: Right. And that's key to explain to people that are new to, to explain that process to them. Cause, again, they're like, "No, they wouldn't be doing that if..." No, here's why. The elite, they are so smart, they set it up where it's gonna cost you billions of dollars to get a product out there. Hence, nobody ever does it because you can't make money off a non-patentable thing. So that's the problem. So that's why you gotta research on your own. Research on your own and go get your apricot seeds, get your cannabis oil and screw the system.

Chris: Yeah, yeah, tell me some of the best. We've talked about diet a little bit, but tell me, if you had cancer, take me through your systematic protocol that you would try first. Like what would say is one for Ian?

Ian: Okay, I've never really dived into this because I have never had cancer and when it comes to other people's lives I don't mess around, I send them to the best. I send them to Dr. Gonzalez; I send them to Oklahoma Camelot Cancer Center because they are very reputable great alternative cancer. And if people don't have money to go to a place, then I send them to Bill Henderson, you buy his book and for 195 dollars he'll be your personal cancer coach. You can call him any time, talk to him and he'll tell you. What I would do, if I had money, I'd go to Dr. Gonzalez or to Camelot Cancer Center. If I didn't, I'd call Bill Henderson and make sure what I had in my mind was okay, which would be alkaline diet, enzymes, laetrile and/or apricot seeds if I couldn't get laetrile intravenously done, apricot seeds.

I interviewed Jason Vale recently, who is like apricot God I call him but he wouldn't like that because he's a hardcore Christian (chuckling) but he's got http://www.apricotsfromgod.info.

His story in a nutshell is, he was using apricot seeds because the chemo and radiation weren't working for him. It was working, so he started selling the apricot seeds to others. It was working for them, FDA caught wind of it, came in, shut them down, threw him in prison for 5 years, totally bogus, the judge lied in the case, it was horrible. But he had to do five years and his cancer came back and I just interviewed him in New York City over Christmas time and his cancer is back because they know it's five years he couldn't follow the protocol and when he got out, he's a little messed up, he admitted it, and he wasn't eating right and now he's fighting it again.

So that was sort of a tangent, but basically, I'm saying apricot seeds are huge natural cancer cure and cannabis oil would be the first thing I would get. I would have no problem getting that in California cause it's legal medicinally here. I may have to make it myself because I haven't found anyone who makes that oil yet. But still, so that'd probably be it, alkaline diet, all the supplements to detox and boost, cannabis oil, apricot seeds and a lot of prayer and meditation, that's the key. Because whatever gave you cancer, especially if you're an adult, you know, it probably came from emotional trauma one way or another.

Dr. Hamer from "German New Medicine", he came up with that theory years ago and just now a lot of people are believing in it. I've seen it myself, the people that don't have it up here and here, they're just sort of like this downtrodden, depressed and they're "Oh' I'm trying to do it."

They don't make it. They never make it. But the ones that are probably like you were, "Hey, I'm fighting this, forget it. I'm researching." And they become a sponge and they cure themselves. I mean they're the ones. And it's the strong powerful mind and the people that have maybe a major, they lost a business, they lost a spouse, they lost a child, you know they can easily connect the cancer to something like that so you have to let go, forgive, forget, move on, maybe not forget, but at least forgive and move on because if you don't, if you're hanging on to that, you know, it's gonna be tough. All the physical stuff you're doing with the diet and everything, if you don't have a free mind, cause thoughts can make you acidic as well. You know, thoughts are acidic, they can be. Same as the food you eat, drinking a coca cola is acidic. Thinking bad thoughts towards somebody or somebody else, that's acidic. So that'd be pretty much it in a nutshell. But again, luckily, I am who I am so I can talk to my friends, they are like kung fu masters of this stuff so I would make sure I'm on the right thing. But anybody out there that wants to connect with me, I become that connection for you and I help people for free, I don't even charge if they can't afford it. It's nice if you buy a video or something, but I'm always online telling people and I don't give them advice, I just say this is what I would do if I was you. Because I'm allowed to do that, you know.

Chris: Yeah, I mean your opinion, you're allowed to have an opinion. (Chuckling) At least as of right now, you are.

Ian: Yeah.

Chris: I love everything that comes out of your mouth is perfect. It's great. I mean, it's like we're sharing a brain. But you're totally right about the stress connection. I mean stress and negative emotions are toxic to the body. They raise your stress... basically, envy, jealousy, hatred, bitterness, resentment, unforgiveness, am I forgetting one?

Ian: Did you have something bad happen to you when you got yours? Cause you're very young to get colon cancer.?

Chris: Yeah. Yeah, I was very young, 26. But you know, the thing is, I did not have an incident. I did not have a major traumatic incident. But most of the people that I coach... I'm a cancer coach on the side, and most of the people I coach almost all of them were in a very high-stress situation, some of them had very traumatic experiences leading up to their cancer, within a few years. You know, I didn't have any of those major traumas, but what I did realize is that I had a lot of negative emotion and low-level stress had a ton of work-related stress and I had negative emotions. Like just stupid stuff like unforgiveness, jealousy, envy and just things that I was carrying with me that I just had to let go of.

Ian: And that makes sense too, cause that second chakra, not to get too mystical, but there are 7 energy centers on the spine, you know, the first chakra is survival, the second is emotional and/or sexual, the third is like, power... do you know these, the chakras?
Chris: Yeah.

Ian: Okay. And then love and then creativity and communication, the third eye are psychic and connection to God. Whether you believe in that or not it's just interesting how almost anybody's cancer you can sort of wherever. Like if somebody gets lung cancer, they probably have issues with love, either giving it or receiving it. Down there, you're saying you were stressed, and you know, that makes sense.

So that's another thing, and I've learned this through the lady that woke me up. J Cynthia Brooks, cured herself of cancer and inspired the film. She had got me into the meditation too, it's Essene, it's a meditation that the Essenes used to do and it's all about energy. Jesus Christ wasn't a Christian he was an Essene. Your body is energy. So, this is good because we're on the same topic. If you have emotional issues somewhere in your body that you're holding onto because of a bad relationship or something, know that those energies, there's seven of them on the spine and they're called chakras. And if you just make them a reality, even if you don't really believe it, just believe it while you're doing your meditation. That's why it's called is grounding, you can sort of visualize grounding that chakra to the center of the earth where it's just gonna, anything that's there is gonna go and when it gets there, it goes out to wherever it came from and not only heals you but heals them.

Again, I don't care if you believe it or not, just do it. And it's a way of, because thoughts are energy and everything is energy, your body is holding energy in different parts of it. You need to release that energy and that's where Cynthia was great with her cancer and she's noticed from all the people that she's helped over the years that people may be perfect on their diet, taking every supplement they need to do but they don't do as good as the ones that do the mental work or the work, work, like really just let it go, you know, it's very important.

Chris: You have to have the will to live and you have to be willing to do whatever it takes to live. You know, there are two components to that. One is, admitting that maybe you have... you may be responsible in and willing to change and then the second part is, you know, not assuming anything. I mean being open to any and all options, leaving no stone unturned. You know, to use a cliché and chasing down every lead. (chuckling) Do you know what I mean?

Ian: Yeah.

Chris: That's just the common trait that I see among all the survivors that I know, they were just, they were determined to live and yeah, when you're determined to live you're gonna do whatever it takes. That means your diet, that means your emotional life, your spiritual life, examining your work environment. I mean, you just have to look at the big picture and make sure that in all these, you know, everything about your life. Something or many things could be contributing to your sickness, so you have to look at it all.

Ian: Yeah, and you see me squirming there a little bit, it's because you know, God bless you if you're in that situation. What if you're the guy who's got the kid that's been taken away by child services and is being forced chemo, what if you're that guy? You're lucky, I'm not that guy, lawyers. I hate the lawyers.

Chris: (Laughing)

Ian: I know that the oncologists, oh man! Again, my heart goes out to Jay Matthews and Eric, my buddy Eric Vigna he's going through it too. They're about to do blood, no, a bone marrow transplant on his kid. Bone marrow transplants don't work. Again, one of the smartest guys I know, Dr. Gonzalez, interviewing him, he was being taught how to do bone marrow transplants. He was doing them. And they were opening up bone marrow transplants like McDonald's in the '80s when he was learning this. He could have been a millionaire, multi-millionaire, and he just saw that first of all, 30 percent of the people that take the bone marrow, die, right away from the transplant. Die! 30 percent, guaranteed.

Chris: Wow.

Ian: And then he basically, I mean he can only say so much because he is an M.D. and he doesn't want to get in too much trouble. But he is basically saying, "It doesn't work." You know, it has worked, like one or two... it's worked... so they have to say it's worked. But it's just horrible and it's not only... cause basically what they do, and I've never known this so I'm glad he told me. When they give you high doses of the radiation and chemo, normally it would kill you, because it kills the bone marrow. So, they get bone marrow from somebody else and hit you with that super high chemo and radiation hoping that it's gonna get rid of it and then they give you somebody else's bone marrow transplant and they hope they can save your life with that. I mean it's just a brinkmanship way of doing things, it's horrible. So, this guy Eric Vigna. he's waiting... I can't believe he got this. He must have a nice social worker or something the child services allowed them to say no to the chemo for the daughter for now because they're trying to build up her strength to get the bone marrow transplant. But that's sort of... you know... ahh... that's still horrible, because ok, granted, nice they let her get off the chemo, 'cause it wasn't working.

That's the other thing too, I would see that a lot as being, "Okay, we're going to try this chemo and see how it works." If it doesn't work, stop using it. But they don't. They just give them more of it, which is horrible. But somehow, he got child services to say, "No, it's ok, she doesn't have to do chemo, let's just get her ready for bone marrow." So, he's doing everything in his power, doing the coffee enemas. She's just a little girl too, like maybe 9 or 12 or something. Every little thing you could think of, they're doing, cause he's praying and getting her meditating and everything. He wants to get rid of that cancer before it comes to bone marrow transplant time which I'm hoping and praying he does. But if he doesn't... I don't know what's gonna happen to that poor little girl, you know.

Chris: Yeah, it's a good thing that they had that window of opportunity to try to build up her body and her immune system and detox and do all those things, you know. Man, I hope it does work for them in the time they have to work with.

Ian: I know, but she's already gone through the chemo, big time. You know, so it's... I mean most alternative places will tell ya, "Yeah, we got an 80 percent success rate, if somebody came to us and has not done any chemo, radiation, surgery. If they've come to us and they've been through the gamut, they don't promise anything. There's only so much they can do. I know a number of cases where they cured their cancer. They had been through so much chemo, radiation, surgery... doctor said, "Go home and die." They went to the alternative and cured it. There was no cancer left in their body, but they died anyway. And of course, be the doctors will write it off as they died of cancer, but they didn't, there was no cancer in their body. They died of the chemo. They died of the cure, supposedly. It's unbelievable.

Chris: Yeah, the side effects are deadly. I mean, the treatments are brutal... it's, you know, it's frustrating as you know to watch people suffer and really not be given, you know, no options. You have one option, you know, and if you don't take this option, you're insane is what the oncologist told me.

Ian: Did you ever confront that scumbag?

Chris: (Chuckles) You know, I didn't. I never went back. He told me I was insane and scared... you know, completely scared... scared me to death.

Ian: Where do you live?

Chris: I'm in Memphis.

Ian: Oh, I was hoping you were in California and I was gonna say, "I'm gonna go grab my camera right now, you and me, we're gonna go to that oncologist office...."

Chris: (Chuckling)

Ian: and I might have to pass... and I'll start, and I'll shoot you confronting him and saying, "Hey do you wanna know how I did it?" And when he says, "No." Then I'll give you the camera, you put it on me and then I'm gonna tear him a new one.

Chris: (Laughing)

Ian: Cause that's what happened with Cynthia, when she went back to her oncologist at UCLA, they called her a medical miracle. She said, "Well don't you want to know how I did it?" "Nope." Scumbags.

Chris: Yeah. They can't do anything with that information. That's the problem. Even if they... even if you told them everything you did and they really liked it and wanted to do it, they're powerless. They can't do it.

Ian: Yeah, I know... but I still they're cowards because they don't have to do what they do. Sure, they gotta... you know, give up their money and stuff, but you know what you're murdering people. I mean, I don't go and rob banks. I could. I'm a pretty athletic guy. I could get a gun. I could probably do alright. I could kill people too and make a lot of money. But that's illegal and against God, you know and against my morals. Well, these guys are legally killing people. And they justify it, well I gotta send my kid to college. What? to be another murderer like you? I mean, these people...

I have had to go on welfare. I have been unemployed. I have scrambled my whole life just to make it. So let some of these guys... the fat cats that are used to being rich and having the Mercedes this and that, let them go and get food stamps for a while, you know. At least they won't be killing anybody. It's just... I'm getting pissed off.

Chris: (Chuckles) Getting all worked up Ian. (Chuckling)

Ian: Little work out (chuckles).

Chris: Well man, this has been really fun. Really great to talk to you. And let's just... again, promote and plug what you're doing. Because of Ian's first film, ICureCancer.Com is a must watch. I give it two thumbs up.

Ian: Thanks, man.

Chris: Buy yourself a copy. Go to ICureCancer.Com. Buy a copy of the movie. Watch the movie. Share it with people that you know. Because all it is its testimonies from survivors and its testimonies from doctors that are treating people with natural therapies and there's so much wisdom in that film and like I said at the beginning of this interview. We learn or we can learn from the experience of others. I mean, that's what life is all about. We learn from each other. And that's everything that I've learned, you know, I've learned from others. When I was desperate to heal myself, I found other natural survivors and I took their advice. So again, now the shoes on the other foot and I'm trying to push as much information as I can on nutrition and natural therapies because I know it helps people. It helped me. I mean, it's helping people that I know, people that are emailing me every day telling me, "Thank you, this is helping. This is working. This is what I did." You know, etc. so it's really an amazing thing. And then, of course, please consider, you know, just buying Ian's first movie will help him. But consider donating to help fund his next project because I know he's shot a lot of footage already; he's still trying to compile all this footage and get this thing edited and get it out there. So that'll be ICureCancer.Com Part II.

Ian: Yeah, basically, you know, I used to have it written on the website, but I got some guys throwing a golf tournament for me and so we didn't want to give out. Makes it look like I was too desperate for money or anything by putting well if you donate this much, you get this, you know. So right now, there is just a donate button. But if somebody throws a hundred bucks in because they can, you know, I send them a copy of part one and an IOU basically for Part II when it's done, you know. And if somebody really wants to come in as a producer and throw in, you know a thousand, or five thousand or more, executive producer stuff, we're open to that and we can negotiate as well. because basically, I have been doing this on blood sweat and tears. And in order for it to get edited properly and then I want it at all the big festivals like Sundance or whatever, whatever we can do. But that's not gonna happen without some help, because we need a little bit of extra, you know. But at the very least, get the movie for the information, that's the thing. Because I say anybody that watches my film is now an ambassador. You're now a teacher whether you wanna be or not, even if that's just giving it to your friend. You've got information in your hands that's gonna probably save lives, because it has been already, you know.

Chris: Awesome. Well thanks, Ian. Appreciate it, man.

Ian: Yeah, thank you brother, you're doing a great job, keep it up, man.

Chris: Thank you, we'll stay in touch for sure. And for everybody watching, thanks for watching. If you like this, please share it. Please like it on YouTube, please like it and share it on Facebook and Twitter. Help us get this information out there. Of course, you can subscribe to my YouTube channel and check me out at chrisbeatcancer.com. I've got a lot of information on nutrition and natural therapies and other survivors' stories besides mine. That's what I'm all about. So again, thanks for watching.

[See photo 1.2]

CHAPTER 2:

BACKGROUND ON YOURS TRULY

Okay, so now for some regular book reading for ya. Hello, my name is Ian Jacklin. I was born and raised in London, Ontario, Canada. I graduated high school as a slightly above average student and took my adopted folks' advice on going to college for electronics technology engineering. Big mistake. I'm a creative and active person so the math and science were much too boring and confusing for me to dig into it, so I dropped out after one semester and started an electrical apprenticeship program. After a few years of that occupation, I knew I had to do something else. It wasn't my idea of a happy, prosperous life going to an extremely cold or hot, dangerous, job site to the 9 to 5 thing for life. Fuck that.

Hold on, let me jump back a bit. Thanks to seeing one of my best friends, Joel get beat up by a couple of bullies. I could not handle watching helplessly and I begged my mom to put me in Karate, which to my amazement, she did because $40 a month was a lot of money in those days! So thus, began that which would become, dare I say, a famous life in the martial arts.

At 14 years of age, I started Kenpo Karate at "The Professional Self Defense Studios" run by my first master Ralph Chinnick. Decades later, Mr. Chinnick followed my holistic advice and extended his life many years saying "no" to chemo and "yes" to nature. RIP Sensei.

By 16, I had my first pro-kickboxing fight. By 20, I was the Canadian I.S.K.A. Champion thanks to Ron Day and Jimmy Fields at Kitchener Kicks. See, very early in my studies, I realized that although traditional Martial Arts were cool, with their Kata's and self-defense moves, I realized Bruce Lee was right in saying "you learn to fight by fighting". So, I did eventually get a black belt, but I knew kickboxing was the key to being able to beat someone down on the street, and that to me was most important. And as it turned out over the years, I not only saved my own life, but a few others as well, thanks to being able to punch and kick really hard and accurately.

An amazing thing happened, not too long after becoming the Canadian champion. Lennox Lewis won the gold medal at the 1988 Olympics and had his first fight in his hometown Kitchener, Ontario, Canada, which was where my gym was, and his designated training spot for the show. So, I got to spar with some of the other boxers that were there, and his trainer John Davenport saw a "white boy that could fight" and talked his manager Frank Mulroney into taking me back to England with them to be their light heavyweight. It was a dream come true especially because I was a kickboxer way before the MMA of today, so we made almost no money at all, but boxers did. I won't get too deep into things now, as I want to get on to why you are reading this book. To learn how to fight cancer.

After about 4 months I knew England was not for me. It rained every day I was there for 4 months. We got "Baywatch" on one of the 4 channels they had, and I knew I had to go to California for some sun. So, I left and went back to Canada with some highly sharpened boxing skills to add to my repertoire as a kickboxer, thanks to the trainers John Davenport and Harold "The Shadow" Knight.

So, back to what I was saying, fuck doing 9 to 5. There I was, 22 years old, and back to working construction. After a summer of that, I was totally miserable! So, with 3 days' notice, I said good-bye to my girlfriend, family, and friends and jumped on my motorcycle with a tent and sleeping bag and headed for Los Angeles, California. I had heard kickboxing was pretty big down there and Jean Claude Van Damme was just hitting it big time in the Martial Art Movie genre in Hollywood. That's all I needed to know.

Well, I achieved my childhood dreams of fighting for the world kickboxing championship against now famous UFC Trainer owner of AKA, Javier Mendez, no less! I got to star in a bunch of karate movies and TV shows. I had some amazing times in Tinsel Town and quite the behind the scenes stories from Madonna's feeding me chicken and Prince almost getting slapped by me for being so weird, just kidding, but he was really weird. Someday I'll write way more about all that but for now, we are on the healing, cancer thing.

That being said. Screw it, here's a Hollywood story for yah.

While I was acting, I studied "Method" by Stanislavsky. I took acting as I did fighting. I studied all the greats, especially Brando. You'd never know it if you have seen any of my films like "Kickboxer III" or "Expert Weapon" because I never studied until after they stopped making these low budget films. But, apparently, I did really good and was told I was like a young Brando and one of my peers told me the teacher said I was the best he had ever seen walk through the doors! So, although I never won an Oscar; I hear I could have. One student who went on to be a respected director actually drew an Oscar on a piece of paper and gave it to me. I don't bring this up to brag, but to show that whatever I put my mind to, I achieve. I did in the martial arts, acting and would do in my next dream of becoming a filmmaker who would make a difference in the world.

Karate films were fun in my 20's but I was now hitting 30 and knew there was more to life than fame and fun. It's called righting wrongs. While doing all that, I also made connections with big money people whom I'd thought would fund my next dream to rid the world of disease, famine, and toxicity. Or at least start with curing cancer, since I just figured out how to do that. But my cries fell upon deaf ears.

So, I still needed them to get my message out there, which at that moment, was "cancer is curable if you stay away from your oncologist. Rockefeller is Draconian medicine designed to kill you and make them richer." Well, no one would fund me. So, I got pissed off and just taught myself how to shoot and edit and soon, as I was good enough, I made "ICureCancer.com" by myself. It was right around the time of the big "dot com" boom and my buddy Brent Beaty of DBR Marketing said I should buy a domain name and we tried "curecancer.com" but it was taken. Then I thought "ICureCancer.com" is better because it puts the responsibility in the person with the disease. Because only they can do it. If you get cancer you have to say, "I" cure cancer!

The way I learned about cancer being curable is because of a woman I was doing a play with back in 1996, J. Cynthia Brooks. She had just cured herself of terminal cervical cancer. This was a woman I had always had a major crush on from the moment I laid eyes on her, 6 years previous while working at the world-famous Roxbury. Well, there she was, rehearsal after rehearsal with me at the Odyssey Theater working on a play called "Spoiled Women." I have always been very shy when it comes to women so just kept to myself until one day, I heard five little words from a whisper behind me, "I just cured my cancer." [See Pic 2.1] [See Pic 2.2]

This was odd to catch that because we were all on break outside having a smoke or whatever and as usual, with a bunch of actors, everyone was vying for attention. To be in the spotlight where I was just there to get my acting up to par so I could go and make more movies that paid well so I could get on with my life. Don't get me wrong, I love acting, but I knew there was a bigger picture and it was about to be shown to me, I heard those now famous words, "I just cured myself of Cancer." I inquisitively spun around and said, "What did you just say?! You can't cure cancer! No one can cure cancer, or we'd all know about it!" Well, long story short, thanks to Cynthia I learned that cancer was not only curable but always had been until Big Pharma came about.

See, in the early 1900's Rockefeller and Carnegie owned the pharmaceutical and textbook companies and decided to take over the medical schools as well, so they could sell more of their drugs. I'll write more on this later, but just wanted to give you a heads up on why I know the information I'm about to give you and your Oncologist probably doesn't. There's no money in curing people. Only stringing them along and draining their pockets. Sad but true, which is why I became so passionate about this and made my documentary and am now writing this book! Must be that Christ-like/bouncer attitude again. Cynthia explained to me that she didn't use the standard treatments of chemo, radiation, and surgery. She did it all holistically. As in, she cut out all sugar, juiced a lot, took supplements and meditated. She actually got me to go to her meditation class at "Center of Light Miracles" in Los Angeles, run by Rev. Lynne Herod-DeVerges. They teach Essene meditation there and if you do your research you will see Jesus was an Essene.

They were all about cleansing the body through diet and mind, through prayer/meditation etc. It's everything Einstein ever said about energy. Everything is energy and our minds are too and able to change or shift energy. Hence, you're hearing so many miracle stories about someone being healed by faith alone. It is no miracle; it is just the power of the mind is very real. Therefore, Cynthia swears by treating the body, mind, and soul in achieving health especially when health is failing to the extent of terminal cancer. The main obstacle she had in convincing and teaching me was that I just couldn't believe that cancer could be curable, and our doctors didn't know about it! So, I let that go on the back burner and wanted to learn about the healing part first and would deal with that later.

I started researching on the Internet in the late '90s. I'd read someone's story and then make sure I called them on the phone too. And time after time, sure enough, I'd get the person who I had just read about and they confirmed it was true. They switched their lifestyles; diets, etc. and were now cancer free!

So, I knew I was onto something and started telling everyone I knew about it and they all thought I was nuts. No one believed me! Which now I see; how could I blame them? I didn't believe it at first either. And this would eventually become a heartbreaking experience I've had to deal with quite a bit since learning this. So many people I see being tortured and murdered by chemo and radiation and I try to explain to them, but they look at me like I'm crazy and just listen to their doctors and usually die. So sad.

What upsets me most is, I never got funding in 1990 and still haven't to this day, other than from my few followers who support me. But never any serious money. By 2003, I was so pissed off, I grabbed a buddy's camera and he let me use his Mac G4 to edit on and made the damn thing myself. With no help other than a friend or two that had a day off here and there to help with the camera. In 2006, I had the Premier in a little old theatre in Elmira Heights, New York. I started showing it at theaters long before the final cut was done. Soon as that first cut was ready, I was playing it every Sunday I could, just in case someone desperately needed that information then! It was cool too because I would take notes at every screening, go home make it better and show the new one the following Sunday. And sure enough, I met this lady April Hart in Elmira who had breast cancer. As she explains in this video, it's a good thing I didn't wait for the final and perfect cut. That first rough cut was just fine! https://www.youtube.com/watch?v=QKFOOuAP9Gc .

I'm not sure how many lives ICureCancer.Com has helped, but I know there are thousands of copies in circulation especially what with pirating so rampant these days, which I don't mind. The more that get to see it, the better! I have never able to get a major distribution deal, as of yet. It's meant to be gritty and passionate and to give information to those in dire straits that could help them cure themselves. And that it does!

I recently called into a radio show that had world-famous holistic healer/author Dr. Leonard Coldwell on, and he not only knew who I was, he said my film was one of the best he's ever seen in this genre! Definitely one of the greatest, if not greatest compliments I've ever received. Right up there with Chuck Norris telling a friend I was the best kicker he had ever seen after one of my fights. And when a commentator/ex-champion – Blinky Rodriguez likened my left side kick to Muhammad Ali's left jab! Only this compliment is even better actually because with my work now people get healed, not hurt.

With all that being said, you now know a bit about me and why I do what I do. I like to right the wrongs I see. I would expect you to do the same for me, if the roles were reversed. So, I must say, I'm not a doctor or an oncologist or claim to heal anyone. Lucky for you, I am not a doctor or an oncologist because then I would be of no use to your well-being. It's illegal for them to cure cancer. But I'm a filmmaker with an attitude.

I've interviewed hundreds of people over the years that have cured their cancers and the alternative doctors/healers that have helped them do it. But know this too: I know some that tried everything and still didn't make it. There are 3 types that can't cure their cancers.

One God calls them—their time is up.
Two, their disease serves them. As in, they like the attention they get and how everyone feels sorry for them and waits on them hand and foot.
Three—those that cannot follow instructions. This isn't a Jenny Craig diet that if you cheat on it you put back on some pounds. Here you die. So, I am bringing to you what I have learned and what I would do if I had cancer right now. I hope this helps you.

Here's an article backing up what I learned in 2003 from Dr. Bernardo at the Cancer Control Society, Los Angeles.
http://www.greenmedinfo.com/blog/why-alkaline-approach-can-successfully-treat-cancer?fbclid=IwAR0WxKeYlvfDVq5jzFULy45Baoygdo-qviRbkEHws96bPnwam1-NsF0CXDA

Article Natural News did on me to give you some basics.
https://www.naturalnews.com/045111_cancer_cures_Ian_Jacklin_natural_healing.html

Seriously, just watch the movie by Del Bigtree, Vaxxed. You will have no doubt after that film vaccines are for big pharma to keep you a customer for life with the horrible afflictions the shots will give you. [See Pic 2.3]

CHAPTER 3:

WHAT I WOULD DO IF I WERE YOU (FIRST STEPS)

I couldn't do what I do without stating to everyone that what I say here is strictly the information about what I would do myself. As it turns out apparently, that's a good thing, otherwise I could get in trouble for giving medical advice and I don't do that. But if it were me, to me, it was a no brainer. I know just because a protocol may work for one, with stage 4 cancer, that might not work for someone that only has stage 2. Everyone is different, and I don't want to give anyone false hope. "Just the facts ma am" as Agent Friday would say.

This brings up a memory from my childhood, which I'm going to share as to the real reason I took such an interest in curing cancer. See, I thought it ran in my adopted mother's family which years later I found out it didn't. Kind of a funny thing and it turned out to be good. Bad, in the sense that all through my childhood my biggest fear was my mom would get and die of cancer. Good, because when I learned cancer was curable, I dove in headfirst and learned all I could about it, made a movie and now writing this book! A lot of people are alive today because of that misunderstanding about my mom. So, like my old acting coach used to say, "Some of the greatest moments in a scene come from a mistake!"

So back to the issue at hand. What would I do if I just found out I had cancer? I will walk you through it. So, in this fictitious scenario, my doctor says it looks like you have a dark spot in your lung, I'm sending you to an oncologist. Here's where you would probably start freaking out, but I just say "cool".

I'd get my test results from the Oncologist and get him to write down his recommendation, which would definitely be surgery, chemo, and radiation. I'd have a cameraman there taping this too. I'd bring up a few other things about alternative medicine, knowing full well he would just scoff at them and probably lose his temper when I would hit him with fact after fact about truly healing the body by alkalizing it, detoxing it and pumping up the immune system. He would stomp out on me—like I've seen doctors do—before I'd say thanks for the tests, and I'll see you in three months to see how it looks then.

I'd have to refrain myself from hitting him with a roundhouse shin kick to the head for just advising me to take a treatment that would make me miserably sick and most likely kill me before cancer would. But I would say, "when I come back, and the cancer is gone you will owe me a huge apology and a promise to start researching holistic medicine" rather than continue to be the mass murdering guy that he is now.

I would, of course, get a second opinion, but start my new lifestyle as if I did for sure have it? Actually, I think to be safe, what with the skies being sprayed, GMO's in food and general toxic overload? Everyone should pretend they have 4th stage cancer every day of the week but one. You can have a cheat meal that day, as if you didn't have cancer. But, just plan for it and probably never get it. Kapeesh?

On the way home, I'd be stocking up on organic lemons and from then on, my only drink (other than juicing & blending) would be lemon juice and water (1/4 lemon per 8oz alkaline water) with a little stevia for flavor. I add cayenne pepper too. It's an old trick I learned from one of my mentors Dr. Bernardo. He was the star of "ICureCancer" the movie and I was fortunate enough to spend some time with him before his untimely death a couple of years ago. RIP Dr. B! Lemons, although acidic, when digested make you alkaline and this is the first and foremost thing for me to do right now. As Bernardo also said, "You don't die of cancer you die of acidosis!"

Any alkaline diet is good but here is **Dr. Bernardo's Diet** basic idea:

Eat as many organic green vegetables & red skinned potatoes as possible (except green peas).

Raw is okay, but you need to break the membrane to get the full nutrition, so steaming is best.

Organic venison, buffalo, lamb and a tiny bit of turkey.

You can eat organic, wild-caught fish (although now that we are post-Fukushima, I personally wouldn't eat anything from Pacific)

Eat 80% vegetables and 20% meat (or no meat) depends on if they have lost a lot of weight. The meat will put weight on them.

A drink that will put weight on a person is organic whipping cream, coconut milk, almond milk, and a little stevia. Tastes like a vanilla shake!

If you bake anything, you use stevia in place of the sugar and gluten-free all-purpose baking flour instead of flour. If you want pancakes you can have buckwheat pancakes and only use organic eggs.

Only organic butter allowed – try to get raw.

As far as oil goes use extra virgin olive oil (in salads, and extra virgin organic coconut oil for cooking).

You also can have a lot of green salads and cabbage. The only dressing you can have is olive oil and vinegar or just squeeze lemon on it.

Sprouted bread mainly, although Dr. B said a little wheat bread is okay, as long as it's homemade without the preservatives.

Drink lots of freshly squeezed lemon in water. Can use little Stevia to sweeten.

Nothing packaged/processed foods of course!

So obviously I'd be on this with absolutely no cheating. Notice there was no fruit or anything with sugar in there other than dark berries and green apple? Cancer feeds off sugar! Had I gone for chemo, all they would have is donuts and cookies in the waiting room? Ridiculous!

Okay, so at this stage, I have denied the barbaric Western Medical treatments and started on my alkaline diet, drinking lots of good water and lemon juice. Time to get even more serious. Figure out if I could afford to go to a clinic or have to go it on my own at home.

CHAPTER 4:

IF I HAD MONEY FOR A HOLISTIC TREATMENT CENTER

You don't need one, if you know what you are doing, but if you can afford it, why not have yourself babied by others for a change. I would call around to alternative medicine clinics. First, one would be,

Camelot Cancer Center Tulsa, OK 74136

http://camelotcancercare.is

Clinic: 918-493-1011

Clinic Fax: 918-493-6589

It is the only clinic in America that I know of that can use alternative methods without being hassled by the AMA or FDA. Apparently, they cured a judge and he told everyone to back off them. I'd find out their exact protocol and prices. OOPS! NEVER MIND THE FBI JUST SHUT THEM DOWN. I think that the judge died. They were only open as long as they were because they cured a judge early on. Lol. And they had a good, 75% success rate was the word on the street. Way too high for Nazi USA, so they got shut down with guns drawn. The stormtroopers roughed up my friend Michael McDonough who was a lab tech guy for the clinic. Medications were literally slapped out of sick people's hands. And they died soon after. Guns were drawn and put to people's heads. I mean just really horrible stuff, traumatizing staff and patients alike. All for what? They thought they had Laetrile. Pffftt! Which they did not have. But even if they did, off label, it is totally legal. Well, Maureen is still fighting to save her house and business. Last I heard, she was opening-up clinics in Mexico! Our hearts and prayers go to all that lost their livers due to the FBI raid. There were several casualties thanks to this disturbance in medicine and care.

Update: Maureen has been on the run from the FBI and police since the clinic was shut down a few years ago! Word has it, her protocol that was curing too many people of cancer is available in Cancun!

Latest News: Migrating the clinic to Cancun had the advantage of moving it completely beyond US jurisdiction and therefore allowed the natural chemo formula M to be weaponized, so it is now even more effective than it was before Camelot was attacked. http://holygrailcancercare.is   ***

Okay, so to Mexico, where it is still okay to practice medicine and my guys at **American Holistic Care** in Tijuana have a great protocol and it is very affordable due to location. As in, it is not on the beach. It is in Tijuana, so you get $35,000 worth for well under $20,000! I met Alessandro Porcella, who for decades has run AmericanBioDental.com in Tijuana, Bio Dentistry: http://www.youtube.com/watch?v=XjoqHLE3tHg and recently attached the holistic cancer healing too: .https://www.youtube.com/watch?v=gumdAjoDCqQ

The main guy is Dr. Andrade https://www.youtube.com/watch?v=RMBZEljHhQQ who is famous for curing Max Factor's kid in the '70s. Well, he's still around and on top of the latest western medicine and holistic when it comes to cancer. He is also a stem cell specialist. Therefore, if I had cancer and wanted to save money I would go to TJ and do the laetrile/DMSO/high dose vitamin c intravenous etc., along with Dr. Bernardo's protocol. They have a 21-day detox and immune boost protocols.

For extreme cases, some do resort to western methods. Now, this would probably never happen to me because I am totally against Western Medicine unless I have been in a car accident and am in the emergency room. But if you just have your heart set on surgery, chemo and radiation then this clinic is the only doctor or person I've heard that uses western medicine on cancer successfully and the reason why is because he has changed the order of the treatment. Everywhere else they do the surgery first, then the chemo and radiation. This is ridiculous! As soon as they cut out the cancer, cancer cells are now flowing through your bloodstream and will settle somewhere and anywhere else. Hence, so many cases of someone being supposedly cured of cancer surgery only to get some other kind of cancer down the line.

What Dr. Vargas at the clinic does is he first will use pinpoint radiation to circle the tumor so if any cancer cells get out it zaps them right there. He also gives a low, low dose of chemotherapy to the bloodstream in case there are any rogue cells that made it past that which kills them immediately.

In 30 years of practice, he has an 80% success rate in curing breast cancer! But you are looking at about $6,000 a week for at least 3 weeks, FYI. However, for any clinic in Mexico, I have found the average price for 3 to 6 weeks of therapy will run you $15,000 to $20,000. They usually send you home with a good supply of oral supplements and diet instructions to continue, on the healing process.

I just saw him recently and he had been in Korea teaching them his secrets. Now he's back in TJ. FYI… I would not do this myself as I'm organic or bust!

So, whether you want holistic or conventional, if I had cancer and $20,000 that is where I would go. A 3-week intensive clinic treatment, then Dr. Bernardo's protocol. Getting and staying alkaline. It is important to note that some clinics in Mexico will take health insurance from America, so make sure to inquire about that.

American Holistic Care and American Bio-Dental do everything: DMSO, high dose vitamin C, laetrile, IPT (Insulin Potentiation Therapy), colon, kidney, liver cleansing, bio dentistry, alkaline diet, etcetera, and he had them all covered. So, any clinic you find that does all these treatments are good in my opinion. If they do not, don't bother with them. For extreme cases, some do resort to western methods.

CHAPTER 5:

TOO BROKE FOR A TREATMENT CENTER

Good, you don't need to be spoiled. Man up. First things first. Try to get a good cancer coach. Someone like me who has done the research for a film or book. Alternatively, someone who cured himself or herself naturally. When I was a pro-fighter, every free moment I was watching old fight tapes of the guys that were champions. So, when someone says, "There is no scientific evidence" that alternative treatments work only anecdotal, I personally do not care. I don't care what studies western medicine have done because I know that most are tainted due to being backed by the drug makers themselves. Of course, they are going to say they work. There has been the case after case where Merck or somebody gets sued for false claims, but they know that's par for the course and the money they make off the drugs before getting caught easily covers the fines! It's sickening. Therefore, I just cut to the chase (like training with the heavyweight gold medalist Lennox Lewis) and learn from those that do it in real life… not those that have not and only do it on paper.

FYI: I have created a forum people can join up and collaborate with others in the same situations called "I Cure Cancer" on Facebook. If you do not know anyone locally that has used alternative medicine to help themselves, this group would be good for you.

 https://www.facebook.com/groups/I Cure Cancer

Another good source and friend is Bill Henderson (RIP) Bill passed during the writing of this book. We will miss him. He is the guy who wrote "Cancer-Free" and he would be your cancer coach if you buy his book and I think, last I heard, pay a couple of hundred bucks for the phone consultations that are ongoing. He would tell you exactly what to do at home to treat your cancer! As a matter of fact, I would probably do this first even if I had the money to go to a clinic because many cancers can be destroyed in no time at all just by getting alkaline and detoxing. You could save some major bucks doing it at home. Alas, he's passed, so you can come to me now. I'll make him proud. FYI, I just spoke to his widow and partner in all his work over the years and she is keeping his light alive and well since his crossing over. So that network is alive and well!

https://www.beating-cancer-gently.com/

I would recommend watching, of course, my film if you have not seen it already "I Cure Cancer" the movie and "Healing Cancer from the Inside Out" by Mike Anderson. Also "Burzynski": https://www.youtube.com/user/BurzynskiMovie "Cancer Is Serious Business" is amazing! It is a film about how Dr. Burzynski found a cure for brain cancer that the FDA and AMA continue to try to bury it because it works. This is a real eye-opener on how the powers that be are evil and are not doing anything but trying to destroy modalities and doctors who have them, in order to keep their monopoly on the medical business. These three films will bring you up to par on what is going on in the cancer business. And that is just what it is, a "business," so do not expect your doctor to help you in this case. You must be your own doctor.

With that being said, now is when the learning can really begin. www.cancertutor.com is without a doubt, the best site on the net for alternative cancer treatment information. My friend Webster Kehr developed and maintains it for nothing. I mean, of all the people on the planet that are in the cancer realm, this guy's information has probably helped more than anyone, if they were lucky enough to come across it. Yet the poor guy still has to drive two hours to work and two hours back every day just to keep the lights on! And here we have mass murdering oncologists, 85% of whom wouldn't take their own medicine or give it to their families, driving around in Porches and sending their kids to top colleges!

Life definitely isn't fair, but I have a feeling Webster will fare much better in the afterlife than any of these low lives. That's the great thing in life. What goes around comes around! Note: Webster sold it to new owners. Word around my campfire, they are legit. So, it's still a good source as of this publication in 2019.

The bottom line key is not doing chemo, radiation… and most times surgery isn't even needed. I would sink my money into an organic diet and as many supplements as I could afford.
Look at Dr. Bernardo's list and get what you can. Check out baking soda cures on YouTube and Food Grade Hydrogen Peroxide! Where there is a will there is a way. If I had cancer, I'd know it was probably because I was acidic, and possibly, had some kind of pathogen in my system. Actually, many times one will test for cancer but really only have pathogens. Ignorant mislead MD's.

My naturopathic friend Dr. Spencer (www.bodyelectrician.com) knows this and will treat his patients with a light dose of **MMS** aka chlorine dioxide which kills all pathogens. **Chlorine dioxide** is the active ingredient in **MMS** after it is activated by acid (see below). The Chemical formula of chlorine dioxide is **ClO2**. That formula shows that there is one atom of chlorine (Cl) and 2 atoms of oxygen (O2) in a molecule of chlorine dioxide. This often renders someone cancer free in no time at all. You just have to kill the pathogens.

For cleaning and as powerful anti-biotic, I use Pure Bio – Hard Surface Cleaner. It's not for internal use, as said on the bottle. But that's because they don't want to sell it as an antibiotic. They don't want the headaches from the FDA. But they do want it for their Hard Surface cleaner spray. That just so happens to be as pure and non-toxic and RO'd water. So, a little secret in the alternative world is to keep this in your medicine cabinet not just cleaning cupboards. ½ ounce couple times a day knocks out most internal infections. Great for cold season.

Pure BioScience formally known as IV-7: This is sold as a germ-killing cleaning product because it does do that too. And due to "mass murdering FDA" rules they can't tell you what else it does. It's the best, natural, anti-biotic in spray bottle ever! It's basically a pathogen killer like MMS (miracle mineral solution) and Colloidal Silver only better. Plus, it does not taste bad and you don't have to mix it.
Here is a video of Ian Clark explaining it:
https://www.youtube.com/watch?feature=player_embedded&v=XmoHPoUgtuQ

There are other products on the market that use silver—but it is important for you to know that they are NOT the same technology as IV-7 Ultimate Germ Defense TM!

Here is the difference: IV-7 contains Stabilized Ionic Silver. The other products do not. Colloidal silver products contain small particles of silver suspended in aqueous solution. The main composition of colloidal silver is metallic silver, but it may also contain silver oxide and other silver complexes.

Silver colloids release minute quantities of ionic silver over time, predominantly through surface oxidation, and dissociation from silver complexes. Numerous complex and expensive processes have been developed to manufacture colloidal silver and this has resulted in large product variability. In comparison, IV-7 Ultimate Germ Defense contains fully active stabilized ionic silver — silver dihydrogen citrate (SDC), at a specific concentration of 30 parts per million – thousands of times higher than colloidal silver but with exponentially less total silver mass. The patented process developed to manufacture SDC provides stabilized ionic silver in aqueous citric acid solution. This economical process results in superior product quality and performance.

- Only stabilized ionic silver, the SDC in IV-7 Ultimate Germ Defense, has been scientifically proven and registered by the U.S. Environmental Protection Agency (EPA) to have quick and powerful broad-spectrum antimicrobial, antifungal and antiviral efficacy.

- The SDC in IV-7 Ultimate Germ Defense works faster than any other silver-containing product on the market today.

- IV-7 Ultimate Germ Defense provides powerful protection while using extremely low levels of stabilized ionic silver when compared to the less effective colloidal silver products that contain much more silver.

- IV-7 Ultimate Germ Defense is stable and will remain efficacious for years when stored properly.

- IV-7 Ultimate Germ Defense has an EPA Category IV hazard rating: the safest rating for any product!

Sold as a cleaner, but I personally store it in my medicine cabinet. Sure, it cleans like no other cleaner, but I take a ½ an ounce for a natural antibiotic. Spray it in the mouth for fresh breath and under my arms since we all know deodorant has toxic aluminum in it. (Wouldn't put it on open wounds, FYI). It kills almost all pathogens, hence it being a great cleaner and since its toxicity level is that of RO'd water, doesn't stop me from using it internally.

Of course, I'm not suggesting anyone do anything that I do. I'm just telling you what I do. I get a chest infection. ½ ounce 2x a day and in a day or two my chest infection is gone. Where, as antibiotics took 10 days. And were really bad for me. I am my own doctor now.

To order: http://store.purebio.com/index.php/pure-hardsurface-products

Ian Clark from Oceans Alive and Adrian Quinn organic farmer chat on holistic health. [See Pic. 5.1]

https://www.youtube.com/watch?v=5lfyuhi0f5Y&feature=share

I could have written a book these guys themselves. Ian created one of the best health products ever called Oceans Alive Phytoplankton and Adrian invented the frosty candle and used his money to build an organic farm which he learned to run himself and produce way more food than any of the Monsanto farmers in his area. Organic grows better! Shame on the farmers that take the easy money from subsidies.

CHAPTER 6:

DR. BERNARDO MAJALCA

(Excerpt from "ICureCancer.Com")

Yeah, my name is Dr. Bernardo. I'm a naturopath and I treat people holistically, which means I treat the whole body. I use no prescription drugs; none of that. What happens, a patient comes to me with cancer, their doctor or oncologist does what he has to do and normally the patient comes to me in the final stage of the disease and many times we can turn them around very dramatically. One of the things that we found out that all cancer patients, their PH is acid. By this, I mean everything in nature has a PH from 1 to 14, 7 being water, blood being 7.2. When we're born all our intercellular fluids including saliva, you have to have, a PH of 7.2 to 7.4. When cancer patients come or anybody, is very acidic, their PH runs around 5. So, what I get the patient, immediately, and I have been called a "quack" for saying this, put the patient on lemon juice and water. Lemon juice is an acid and when you drink it, it helps to an alkaline tide in the body. So, your PH starts going up. It might take three weeks to four weeks, cause, you are approximately 80 percent water. So, if you weigh 200 pounds, there are about 160 pounds of water; we have to raise the PH to 7.2, and it's been my opinion that all cancer ceases at PH 6.8 and it dies at PH 7.

I have many patients that came to me that were told, "Go home and die. You got four weeks, five weeks." But I have many other people who come to me they have been written off and I've been Arrested, because I was treating patients in this country and I'm not supposed to treat patients.

I treated only patients that have been written off; they'd had chemotherapy, they've had radiation, they had countless surgeries and yet they, they never address the problem! You only have cancer, because you have acidosis! That means your cellular fluids PH, are in the neighborhood of 5, and that's why you have pain. Why do you have pain? Cause vinegar is a PH of 5.3, if I inject vinegar in you, you're in excruciating pain! And that's why you have pain, cause you're very acidic!

Cancer is on the rise. We've spent trillions of dollars. You know, we're winning a war! Hell, we're not doing a damn thing except losing our ass! One out of two people, that's 50 percent of the people have cancer right now. Fifty percent! I had cancer, all my nurses were crying. I said, "Why you girls crying?" "Well, you got cancer, you got cancer, you're gonna die and I'm gonna lose my job!" I said, "If I can't get rid of my cancer, I deserve to die!" A month later, my cancer is normal, everything is fine. My PSA which had been 48 and then it was 0.0. It's been 0.1 or something like that in the last five years. And I tell patients when they come to me, "Well, my doctor says I got two weeks, or I got a month or 3 months." I said, "Unless he gets a phone call from God and God tells him Mrs. Such and such has only got two weeks or a month," then you can believe it. What the hell, he is just a man; he goes to the toilet like every other man. He's not God. He may think he is God. He's arrogant, most of them are. I have been in medicine 51 years and I can tell you 20 percent of the doctors are fantastic, the others, unfortunately, are in it for the money.

Look, they're talking about prostate cancer, we've got to freeze it, we got to do this. It needs some nutrients. I've never had anybody that died of prostate cancer. I've had Strips Lahoya, a doctor in France, who sent me a patient six, seven years ago his PSA was 4,280. Anything over 4 is cancer. Normally at around 1,200, you die. This was a mean ole' crabby guy and I should have let him die! But anyway Dr. LaChance said, "Can you help him?" I said, "Well how much time you give him?" He said, "A week!" I said, "Oh, hell that's plenty of time!" He said, "Bernardo, get serious, his PSA is 4,280!" I said, "Well hell that's no big deal!" He said, "Get serious, you understand English?" I said, "I'm an American dummy, 4,280!" I said, "Send him to me!" He said, "He also got bone cancer!" I said, "Oh, of course, it comes with the territory!" I said, "What's his alkaline phosphatase?" He said, "It's over 2,000!" I said, "No, big deal!" He said, "Bernardo, are you for real? Are you a mad man?" I said, "Call me whatever you want! Send me the guy."

When the guy came, he could barely walk, he walked like a hundred-year-old guy. Pain, we had to put like five pillows under him because of the pain. A week later his prostate-specific antigen called PSA, which is a marker that identifies cancer in the prostate had dropped by a thousand points, in five weeks his PSA was 0 point something. Five weeks; Dr. LaChance told me, he says, "I find it hard to believe that you can do this and over here we can't do those things." His PH, when he came, was like 4.8; at 4 and a half, you die! Slowly, within three weeks, his PH was 7.2. And in five weeks, he was completely free of cancer!

Testimonial for Dr. Bernado:

Hi, I'm Lucica Brensensky, I am 57-year-old and I'm self-employed. I was diagnosed with cancer in Russia. I came to the United States and went through conventional treatment and the first time it was successful. Like in couple years I got a new episode of cancer and was introduced to Dr. Bernardo and got this treatment and his protocol, how he does it. And since then I am in remission. That's it.

Dr. Bernardo: You know, I'm not a diplomat, I call it the way it is. When I was a young man, I went to Korea with 4,000 men, a year later, only 7 of us came back. That changes your priority in life. When you see fine young men torn to pieces [tears in eyes] you know you've got to do something when you get back. If you get back alive. That's what I've devoted my life, 51 years. You would say, "Well hell, that guys gotta be rich!" Hell, I'm in the hole over $270,000. But I saved a lot of lives and that's what it's all about. Doctors used to chew my ass out, "Well you gotta get a Mercedes?" Hell, I can barely afford to drive my Chevy, what the heck are you talking about, Mercedes?

You know, once you've seen death, and I've seen enough death to last me 10,000 years [tears in eyes]. I've seen pain. I've had pain for thousands of years, more than I can ever handle. In fact, I lost a girl once and I told God, "That's it! There's nothing you can do cause, I'm gonna go home, get my 45, go in the backyard and blow my brains out and there's nothing you can do!" So, I drove home, I lost this beautiful girl just hysterical cause I used to get very, very, depressed, suicidal, every time. So, I drove home, ran upstairs to get my 45, it had 7 rounds of armor piercing. I'm gonna go in the backyard and just go. Just like that. And I went in there and someone had stolen my pistols. That's right!

Lucica: The first day I came, and I had the tumor in the shape of a pancake, so it was obvious the size then. So, he put a circle around it on the first day and in couple days he compared the results how it shrunk. So, he put another smaller circle and it was quite an experience to look at the mirror and see how it change. Yeah.

Dr. Bernardo: And I made that resolve when I left Korea alive that nobody would ever die in my presence! Ah, I have a naturopath license in the United States. I also had a license from Mexico. Now, licenses in Mexico are not recognized over here. So, people would call me to say, "My father is dying, and my mother is dying, or my son is dying, can you please help me?" I said, "Well you know I can't treat over there!" But I'd go over there and of course the patient is dying, and of course, I treat the patient! And I had 30 patients that I treated, and one died. When I got there, she weighed about 65 pounds. And I told her husband, "It's too late for her! There's nothing I can do!" So, anyway, she died the next day. She called, he called the AMA said, "Well I think a doctor here killed my wife."

Well, they raided me; they came in with shotguns and everything else. And luckily, I wasn't there. I was in Mexico. And my secretary called me, he says, "All the cops in the world are over here!" I said, "What do they want?" He says, "They want to arrest you!" I said, "For what?" He said, "You treated patients over here?" I said, "Yeah I treated them! They're alive!" He said, "Well you can't treat them over here!" I said, "They were gonna die, dummy!" He says, "I don't care!" He said, "You show up here and we need to talk to you!"

So, I went up there about a week later. And she said, "Tell us everything you did." So, I did. After I finished, they said, "Get up! You're under arrest!" I said, "For what?" He said, "You treated patients over here!" Next thing I know I'm charged with 25 felonies. TWO MILLION DOLLAR BAIL! TWO MILLION! I said, "Jeffrey Dahmer only ate 18 people, and he was only a million-dollar bail!" He said, "Well you are more dangerous!" Next thing you know, they had my picture in about 30 newspapers around the world. I mean, in the United States. They had me on a two-million-dollar bail. Captured Doctor Death named as Dr. Bernardo. Their Assistant DA, "We have to make an example of this man. He's dangerous because he practices alternative therapy and even though he is a naturopath that doesn't call for him to be giving IVs to people that are dying." So, on and so forth. Well, they were right. But I CANNOT stand, and watch people will die... if I can do something about it. Make a long story short, the trial goes on for about two weeks and it's on ABC, CBS, and NBC every night for about two weeks and the guys in jail would say, "Hey doc you're on television again! Come see ya!" [chuckling] Her lady's doctor came, he said, "She was terminal! She wanted to die. She was down to 65 pounds because her husband treated her like a dog." And she told me, "Don't save me. I want to I want to die!"

I said, "You're dying anyway."

So anyway, the Judge says, "Counselor, I have great news. I've finally got a cell for Dr. Bernardo in Folsom Prison and he's going to serve twenty years. Not a day off for good behavior or early parole. He will serve twenty years. So, I told him, "Your honor, hell, make it 40 years but I'll make you a promise, I'll make you a solemn promise, like McCarthy, said, 'I shall return'. And you listen, when I get out of prison, you listen for a truck and trailer coming up the front door!" He said, "What truck and trailer?" I said, "The one I got loaded with gasoline and composite C, composite C is several hundred times stronger than dynamite and I will turn this building into while talcum powder, your honor, including you and I'll be happy to drive that truck!" So, the guy went berserk, [motions hand like gavel slamming], "Put this man in the cooler, get him out of here!" I was hoping he'd have a stroke, but it didn't happen.

Finally, the Judge says, "Well counselor, we're ready to sentence him." He said, the Judge says, "Any last words?" I said, "Well you gonna take me out and shoot me?" And he said, "No, you're gonna serve 20 years!" I said, "Okay, I did my duty as God gave me the light to do this duty! What is my crime? There are 29 people whose lives are saved, and you can send me to a hundred years I don't give a damn and, probably, unless I go to solitary, I will be treating prisoners over there. I said, "People will not die in my presence!"

So anyway, he said, "Okay. Counselor, I'm ready to sentence your man! Ah, Bernardo..." About this time this guy busts through the front door, he said, "Who are you?" "A friend of the court, your honor, Amicus Curia." "What do you mean, what do you mean busting in here?" He said, "Your honor, we've checked this man's record!" He said, "What do you mean checked his record? Who are you?" He said, "I'm Chief of Psychiatry at the VA Hospital in LaHoya. Matter of fact that you people say that he didn't serve in the military! Wrong! His record shows above and beyond the call of duty time and time again with complete disregard to his personal safety. We feel it is a great injustice if you send this man to prison. He is mentally unstable your honor. He has post-traumatic stress." So, I said, "Post-traumatic stress that's a cop-out for a bunch of god damn cowards what are you talking about post-traumatic stress. Don't give me that brush crap." He said, "You see your honor he refuses to believe that he is sick!" I said, "I am not sick! I just saw so much death that nobody's ever gonna die in my presence. If it means my life; do it!"

So, anyway, he said, "Your honor, you must release him to me in the fairness of justice!" He said, "Well what are you gonna do to him?" He said, "Well we're going to make him halfway balanced. As you can see, he is way off kilter. He's very unstable." So anyway, he said, "Alright, you got him for 90 days. You bring him back, make sure he is stable because I want him to realize the gravity of the twenty years, he is gonna spend."

So anyway, they took me up to Palo Alto and I was tortured mentally, terrible. It was the worst time of my life [eyes tearing]. They wanted to know what I saw there, and I wouldn't tell them. So, they finally made me break down. "You have to tell us what you saw!" I said, "You weren't there [crying] you don't have a right to know what happened over there. "So, anyway after a few days, they broke me. I told them.

Ninety days later they brought me back. And my attorney picked me up at the airport. He said, "Well, they are going to sentence you tomorrow morning." I said, by this time I had a prayer chain of a couple of thousand people, I said, "I'll leave it up to God. If he wants me to go to prison, I'm ready to go. If he wants me to stay out there for 100 years, I'll go. Take me out back and execute me, I'll go!"

The Judge says, "Is this Bernardo?" "Yes." "Are you the Counselor from Texas?" "Yes." "Did you pay your fees?" "Yes." Well, I've been reading this report, there's no question that this man is obviously mad. His desire to save lives, whether it was due to what he saw in combat or his mental illness, whether its post-traumatic stress, I'm not gonna say. But I will do no good to send this man to prison. So, I'm gonna dismiss him and I'll put him on some type of probation." And that was it. That was it.

I've got doctors that practice in Mexico and I tell them what protocols to use and we're doing great! We're doing great. I think there's at least one patient here, that came to me and I told him, he had colon cancer. I said, "Get rid of the colon cancer get back, because if you have surgery for the colon cancer it will ALWAYS, ALWAYS, come back within three to four months. No ifs, ands, or buts about it. Why? They did not address the problem; your problem is ACIDOSIS.

You can take out all the tumors, you can give all the radiation, you can do all the surgeries, you have not corrected the problem, which is acidosis and that's what activates cancer. "Well, we'll give you radiation." What the hell is that gonna do? Except for screw, you up.

Testimonial by DeWitt Bell:

My name is DeWitt Bell, I'm 64 years old, my occupation is a designer, writer, businessman. About a year ago, a little more than a year ago, I had gotten very sick, and I'd lost about 30 pounds. And I said, "Okay, I'll surrender. I'll go to AMA. I'll go to conventional medicine and I will see what they say. I come out of the colonoscopy and they say, "Here's a picture of your problem. You have a stage IV Tumor, your colon is almost completely blocked and if we do not operate you'll be dead within three weeks. "So, I said, "Well I don't have much choice, do I? Go ahead." Then they come in and they said, "Okay, now you have-to-do chemotherapy because people who have what you have will be dead in five years, but the chance is, 60 percent chance you'll be dead in five years if you don't do that." And I said, "Well, honestly, I've never seen chemotherapy cure anybody. "You know, I've seen a lot of people take it, I've seen their hair fall out, I've seen them get nauseous, but I've never seen anybody get well. So, I'm gonna have-to-do a little research on this.

So, I got out of the hospital and I called a doctor, a naturopathic doctor whom I knew, and I said, "Do you know any alternative cancer treatments?" He said, "I've heard of one guy, Dr. Bernardo, but let me check." So, he called, said, "Yeah, he's probably 'the' guy." So, I called wept over the phone and said, "He saved my life." "Everybody had given me up so, I called Dr. Bernardo, and I said, "What is it you do?" He said, "Call these numbers." And he gave me three numbers to call. Everybody said they were going to be dead and he saved me." And so, I called him back up said, "Well, okay, what do you want me to do?" He gave me three things to do and he said, "As soon as you can travel," cause, I was just out of the hospital, could hardly walk, this was last May. He said, "Come down and see me." So, I went down to see him, I walked into him, he took one look at me and he says, "Ah, you're easy, you'll be cured in six months." Actually, I was cured in three months.

[See Pic 7.1]

Dr. Bernardo: My father was a country doctor; he practiced for about 40 years. If people had money, he charged them. If people didn't have money, "Well, today is Thursday. I don't charge on Thursday." Twenty years after he died people were still bringing vegetables to the house. Twenty years after he died. That's what being a doctor is.

CHAPTER 7:

DR. BERNARDO'S PROTOCOL WITH SUPPLEMENTS!

Okay, with all that being said, this is the most important part of the book! This chapter is broken into two sections. The first section provides a high-level overview of Dr. Bernardo's Protocol and includes the full list of supplements. The second section goes into much more details regarding how to execute the protocol into your daily routine and dives deeper into how the protocol addresses every aspect of your life on all levels; physical, mental, emotional, and spiritual. Let's get started!

Section One - Dr. B's protocol.

He told me he had a 95% success rate with folks that came to him before doing any chemo, radiation or surgery. Of all the folks I interviewed over the years, I believed him.

Dr. Otto Warburg had it all understood in the early 1900s by figuring out cancer can't live in an alkaline state. Using EFA's and dark cruciferous vegetables and becoming alkaline / oxygenated people are curing themselves of every stage of cancer of 1 to 4. It's simple science. Your average person has a PH of 6.3. Cancer is 5. 4.5 you die. If you get to 7.2 or 7.4 cancer not only stops growing it dies. Dr. B would say if your PH is 7.4 for 3 months you are cancer free. The tumors will be calcified/dead. As long as you keep on this program, your cancer never comes back.

Now it can take 18 months sometimes but usually within a few months of a strict alkaline diet and juicing and as many of the supplements as you can afford people get their PH's to 7.2 and boom, their body is finally running correctly again.

Some people like to use baking soda and maple syrup. Dr. B used that especially for the lung cancers I remember.

NOTE: I am not a doctor, and this is not meant to diagnose or treat disease. However, this is intended to share my healing experience and to show that there are foods and plant-based

sources that can and do facilitate health and healing even in extreme disease situations such as I experienced observing for 2 decades.

RE: Dr. Bernardo's Anti-Cancer Protocols & Regime

Introduction:

The first thing anyone diagnosed with cancer must realize is that it is not a death sentence! As Dr. Bernardo says, it is a major inconvenience but not a death sentence! Dr. Bernardo's program with the juicing and super-supplements takes work and must be maintained. If you go off and become acidic again, cancer will come back.

THE HEALING PROTOCOLS

There are four basic components of the protocols:

> (1) ingesting only highly alkaline food, water, and juice;
>
> (2) juicing,
>
> (3) essential fatty oils with a 1:2 Omega 3: Omega 6 ratio, and
>
> (4) supplements.

The first and third components are the nutritional derivative of Nobel-Prize winning research, which has largely been ignored. The first, "alkalinity," is the attempt to turn the body's acidic chemistry around to alkaline, since the research shows that disease cannot live in an alkaline body. Buy the alkaline strips at Whole Foods, testing your saliva each morning under your tongue when you wake up before you eat or drink anything. The third, "essential fatty oils", is based on scientist and Professor Brian Scott Peskin's work. Peskin interpreted into a nutritional format the theories of oxygenation which won Otto Warburg a Nobel Prize (you should read "The Hidden Story of Cancer" by Scott Peskin available at www.brianpeskin.com as soon as you have a chance! If you cannot afford the book, he has many informative articles right on his website).

STEP #1: ALKALINITY

Begin by what you can eliminate from, and add to, your diet. Eliminate all acidic intake, carbohydrates, and stimulants such as coffee, sugar, wheat, rice, potatoes. The goal is to return the body to an alkaline state since Nobel-prize research shows cancer cannot live in an alkaline body.

Drink only highly alkaline water meaning water infused with fresh lemon juice, as much as possible. Each "superfoods" such as lemon, which is acidic outside but, when mixed with your saliva, becomes very alkaline to the body. Obtain a list of alkaline foods to eat, such as; greens, wheatgrass, fresh organic salads without sugar dressing (I now mix freshly squeezed lemon juice, a small amount of virgin olive oil with some stevia sweetener). A must-read book resource is Dr. Young's. The PH Miracle, which explains the healing power of alkalinity and much more.

As I am writing these words, Dr. Robert O Young is being attacked for this book PH Miracle and is facing prison time. Once again, apparently, it's illegal to cure people of diseases. NOTE: As we go to press Young was going to be sentenced to three years and eight months in jail in June 2017. He did 40 days and was let out. His protocol and products would make Dr. Bernardo proud -- https://phmiracleproducts.com/?aff=21

The AMA and FDA medical mafia owned and run by the Rockefeller Illuminati scum are also taking away Louis Smith's freedom for selling the MMS I spoke about above that cures Malaria and Herpes and cancer. "A federal jury sat through seven days of testimony, alleging Louis Daniel Smith, 45, of Spokane, sold the toxic MMS liquid as a miracle cure for cancer, AIDS, malaria, hepatitis, Lyme disease, asthma, the common cold, and other diseases and illnesses. Evidence at the trial showed Smith operated 'Project Green Life' (PGL) from 2007 to 2011. PGL sold MMS over the Internet, according to Consumer Affairs."

This family man can help those cure themselves of terrible afflictions, but our leaders lock him up. Unreal. But the CDC can force formaldehyde, Windex, and monkey nuts in our children's veins. Okay back on track after that dose of reality.

Another example of a superfood is Almonds. I have never heard anyone say anything adverse about them, they are always recommended as high in nutrition and protein (proper protein is highly beneficial in fighting cancer). Have snacks handy such as Granny Smith apple slices combined with raw almonds (Note: must be Granny Smith, all other apples are too high in sugar). Garlic is another superfood (fresh) which boosts the immune system. It's all about eliminating toxins, boosting the immune system and increasing killer cells when it comes to cancer recovery.

STEP #2: JUICE

"Juice," at any time, is a recipe from Dr. Bernardo, as follows. Now, I'm not talking about bottled or canned fruit juice sold in stores! I'm talking about organic fruit juiced with a juicer at home. Juicing is effective because (1) it is super nutrition right to the cells, (2) it contains live enzymes which ordinarily would be used to break down food, but when ingested without the pulp will go directly to the cell. Everything is always organic. Also, ingredients like carrots have anti-fungal properties.

Dr. B Cancer Cure Special: 1 granny smith apple (no other apple will do, others are too high in sugar content) 1 carrot, 1 lemon, 4 florets of broccoli. 4 florets cauliflower 1/2 cucumber, 1/2 beet, 1 slice ginger root, 1 slice pineapple, 1 slice papaya, 1 slice daikon radish (I add kale).

Note: The above juice is an emergency juice. If you're healing progress, and you need a mental "break", try just juicing the tasty fruits: granny smith apple, carrots, papaya and/or pineapple, ginger and cauliflower for a day. They are all very healing and without the green taste and include the cauliflower which is not as potent as broccoli but still cruciferous. Then get back on the full drink.

Keep reminding yourself that you want to live, and that is what this is all about!!! NOTE: To the extent, you can add wheatgrass whenever you can stand and afford it, DO IT!! It is one of the most potent healing juices ever. I worked up to 4 oz. once a day, substituting for the mid-day juice. Its healing properties are amazing.

STEP #3: ADD SUPPLEMENTS including PLANT OMEGA OILS and ESSENTIAL OILS (internal and topical)

Dr. Bernardo's Vitamins with my juice and/or food, divided into three times during the day. The brand you take is VERY important, since the FDA does not regulate, and Dr. Bernardo has found that some brands are ineffective (he has over 300 cancer patients he treats at one time, so he knows). All products can be purchased on the internet.

As we go to press I have just had the honor to meet Dr. Robert O Young who's protocol like Dr. Bernardo's has a 9o + % success rate using the pH balance method. As it turns out they learned the same things from different parts of the world. Dr. Robert O Young took things a step further with creating his own supplements designed to balance one's pH and I highly recommend them. https://phmiracleproducts.com/?aff=21

Supplements

Beta Glucan – Immune System Support: WGP Beta Glucan 500 mg. 2 tablets/2x a day. Priority One Brand (www.priorityonevitamins.com)

Boswellia Extract (700 mg 2x a day): use Source Naturals (www.sourcenaturals.com). This is an affordable tablet derivative of frankincense (see below).

QH Absorb UBIQUINOL: Q10 (200 mg 2x a day): must be UBIQUINOL. Unfortunately, this is a little costly, but it is worth it. I have learned the hard way that Dr. Bernardo knows what works. People will tell you otherwise, but they don't have a history of healing cancer as Dr. Bernardo does. Jarrow makes this (www.jarrow.com).

Active Selenium: (600 mcg 2 x a day):
Source Naturals is a very good brand (www.sourcenaturals.com). VERY important to cancer patients, this is one of the first supplements researched. My friend whose husband is a cancer doctor at MD Anderson Cancer Clinic in Houston had clinical trials going to show how effective this was treating cancer until his funding was pulled from him.

Vitamin D: I buy from my chiropractor's website (which has many interesting cancer articles) which is: www.dcnutrition.com. Dr. Geene used to be a pharmacist with MD Anderson Cancer Clinic in Houston, TX and says these supplements are pharmaceutical grade. The Vitamin D drops are immediately absorbable and dropped on the tongue. Vitamin D 4000-6000 IU

MSM: this is sulfur, dissolvable in water. The powder form is the most effective according to my chiropractor who used to be employed by MD Anderson Cancer Clinic and observed cancer clinical trials (not tablets for some reason). Very healing, known to be anti-cancer. Also get this from Dr. Greene's website: www.dcnutrition.com.

MSM SUGGESTED USE: 1/2 rounded teaspoonful 2 to 4 times daily (after meals)
this is from a 16-ounce bottle, from website DC nutrition
(MSM you want at least 1000 mg per day)

Plant-based Omega Oils and Essential Oils: both are "oxygen magnets" to the cells. The Omega oils are available at YES Supplements website: www.yes-supplements.com (organic evening primrose oil, organic safflower & sunflower oil, organic flax oil, organic pumpkin, organic extra virgin coconut oil): 1,450 mg in 2 capsules: take 5 capsules 3 times a day).

The essential oils are amazing concentrated plant and fruit oils. They are antiseptic, antibacterial, anti-viral. There is the equivalent of 500-800 plants or Fruits to a bottle, so you need the purest available which are Young Living and DoTerra Oils.

One can use Frankincense topically over cancer and it would create a rash EXACTLY over and outlining the cancer. Then, when the cancer went dead – NO MORE RASH! That is consistent with medical research that the oils enter the cell Membrane, pull out toxins/poisons and oxygenate/regenerate the cell. Frankincense, in particular, help apoptosis which, as I understand it, helps eliminate damaged cells before they become cancer. Incorporate these oils into your lifestyle on a regular basis and feel younger and stronger all the time!

Graviola (Therapeutic Laboratories brand, red bottle). This is an herb from the rainforest, which has been studied as very anti-cancer. It is very affordable. 2 tablets, one dropper or two capsules/2 times a day.

AHCC: promotes killer cells. 1 tablet, 3 times a day.

Vitamin C: Here is a chiropractor's website (which has many interesting cancer articles) which is: www.dcnutrition.com (Vitamin C - 5000 Mg would be the least.)

Turmeric: VERY important: You can buy this in bulk very cheaply over the internet or at an Indian food store. It is an antiseptic. A scientist that works for an oncologist lab told me her mother in India used to use it to heal external sores. It makes an easy paste with a little water, and if you drink 1 T. w/ 1/4 black pepper in water it is an incredible anti-cancer formula (it all mixes to equate to chemo). It contains curcumin, which stops the spread of cancer pathways, according to research articles. Drink in the morning and again at night. If you want tablet form, buy Planetary Herbals brand (www.planetaryherbals.com).

Coral Calcium w/ magnesium, zinc, and vitamins A & D (775 mg 3x a day): Vita Source brand is good (1-800-576-2471 or www.myvitasource.com). 3 tablets a day or more. Be very careful with the brand, because Dr. Bernardo says some companies add sand since this isn't FDA regulated, which can be very harmful.

Probiotic Master Supplement (5 billion CPU) (better ones now offer 50 billion live probiotics per capsule). E.g., see: https://store.draxe.com/products/organic-sbo-probiotic

Iodine drops: the cheapest is Lugol's Iodine drops distributed by various distributors including McAdam health Inc. (406-223-9949). You can overdose on this so be VERY careful only to take 4-5 drops a day.

Note: the above food-based supplements are missing in every cancer patient's body and/or help multiply killer cells to attack the cancer. That is why they are part of the protocols. To the extent you can't get or afford them all, DO WHAT YOU CAN. Some of them are VERY inexpensive, such as the Iodine, Turmeric (especially if you buy in a bulk container from an Indian spice store and just dissolve in water and drink), graviola, etc.

HERE IS A SAMPLE OF A DAY'S DIET:

Breakfast: Breakfast Tea (preferably chamomile) Organic eggs, Breakfast "Dr. B Enzyme juice", supplements.

Lunch: Salad with salmon (lemon and olive oil dressing), includes almonds and avocado Juice, supplements.

Dinner: Fresh salad w/ lemon and olive oil dressing Juice, supplements.

Break: Pectasol (a drink made of dried citrus pectin, to encapsulate the cancer and prevent metastasis or growth). NOTE: this is modified citrus pectin, which scientifically was advanced by scientists in recent years to be able to inhibit cancer growth not only in the colon but the rest of the body. It is made here in Santa Rosa (www.econugenics.com). It encapsulates the cancer and prevents it from metastasis. You can use this product during the first several months to give peace of mind.

The research scientist at econugenics said it should not interfere with the nutritional value and effectiveness of the other protocols.

Conclusion

There are many ways people have completely healed themselves of cancer. Being a researcher, I have researched many of them. I can tell you that the healing foods are usually plant-based and anti-fungal. Before your body can completely accept these nutrients it is important to detoxify the poisons in the body which have lead up to the disease, so anything which is detoxifying is helpful: dry hot saunas and bike rides to sweat and build the immune system (NO wet saunas which use chlorinated water), colonics or enemas, organic foods and juicing all slowly help the body detoxify. These plant-based protocols fit the medical community's knowledge which tries to replicate natural healing only with artificial drugs which have many guaranteed negative side-effects (actually direct effects!). The above are the basic natural plant-based healing protocols. Juicing is a must.
[See Pic 7.2]

Section two – Bernardo's Protocol

Authors Note: Thanks to Burton Goldberg and many of Dr. Bernardo's patients, we compiled an old letter accompanying his coaching. Enjoy everyone.

Introduction:

Cancer has been and continues to be treated and cured worldwide in countries where economic and political considerations do not restrict an individual's right to freedom of choice for medical treatment. Our treatment protocol requires strict adherence to your physician's instructions. Diet, juicing, teas, and supplement protocols must be followed exactly and may be a radical change of lifestyle for you. The protocol may not be easy to implement in the beginning, but the rewards of recovery and health will ease your hardships. Remember, there was something in your previous lifestyle that caused your Hypoxia (low oxygen concentration). Perhaps your diet, stress, toxic substances, abuse of your body and/or negative emotions caused the cancer.

Hypoxia, 35% level, is the only cause of cancer as proven by the brilliant biochemist and two-time Nobel Prize winner, Dr. Otto Warburg. All your systems, organs, blood, bones, and tissues are intricately and complexly affected by each other, and your emotional state will have a great bearing on your well-being. This book is not intended to be a guide for self-treatment but is provided for educational purposes by your physician who employs our protocol. New research and discoveries are constantly being incorporated into this program's protocol to improve the speed and quality of recovery for cancer patients. As new information is received, this patient guide will be updated.

It is critical that you follow the instructions in this book and those of your physician, exactly. You must never deviate from the program's protocol without consulting your physician. Your diet is very important - your decision to take one bite of something prohibited on your diet could be the mouthful that results in severe pain due to increasing the acidity in your body. Do not even consider "binging" or "cheating" as your life depends on following this protocol.

Read this entire book several times carefully, and make sure you understand ALL instructions. If there is anything you do not understand, ask your physician immediately. Your success with this program's protocol will depend on you and your commitment to health.

1. Following your diet
2. pH Testing
3. "Muscle Testing" everything before ingesting
4. Keeping a positive attitude
5. Resting peacefully in the sun before 11 am or after 3 pm

This protocol has been developed by the dedicated physicians, hematologists, bacteriologists, pharmacologists and other professionals in the healing arts who follow Hippocratic first law: "To do the patient no harm" and whose only motive is to heal. Drawing upon the latest research and proven, safe and effective therapies, these professionals will lead you to recovery.

PROGRAM SUMMARY

This protocol addresses every aspect of your life on all levels: physical, mental, emotional and spiritual. All are interdependent and must be followed to ensure a complete and speedy recovery:

- pH Testing
- Muscle Testing
- Diet/Nutrition
- Oral Supplements
- Exercise

- Heliotherapy (Full spectrum/sunlight)

- Non-toxic pain management

- Eliminating Stress & Negativity

- Physical, Emotional, & Spiritual Support

- Mental & Attitude discipline

- Removing Toxins

- Avoidance of negative electromagnetic fields

- Avoidance of toxic products for personal hygiene

- Avoidance of toxic products in the home

We believe that your recovery will be additionally benefitted by self-education. The more you know and understand, the more likely you are to follow the program's protocol to your greatest benefit. Always follow your physician's instructions and this protocol. If you have any doubt whatsoever about ingesting or initiating any therapeutic practice - ask your physician before you do it!

CANCER (TUMOR) MARKERS

Results of your blood tests are carefully examined and evaluated and will assist your physician in monitoring your condition. Cancer markers are an indicator of cancer's activity; the higher the marker, the more active the cancer. As a person improves, the cancer markers will be lower.

Test Name and Type of Cancer in which Marker may be Found

CEA (Carcinoembryonic Antigen)

Colon, lung, metastatic breast, pancreas, stomach, prostate, ovary, bladder, limbs, neuroblastoma, leukemia, osteogenic carcinoma

CA 125 (Ovarian Cancer 125)

Ovary, fallopian tube, cervical, endometrial, vulvar, pancreas

PSA (Prostate Specific Antigen)

Prostate Cancer

ALP (Alkaline Phosphatase)

Osteosarcoma, hepatocellular carcinoma, metastatic tumor to the liver, primary or secondary bone tumors

CA-BA (CA Associated Breast Antigen)

Breast Cancer

PAP (Prostatic Acid Phosphates)

Prostate, leukemia

LDH (Lactate Dehydrogenase)

Acute lymphocytic leukemia, non-Hodgkin's lymphoma, Ewing's, sarcoma, neuroblastoma, carcinoma of the testis, liver cancer

TPA (Tissue Polypeptide Antigen)

Gastrointestinal, genitourinary tract, breast, lung, thyroid

CT (Calcitonin)

Thyroid, lung, breast, pancreas, liver, kidney, carcinoid

CA 10-9 (Cancer Antigen)

Tumor Marker - Colon, lung, gastrointestinal

CA 15-3 (Cancer Antigen)

Tumor Marker - Breast

IMPORTANCE OF PH TESTING

Your body has cancer because it has become acidic. Every living thing in nature has a pH range from 1 very acidic (example: fuming Hydrochloric acid) to pH of 14 highly alkaline (example: Drano). Blood has a pH of 7.24. The normal body pH should be above 7.2 to 7.5.

First thing in the morning upon awakening, test your pH by checking your saliva. The lower your pH, the more active your cancer is. All terminal patients have a pH at or below 5. At 4.5 you die.

It becomes imperative to raise an acidic pH to a range above 7.2. Being acidic will cause the cancer patient severe pain, to lose their appetite and to feel extremely weak. This pain is comparable to being injected with vinegar, which has a pH of 5.3.

To combat the pain of being acidic, the cancer patient is given painkillers such as morphine, codeine, Vicodin, etc. Painkillers may alleviate severe pain but will make the cancer patient even more acidic. Normally, it takes 12 weeks to get a so-called terminal cancer patient to reach a pH of over 7.2. However, with our recent discovery by our filmmaker Ian Jacklin... of a liquid supplement called ASEA, the cancer patient will usually reach a pH of over 7.5 within 7 to 10 days.

In many instances, a change in saliva pH will bring relief from pain. In the body, the pH of saliva is an indication of its acidity or alkalinity. The pH is expressed in terms of numerical value with 7 being neutral (neither acid nor alkaline), less than 7 is acid and greater than 7 is alkaline. The quantity of fluids ingested, the metabolism of food, the amount of physical exertion, one's emotional state, and the time of the day can alter the degree of acidity of your body. the pHydrion paper provides an instant method of determining acid-alkaline pH in the 5.5 to 8.0 range.

Another way is to check the urine. Not your first urine of the day but one later and a couple hours after your meal. This is closest to the interstitial fluids Robert O Young speaks about. Your goal is for it to be 7.2 or 7.4. It takes most people 12 weeks so don't' stress out. Some take 18 months.

Lemons (even though they are "acid") will cause an alkaline reaction. If you have cancer pain, a great way to reduce your pain is by drinking water with fresh lemon juice, therefore causing an alkaline tide (release of sodium bicarbonate). Also, taking a teaspoon of baking soda in 4 ounces of water will reduce pain by neutralizing the lactic acid.

REMEMBER feeding the cancer sugar causes most cancer pain! Sugar is converted to lactic acid, which nourishes cancer. ALL natural and artificial sugars, including honey and agave, are prohibited in the cancer patient.

HOW TO TEST YOUR SALIVA

You will need pHydrion paper (strips) to test your saliva

We prefer the strips that have a range from 5.5 to 8.0 [See Image 7.3]

http://www.phreshproducts.com/beststrips/

1. First thing each morning and before drinking water or brushing teeth.
2. Tear off 2 inches of pH paper from the roll
3. Place paper on top of the tongue for 10 seconds
4. Compare the color of pH paper with the color chart on the pH paper roll dispenser
5. There is a number above the color - write the number and date on your calendar and inform Dr. Bernardo of the pH number

Charting your pH is very important to your health. Make sure to do this every morning until told otherwise.

DIETARY GUIDELINES

ALL food and supplements must be muscle tested prior to ingesting

Eat foods as close to their natural state as possible. Processed adulterated and altered foods are diminished in their health-giving properties. The immune system cannot be sustained by "dead" food. Eat organically grown foods as much as possible. Foods grown on chemically fertilized soils fed and sprayed with pesticides will not benefit you as much as organically grown foods on highly mineralized soils with good organic matter content.

At least 50% of all the foods you eat should be raw. Read food labels carefully. Prepare food as close to the time of eating as possible. Prepare only the amount you can eat. No leftovers as they are dead food. Make mealtimes as enjoyable as possible. Take the time to relax and enjoy your food to help in the digestion.

Do not drink large amounts of water at mealtime. Water has no food value instead of sub fresh vegetable juices or teas (Essiac, Purple la Pacho, pH Tea, Green Gunpowder). If unfamiliar with using natural foods, purchase a cookbook from PMR or find a natural food cookbook for recipe ideas.

Always eat breakfast within 1 hour upon waking.

If in doubt - DON'T EAT IT. Consult your physician.

Do not allow more than 3 hours to elapse between eating and drinking something.

DAILY FOOD CHECKLIST

6 oz - 2 times daily of fresh vegetable juice. Make sure to drink with a straw

2 - servings of green leafy vegetables

1 - sea plant and/or daikon radish

8 oz - 2 times daily Tea (Essiac, Purple la Pacho, pH Tea, Green Gunpowder)

1 - Fresh raw vegetable salad

Protein (ie. meat, fish, legumes, etc.) keep to a minimum

NOTE:

If Imuplus is recommended in your protocol, make sure to drink 2 packets 2 times a day in goat milk or water. If you like, you may add cinnamon, nutmeg, or 100% pure stevia.

FOOD PREPARATION

Prepare foods by using the least amount of water possible for steaming or juicing.

Wash all vegetables/fruit with non-toxic cleaning products

Broiled - food may be lightly broiled

Oven roasting at low temperatures and hot, dry air are also recommended.

USE THE FOLLOWING PRODUCTS:

Stainless Steel

Cast Iron

Glass

Corning Ware

Pyrex

Enamel ceramic ware (lead test first)

Juicer, Triturator or press (Recommended: Champion, Norwalk, Juice Man & Jack LaLanne)

Food Processors

Graters

Grain Mills

DO NOT USE THE FOLLOWING PRODUCTS:

Microwave

Aluminum foil and/or pans

Teflon or Non-stick coating pans

Electric blenders (kills enzymes), use juicer

Excessive heat or smoke: Frying, charcoal broiling and/or barbecuing

RECOMMENDED FOODS - "DO EAT"

(*) Especially Important to Eat

(+) Eat only if approved by a physician

(#) Eat Sparingly

WATER - Distilled or Spring Water ONLY

MILK - Almond Milk and/or Goat Milk

SOUP (*) Fresh Homemade

Bread - Ezekiel Only

(*) SALADS - Green Leafy

(*) TEA - Sierra Madre, Purple La Pacho, pH or Green Gunpowder

(*) SEA PLANTS

Agar-agar

Arame

Dulse

Hijiki

Kombu

Nori

Wakame

(+) BEANS & LEGUMES - only

Azuki (adzuki)

Black Beans

Lentils

JUICES

(*) Fresh Grapefruit (6 oz)

(*) Fresh Mixed Vegetables

(*) Carrot Juice with Avocado

CHEESE - MADE FROM GOAT

Goat Cream

Brie

Havarti

(#) SALT - Sea Salt only

SPROUTS (Not more than 5 days old)

SEEDS - Fresh, raw and unsalted

Flax

Pumpkin

Sesame

Sunflower

POTATOES

Red - baked or steamed (eat the skins)

Yams

FISH - Fresh, Salt-water, non-scavenger

Cod

Shark

Snapper

Sole

Trout

Tuna

(+) MEAT - Only

Buffalo

Deer

Goat

Lamb

NUTS - fresh, raw, and unsalted

Cashews

Walnuts

Almonds

Hazelnuts

Pine Nuts

Macadamia

Pecans

NO PEANUTS

(*) GRAINS - whole grains only

Amaranth

Brown Rice

Buckwheat

Millet

Triticale

Wild Rice

FRUITS - NONE except the following

Avocados

Berries, all berries, all you want every day

Green apples / Granny Smith

Japanese Pickled Plums (Umeboshi)

Lemons

BAKING POWDER - Non-Aluminum ONLY

SWEETENER - 100% pure Stevia ONLY

VEGETABLES & HERBS - Fresh ONLY

Artichokes

Asparagus

Avocado

Bamboo Shoots

Bean Sprouts

Beets

Beet Greens

(*) Broccoli

Bok Choy (Greens, Stems)

(*) Brussel Sprouts

Cabbage

Carrots (only with Avocado JUICED)

(*) Cauliflower

Celery

Chard

Chicory

Chives

Cilantro

Collard Greens

Cucumber

Endive

Escarole

Garlic

Ginger

Green Beans

Green Onions

Jicama

Kale

Kohlrabi

Leeks

Lettuce

Mushrooms

Mustard Greens

Okra

Onions

Parsley

Parsnips

Peppers

Pimento (fresh)

Potatoes (Red Irish ONLY)

Pumpkin

Radishes

Rhubarb

Rutabagas

Spinach

String Beans

Squash (Acorn, Butternut, Yellow Winter, Zucchini)

Swiss Chard

Turnips

Turnip Greens

Water Chestnuts

Watercress

Yams

NOT RECOMMENDED FOODS - DO NOT EAT!

Bread - NONE except Ezekiel

Baking Powder with Aluminum

Beans and Legumes - except Sprouted under 5 days old

Carob

Cereals - NO CEREALS - including Oatmeal (Nothing in a Box)

Chocolate

Cornstarch - use arrowroot instead

Fish - smoked or salted

Flour - refined

Pasta, noodles - made with refined or processed grains

Refined or Processed Foods

Salt - except Sea Salt

Shellfish - ALL

Sprouts - over 5 days old

Sodas - NONE AT ALL including unsweetened & Ginger Ale

Tomatoes - except Cherry Tomatoes

Vinegar

Water - Fluoridated or Tap

Wilted Fruits or Vegetables

DAIRY PRODUCTS - except Raw Goat Milk and Cheese made from Raw Goat Milk

Cheese - Eat only what is on the RECOMMENDED LIST

Butter

Margarine

Milk

Yogurt

DRINKS

Alcoholic Beverages

Cocoa

Coffee

Iced Drinks

Soft Drinks/Sodas

FRUIT - ALL except

Avocados

Granny Smith (Green) Apples

Japanese Pickled Plums

Lemons (Fresh)

SUGARS ALL including

Agave

Brown Sugar

Corn Syrup

Honey

Maple Syrup

Molasses

Sugar Substitutes

White Sugar

SWEETS ALL including

Cakes

Candies

Cookies

Custards

Gelatin

Ice Cream

Pastries

Sauces

GRAINS

ANY Refined or Processed Grains

White Rice

JUICES - ALL Fruit Juices (Canned, Frozen or Sweetened)

MEAT

Bacon

Beef

Luncheon Meats

Sausages

Pork

Veal

POULTRY ALL including

Chicken - ONLY Range Free is OK

Duck

Goose

Pheasant

Turkey

JUICES

Use fresh organic fruits and vegetables for optimal results. Juicing contains enzymes which are beneficial in assisting to repair the body

DR. B's Cancer Killer Juices.

#1 ENZYME JUICE

1 Granny Smith Apple

1 Carrot

½ Cucumber

½ Beet

¼ inch Daikon Radish (Looks like a White Carrot)

7 Asparagus Stalks (COOKED)

1 cup Broccoli

¼ inch Fresh Ginger

2 Brussels Sprouts

½ inch Slice of Fresh Pineapple

Drink Enzyme Juice within 20 minutes of making, with a Straw ONLY

#2 AVOCADO - CARROT JUICE

½ Avocado, place in a bowl and mash well

Add 8 ounces of Fresh Carrot Juice to Avocado Mixture

Let Avocado - Carrot Juice sit for 30 minutes and drink with a Straw ONLY

The benefit of Avocado - Carrot Juice contains abscisic acid, which helps to build the body's immune system.

#3 ASPARAGUS JUICE

Place fresh cooked Asparagus in a juicer, enough to make 4 ounces (Approximately 8-10 stalks)

Drink 4 ounces of Asparagus Juice twice daily, with a Straw ONLY, as soon as it's made

Do not drink more than 8 ounces per day

OR

Eat 1 small can of Asparagus Daily

#4 WHEATGRASS JUICE

Place fresh Wheatgrass in a juicer, enough to make 4 ounces (START with 2 ounces)

Drink 4 ounces of Wheatgrass Juice twice daily, with a Straw ONLY as soon as it is made

Do not drink more than 8 ounces per day

If you find the Wheatgrass makes you ill, do not drink it

The benefits of Wheatgrass Juice - Cleanses the blood, organs, and gastrointestinal tract of debris; stimulates metabolism by enriching the blood, and aids in reducing blood pressure by dilating the blood pathways throughout the body.

Resources for Wheatgrass - Java Juice, Health Food Stores that have a juice bar, Henry's (in most California Stores), Evergreen Juices Inc. (Canada) wheatgrass can be ordered and delivered to your home.

SUPPLEMENTATIONS

Follow your individualized protocol, which may include taking many oral supplements daily. Some patients find that their individualized protocol included taking what they consider an impossible number of supplements on a daily basis! Our patients have reported, what initially seemed impossible or significantly annoying at the start of their protocol, soon became almost a pleasure. As taking the supplements created an influx of nutrients to the body, and brought about increased feelings of strength and well-being.

Taking the supplements recommended in your protocol is crucial to your recovery. You must never miss nor forget to take a single supplement.

This also means you, or someone assisting you, must be responsible for making sure you always have the needed supplements on hand. Make sure you have an adequate supply of all your recommended supplements. Never wait until the last minute to order your supplements.

DO NOT assume that your pharmacy nor supplier is always going to have what you need on the shelf when you need it! PLAN AHEAD!

DO NOT purchase any supplements from your local health food stores, unless they are identical to what is provided with your protocol.

All of our supplements have been tested for electrical energy. Many similar brands are toxic with traces of benzene or other elements which will deplete your body of its electrical energy, therefore making you feel weaker.

"The human body heals itself and nutrition provides the resources to accomplish the task."
-- Roger Williams PH.D

MUSCLE TESTING

Physicians have found a very simple and accurate method to determine if you are sensitive to any food or substance or if that substance might be harmful to you called "Muscle Testing." This process is also known as "Kinesiology" and such a simple process that many people find it difficult to believe it actually works. Do not be fooled by the simplicity - "Muscle Testing" is not superstitious ritual - it is a scientifically proven procedure.

"Muscle Testing" is critical to your therapy. It will ensure that you ingest no substance nor food that may be harmful to you. You must "Muscle Test" everything. As your condition changes, so might your body's reaction to various foods and substances. Just because you test "Good" on a substance today, does not mean it won't test "BAD" or be harmful to you tomorrow.

ALWAYS TEST EVERYTHING before ingesting!

For further information on the "Muscle Testing" process, please read the book Your Body Doesn't Lie, by John Diamond.

"Muscle Testing" Procedure

1. Stand with your right arm relaxed at your side, raise your left arm out to your side and hold it parallel to the floor with the elbow straight.

2. Have a friend face you and place his/her left hand on your right shoulder to steady you.

3. Have your friend place his/her right hand on your extended left arm just above the wrist.

4. Prepare to resist having your arm pushed downward. Place your right hand in the center of your chest with your palm flat against your chest.

5. Have your friend push down on your left arm quickly and firmly. The idea is to push just hard enough to test the spring and bounce in your arm. Not so hard that the muscle becomes fatigued. It is not a question of who is stronger but of whether the muscle can lock the shoulder joint against the push. Notice how you resist and how far down your arm goes. This is your baseline measure. Start with fresh lemon and notice how strong your arm is. Repeat with a piece of candy and notice how your arm drops. Your arm dropping is indicating that what you are testing is "NOT GOOD" for you.

1. Now take the food, injection, or supplement you wish to test in your right hand. Hold the item against the center of your chest.

2. Repeat steps 1 through 5.

If you are unable to resist and your arm goes down easily or lower than your baseline measure, this means the item is "NOT GOOD' for your body - DO NOT EAT or TAKE IT!

If you can resist with equal or greater strength as when you tested without anything (your baseline measure), then the substance will not harm you and you may use it.

NEVER INGEST ANY FOOD OR SUPPLEMENTS UNLESS YOU HAVE "MUSCLE TESTED" IT FIRST!

Remember: Your body is changing daily, and food or substance may test "GOOD" today and test "BAD" tomorrow.

"All of life is a journey, which paths we take, what we look back on and what we look forward to is up to us. We determine our destination, what kind of road we take to get there and how happy we are when we get there." - Steven Tyler

MERCURY

In 60 years of treating so-called "terminal cancer patients," we have never seen a case where patients were not contaminated with mercury.

Amalgam fillings contain 51% mercury, one of the most toxic elements in the world. This has been known since 1920. Over 12,000 plus articles prove the highly toxic results of mercury amalgam fillings.

Mercury paralyzes the lymphocytes, the part of the immune system which is responsible for collecting the cancer microbes in the bloodstream and feeding them to the red blood cells for their destination.

The older a person gets, the greater the toxicity. People chewing gum are exposed to mercury vapors from amalgam fillings. Also, breathing in about 17,000 times per day, this mercury poisoning affects every part of the body. This explains to us why we see so much mercury in urine and hair samples in people with severe chronic illnesses.

Cancer, chronic fatigue, fibromyalgia are a few of the illnesses that can be attributed to mercury poisoning.

We had a case where a patient had gone blind. A major university in California told the patient that she had hysterical blindness; her mercury levels were never tested.

When the patient came to our office after a hair analysis test, we discovered industrial levels (mercury levels over 2.5 ug/g) of mercury in her body. After her amalgam fillings were removed she was given 100 grams of Vitamin C orally for 2 weeks and then 5-8 grams daily for another 12 weeks. After four months, her vision was restored to normal and the highly toxic levels of mercury were decreased by 98%. The lab that performed the hair analysis stated that this was the highest level of mercury they had ever recorded and were surprised that the patient had not died of mercury poisoning.

SUPPORT

Your support system is very important to your recovery.

At all times, avoid negative people or people who do not support you and the decisions you are making regarding the therapy process you have chosen.

It is critical and crucial to your healing process to only surround yourself with loving people who will be supportive of you (ie - loving family, friends, coworkers, your church or spiritual advisor) and the therapy process you have chosen.

Many cities have cancer support groups that are uplifting, inspirational, and provide activities that you can participate in.

If you find your new protocol difficult, we will provide you with the names of other cancer survivors we worked with that you can team up with. Cancer survivors are a great source of support as they too have been through this process and survived.

"Eventually you will come to understand that love heals everything, and love is all there is."
-- Gary Zukav

ANGER

It is imperative that any/all strong, negative emotions (ie. anger, hostility or resentment) are dealt with IMMEDIATELY, no matter what the cause!

You must search and identify the underlying problems causing these feelings. Negative feelings and all the associated emotions are highly destructive to your health and healing process.

Negative emotions will feed your cancer and can increase tumor markers dramatically, sometimes as much as 200 points per day. Failure to let go of hate, anger, hostility, resentment or past pain will not only hurt you, but it will also kill you. It does not take long to reach the point of no return "DEATH".

Whatever has happened in the past is over, you cannot go back - it is beyond your control. All your hatred and all your negative emotions are water over the dam - IT IS OVER - and crucial to your healing process. These negative feelings must be put aside so you can move on.

YOU HAVE TO LET GO!
YOU MUST MAKE PEACE WITH YOURSELF AND OTHERS!
YOU MUST FORGIVE!

Treat negative emotions as vile poisons that will feed your cancer and guaranteed to cause your death. Stay away from those people that you hate, feel anger or resentment towards, and resolve your feelings NOW! Let it go and move on.

In two years, out of 21 women that came to our office with breast cancer, seventeen cases were due to anger from their husbands or boyfriends. If you cannot resolve your problems and remove the anger, then you may want to consider a separation or divorce. The women who divorced their husbands are alive and well, and the others died within six months after returning to the same negative, hateful relationships.

You must NOW call on every survival method you have or search out new tools to deal with and rid yourself of negative emotions. Where there was hate, anger or hostility, there must now be love, peace, forgiveness, and compassion.

Love with Passion
Live life in the now
Live each moment to its fullest
Forgive and forget

ATTITUDE
Your positive attitude and emotional state is just as important as your diet and just as critical to your recovery and continued health.

Enjoy what you eat and make mealtimes pleasant. Take your time. Chew well and slowly. Pay attention, savor, and enjoy the flavors and textures. Be grateful. Make your environment as pleasing as possible. Let the light in; invite your friends to mealtimes. The food you eat is critical to your recovery - how you eat your food can affect how your system utilizes it.

Many cooks will swear that using the same ingredients, the same amounts, and the same recipe they will get different results. A meal prepared when a chef is angry cannot compare (nor will they receive any compliments) with the same meal prepared with joy.

Maintain positive thoughts and feelings. Use all your strength to eliminate your negative emotions and thoughts. Take at least ½ hour each day as your special, quiet time to meditate or pray, leaving all your worries behind and concentrating on that which is positive and helpful. Training your mind to focus on positive thoughts may not be easy. Treat your negative thoughts and feelings as the devil. Be a warrior and win!

Remember to laugh each day; "A heart of joy does good like a cure". Try to find something joyful in what may appear as tragic. Research has shown that certain chemicals (endorphins) are released in the body when we laugh and will stimulate your immune system. Many health care professionals suspect that many positive, health-giving effects of joy and laughter are as of yet, undiscovered. Norman Cousins, in his book "Anatomy of an Illness as Perceived by the Patients" states he watched old comedy movies and laughed to combat a life-threatening illness, and that this laughter played an essential part in his recovery. Take a laughter yoga class and enjoy the laughter.

Researchers have proven that our posture, facial expressions, thoughts and emotions all have a real effect on our body's health. When we experience pain or illness, we can help make beneficial changes to our immune system by simply simulating joy and happiness in our body language. It appears that even though we might not really feel happy, the result is that through smiling, standing erect, whistling while we walk and other bodily expressions of happiness, many systems in the body are receiving messages of health and begin to follow these instructions.

Many worshipers, after singing with heads held high (arms swinging and raised upward), in expansive expressions of joy and gratefulness, experience a sense of well-being and a healthy glow. No one has found any toxic side effects to the practice of smiling, laughing or "Jumping for joy." Could it be that if we took the time each day to express happiness through body movements and expressions (even if we don't "feel" like it), we might improve our health and later really feel the joy of well-being?

It may be helpful to create for yourself a short and simple prayer or affirmation to memorize and use whenever you find yourself bombarded by negative thoughts or feelings. One patient, who is now fully recovered, wrote this for himself.

"At this moment I am alive and have many things to be grateful for. My body quickly ELIMINATES anything harmful that it encounters, and I now imagine and feel exactly how I would feel when I first realized I am truly in perfect health. It is a feeling of incredible relief, unbounded gratitude and an intense desire to enjoy and maximize each and every moment of my life. With each breath, thought, and action, I thank God for this great and glorious gift of life."

Attitude is a little thing that makes a big difference
-- Winston Churchill
[See Image 7.4]

EXERCISE, FRESH AIR & SUNSHINE
Exercise, fresh air, and sunshine are prescribed for very important reasons.
Daily movement or not moving your body can directly affect the speed and completeness of your recovery, along with the quality of the air you breathe and the amount of sunshine you receive on a daily basis. These things are not just something you "should do" but something you "must do".

Exercise (always ask your physician before starting any exercise regimen)

While exercise is known to have positive and beneficial effects on the body, other simple activities such as gardening, house cleaning, stretching, yoga, or any positive body movement, are also just as beneficial to our bodies. In movement there is life, in stagnation there is death.

As you begin to feel stronger and more comfortable, start adding other forms of exercise to your daily routine. Any recreational activities such as swimming, badminton, ping-pong, even horseshoes can be beneficial. Keep as active as possible. Get a treadmill or stationary bike and pedal away while you watch your favorite TV show. With regular bicycling, you will enjoy the outdoors (Fresh Air) and get back the feeling of when you were a kid riding their bicycle.

Walking

Walking daily, you will receive two benefits: exercise and fresh air. Walk at least twice a day outdoors in a park away from streets and fumes for 20 minutes. While walking, do some deep breathing where the air is fresh and clean. Keep your head up, enjoy your walks, and build up to where you are walking briskly with a "happy gait". You should be able to say your ABC's while walking and not be winded.

Fresh Air

Now that you've gotten your daily doses of clean air on your walks, try to improve the air you breathe inside your home and workplace, you may want to purchase an air purifier.

Sunshine

Sunshine on our bodies helps us to metabolize and better assimilate many needed nutrients. Remember Vitamin D? The Sunshine Vitamin!

Daily, get at least 16 minutes of sunshine on your entire body, both front and back. 8 minutes on each side, BEFORE 11:00 AM or AFTER 3:00 PM.

Make your exercise periods enjoyable and joyful!

STRETCHING

Each morning, take 15 minutes to stretch.

Depending on the condition of your health, you may or may not be able to stretch your entire body. Start slowly by stretching as many limbs and joints as you can without experiencing pain.

Daily stretching of your entire body will keep your body flexible. Stretch and move your toes, legs, hips, arms, fingers, neck, and spine. Stretch your facial muscles too. Make funny faces.

There are many books and youtube videos you can obtain which will provide you with simple and effective stretching exercises.

Beginning/gentle yoga stretches are highly recommended. You may also consider visiting a physical therapist to assist you in establishing a stretching routine that is best for you.

In addition, always change your lying or sitting positions and stretch if you have remained in one position for 15 minutes or longer. Many animals do this instinctively - watch a cat stretch. "Do a cat" stretch every morning before you get out of bed.

Stretching in a swimming pool is a wonderful way to begin increasing your flexibility and many people whose bodies are particularly inflexible find stretching in the water the easiest way to begin.

"If you have only one smile in you, give it to the people that you love." -- Maya Angelou

PERSONAL HYGIENE & YOUR ENVIRONMENT

Many cosmetics and cleaning products contain substances such as benzene, which are carcinogenic or toxic to our bodies. Use hygiene and cleaning products that are as natural as possible.

Avoid the following:

Personal Hygiene Products: Hair color or permanent wave solution, toxic hair sprays, synthetic cosmetics, lipstick made out of coal tar dyes and antiperspirants that contain aluminum. Use only natural non-allergenic cosmetics and deodorants.

Microwaves: If there is a microwave in the house, get rid of it IMMEDIATELY. If you are in a location that is using a microwave, leave the room while it is on.

Radiation Emitting Items: Avoid prolonged exposure to radiation emitting items such as computer screens, color televisions, electric power lines, and cell phones.

ELECTRIC BLANKETS/HEATING PAD - DO NOT USE under any circumstance. Research has shown an increased incidence of cancer with persons using electric blankets. You may heat your bed with an electric blanket but turn it off prior to getting into bed. If you want to use a hot-pack, we recommend using SNAPHEAT.

Environment: Keep your home clean and free of dust and mold. Avoid carpets as they provide a great home for mites and pollens. AVOID cleaning solutions, solvents, paint remover, and insect sprays.

Noise: Remember that noise can also affect your health. Make your household environment as quiet and peaceful as possible. Play soft soothing music.

Air: Using an air purifier will enhance your indoor air quality. Make sure you have the device on at least 12 hours per day.

PAIN MANAGEMENT

NEVER ALLOW ACUTE PAIN TO CONTINUE WITHOUT NOTIFYING YOUR PHYSICIAN.

Our protocols preferred the method of pain management and reduction is pH management. Importance of pH Testing. In many instances, a change in saliva pH will bring relief from pain. The pH of saliva is an indication of its acidity or alkalinity. The pH is expressed in terms of a numerical value with 7 being neutral (neither acid nor alkaline) less than 7 is acid and greater than 7 is alkaline. Virtually everybody activity - the quantity of fluids taken in, the metabolism of food, the amount of physical exertion and even one's emotional state and the time of the day can alter the degree of acidity of saliva. Urine should have a pH of about 6 to 6.4 (slightly acid). pH provides an instant method of determining saliva pH (See chapter 5 on pH Testing) Your saliva is ACID if the color of the paper matches a color on the chart (YELLOW), which is less than 7. Your saliva is ALKALINE if the color of the paper matches a color on the chart (GREEN), which is more than 7. Eating cranberries will cause an acid reaction. Lemons (even though they are "acid") will cause an alkaline reaction.

If your saliva is ACID:

Take 1 Tablespoon fresh lemon juice in 4 ounces of water, three times daily and drink 6 ounces of **ASEA** (2 ounces three times daily) on an empty stomach until pH changes.

(Personal note: I turned Dr. B on to the **ASEA**. Yes I'm bragging. It's great for pro athletes too.)

Your saliva should be ALKALINE

Remember, feeding cancer carbohydrates (which will cause a drop in pH) causes more cancer pain. These carbohydrates then turn into lactic acid, which is the main food or nourishment of cancer.

THIS LACTIC ACID BUILD-UP IS THE FOOD THAT NOURISHES CANCER.

OUR JOB IS TO STARVE THE CANCER BY COMPLETELY ELIMINATING LACTIC ACID FROM THE BODY, AND BY DOING THIS MOST CANCERS WILL GO INTO REMISSION.

Do not let your pain levels get out of control. On a scale of 1 to 10, if your pain is over 6 contact your physician.

REST AND RELAXATION

Try to maintain regular sleeping periods. Notify your physician if you are having trouble sleeping.

Take at least a half hour daily for relaxation. Do something which gives you enjoyment and produces inner peace, calmness, and contentment.

This may be a quiet time you spend in your garden or workshop, listening to music you enjoy, reading a favorite book, or whatever brings your joy.

The more activities you can participate in which are positive and enjoyable, the faster your recovery will be.

During the day, observe your body. Are you tense? Are all your muscles relaxed? How can you change your position to make yourself more comfortable and relaxed?

Many people have found swimming or yoga (gentle or laughter) to be helpful.

Laughing three times every day will build up your immune system. Have a loved one tickle you!

Hug and kiss each other as this too will build up your immune system; it's simple to do and a joy to give and receive.

Joy and gratefulness can do much to assist in your healing process.

"Love is the great miracle cure. Loving ourselves works miracles in our lives."
-- Louise Hay

REMOVING TOXINS

ONE (1) HOT SALT BATH DAILY

Take one (1) hot salt bath daily (at bedtime), to increase circulation and encourage the discharge of toxins.

Place 4 cups of salt into your bathtub. (DO NOT use Epsom Salt).

You can purchase a 20 lb bag of Morton's Salt at any grocery store.

Add water, which should be as hot as possible.

Soak in the tube for as long as you can or until the water becomes cool (about 15 minutes).

Make sure that your entire body is completely submerged, all the way up to your neck in the saltwater.

Do not completely rinse off your body as this will assist you in falling asleep.

Also, saunas are good for sweating and removing toxins if you have one available to you.

Sweating is very important to the bodies healing process; it increases circulation and facilitates the elimination of harmful toxins.

And making peace with our past creates a sense of lightness and freedom within our mind, body, and spirit." - Craig Townsend

ENEMAS

Coffee enemas are to be taken for additional removal of toxins in the body and will markedly decrease nausea. Coffee, when taken in a retention enema, enters the liver directly through the mesenteric vein and stimulates the liver to excrete toxic substances into the bile system. This periodic build-up in the liver of toxic materials may largely account for nausea.

It is best to do the coffee enema first thing in the morning or whenever you begin to feel sick to your stomach.

Place 3 Tablespoons of ground coffee in 1 quart of water in a glass or stainless-steel container.

Bring to a boil and turn the heat off immediately and let steep for 5 minutes.

Place coffee mixture in an enema bag - it should be as hot as you can tolerate on your hand

Place nail 42 inches above the floor and hang the enema bang on the nail.

Lie on your left side on the floor with your knees drawn up, holding the on/off switch next to your buttocks.

Allow the coffee mixture to flow into the colon, taking in as much of the coffee mixture as you can hold.

Wait 1 minute until distension (fullness) is gone.

Repeat the process

After 3 minutes on the left side, roll over to your back.

Stay on your back for 3 minutes and then roll on to your right side.

If you must evacuate, do so.

You initially may only be able to take in a few ounces.

Build up to ½ to 1 quart per day (1 time a day) - It is best to do the coffee enema first thing in the morning.

TESTIMONIALS

LB

I first became ill with cervical cancer in 2003. I refused chemotherapy and I was fine until 2006. Doctors told me I had a tumor in my left lung and it was probably cancer that had spread from cervical cancer from before. I went to see Dr. Bernardo for it and 6 months later my tumors were gone. LB

KS

I want to thank you for all you've done throughout 2009 to help me regain my health. When I contracted a rare mold that attacked my lungs while on a business trip to S. Korea, you were able to both find and treat my malady while conventional medicine remained baffled. Gratefully, KS

PS

This is a summary of my experiences with my diagnosed illness of Leukemia and the successful treatment that you put me on that brought me back to health.

In 1998, I was set to have a fibroid operation. As part of the pre-op tests, they discovered leukemia. I was sent to a specialist who wanted to start chemotherapy the next day. I refused. I researched and went to a nutritionist. I began a special diet, Acupuncture - Korean and Chinese - a Qi Gong Master and Acupuncturist.

My daughter's schoolmate's father had been diagnosed with Lung cancer at Cedars and had been declared terminal 5 years before. (RL) journeyed to Mexico searching for treatment. While there, he was referred to Dr. Bernardo, whose clinic he went to. Under Dr. Bernardo's care, his 42 lung tumors cleared up in 12 months. CAT scan and MRI detected no traces of lung cancer. I talked to (RL) for two hours; he told me about his treatment and gave me Dr. Bernardo's phone number.

I called Dr. Bernardo, and within four days, I was in his clinic in Mexico. I work in the film industry and I told Dr. Bernardo that I could come in four months because of work. He said I must start treatment if I wanted to survive. I did, so I went immediately to his clinic.

As part of the condition, I had a spleen that weight 15lbs 9ozs. That was we eventually removed after my blood counts became normal and I stabilized. I started treatment the morning after I arrived in Mexico. My blood eventually stabilized, and I was able to continue my treatment at home. That was in 1998, it is now 2010. I am still on this earth because of Dr. Bernardo's dedication to his patients and his ongoing research. My family and I are in his debt. PS

BN

To say that (J) & I are glad you came into our lives would be the biggest understatement of our lives! Without your guidance (J) would not be here today. Here is a summary of our experiences with (J's) illness for you to pass on to other people who may not yet understand how God's food can heal a diseased body.

After months of agonizing symptoms in February 2008, our eight-year-old daughter was finally diagnosed with Medulloblastoma...brain & spinal cancer. She immediately underwent brain surgery to remove a massive tumor that was against her brain stem. She had another small tumor on her spine that would be left there due to high collateral damage she would suffer from surgery. After recovering from her brain surgery, she began radiation & chemotherapy for about six weeks. After a one-month break, she began a six-month schedule of additional chemotherapy. That was already destroying her little body. Nausea, constipation, abdominal pain, severe anemia, leg paralysis, constant infection, and fear were major side effects that greatly overshadowed the expected ones like hair loss, burned skin, and extreme weight loss...At the fourth month, her spinal tumor had disappeared, however, she had relapsed with a new brain tumor. Clearly, this was not working for her. It was recommended to us that we make arrangements for hospice and make the best of her final days. There were a few big options: additional surgery, bone marrow transplant, stem cell implant, or additional chemo and radiation. However, admittedly, there would be only less than a 3% chance of success for (J).

Through some great friends (B & LW), we were put in touch with you. I remember you telling me that (J) was NOT dying of cancer but acidosis. We immediately started your recommendations. When we first measured (J's) pH, it was 5.5 or lower. The pH even began moving upward. At exactly 8 weeks, her pH finally made it to 7.2. We had been scheduled for another MRI when we were released because of her relapse. To everyone's astonishment, the results of the MRI showed that the tumor had shrunk by 75%!!!! We continued your detoxification and fresh vegetable recipe regimen. We recently had another MRI to find that the tumor is COMPLETELY gone! Praise God! Thank you for all of your hard work. Thank you for coaching us through this most difficult time. Thank you for dedicating your life to saving people's lives by pointing us to God's food. Thank you for enduring criticism by those who just don't want to be open to how God heals through his food. Thank you for constantly being available for advice. Thank you for helping us and (J's) life.

Please forward our contact information to anyone that would like more details about our experience with (J). Warmest Regards, BN

LP - May 3, 2010

I would consider it a privilege to let others know what you have done for me. It is with great pleasure that I write this letter and hope the information herein will be helpful and encouraging to others.

I had been diagnosed with breast cancer in the fall of 2000. I had a mastectomy and no chemo or other treatment as the doctors anticipated only a 3% chance of recurrence. In fall 2008, the breast cancer had metastasized to the spinal column and I had emergency surgery with radiation. I was told that I should follow a regimen of drugs to prevent the recurrence, as there is no cure. None of the treatments agreed with me and I had a series of serious infections as a result of them.

I was exploring Brian Peskin's website and contacted him about his treatment regimen for metastatic breast cancer. He referred me to his friend, Dr. Bernardo, in California, who had a much more stringent regimen and a record of success with a serious cancer diagnosis. That chance referral has changed my life. I started with Dr. Bernardo in November 2009. I did the juicing, modified my diet as he prescribed and took the supplements. After getting off all other cancer medications and following Dr. Bernardo's directions, I had not one more infection of any kind. All my blood chemistry numbers are now normal and my oncologist, after my last CT scan, in April 2010, was amazed that he could find no signs of cancer. He said, "I wish I could take credit for this, but I know you didn't follow any of my advice." This statement is true, as I followed Dr. Bernardo's instruction and forsook any of the typical drug therapies. My statement to my oncologist was that if I could not fight off the smallest bacterial that doesn't affect others, how could I fight off cancer. He agreed with my logic.

I am now down to ½ an Aleve twice a day. Expect to soon not need any. The pain in my back is minimal and probably due only to the rods they put in at the time of the surgery to stabilize my spine. Medicine has its place, but I believe your approach to God's healing power is the key in my recovery.

Dr. Bernardo, you are always upbeat and encouraging. Your caring association is rare and it is a pleasure to work with you in the healing process. God bless you and your work. LP

RL

An oncologist at a major prestigious hospital in Los Angeles advised me to get my affairs in order. "That I had less than a week to live." I went to see Dr. Bernardo at his hospital in Mexico. I showed him my x-rays with 42 tumors. I had expected him to say no hope.

On the contrary, he told me, "RL, you are very sick and you have just won the Olympic Gold Medal for the most cancer tumors in the lungs; however you are not going to die if you start on my protocol immediately." I smiled and thought this poor doctor doesn't want to tell me that I am dying. I started Dr. Bernardo's protocol and in 12 months, I was in complete remission.

Sometime later when I met Dr. Bernardo, I told him that you are a maverick, a mad scientist, and a madman, but most of all a genius. Thank you for saving my life. RL

"Love cures people - both the ones who give it and the ones who receive it."
-- Dr. Karl Menninge

CHAPTER 8:

INTERVIEW WITH RHONDA MAJALCA AND CONSTANTINE KOTSANIS M.D.

(by John M. Forrester john@johnforrester.com) [See Pic 8.1]

John: We are thrilled to present this exclusive interview with Dr. Bernardo's wife Rhonda, who worked alongside Dr. Bernardo for many years, and Constantine Kotsanis MD, who was working with Dr. Bernardo at the time of his passing. Dr. Bernardo dedicated his entire (60 year) career to helping patients recover from degenerative diseases and to achieving healthier lifestyles through immune system boosters, antioxidants, vitamins, minerals, and a change in diet and fresh juices. His results were legendary, and Burton Goldberg, the 'Voice of Alternative Medicine', has described Dr. Bernardo as "the greatest naturopath in the world."

This interview with Rhonda and Dr. Kotsanis serves as an addendum to Dr. Bernardo's Patient Guide, which was last updated in 2011. It is designed to help give the patients a deeper understanding of the protocol, to understand the rationale, and to learn what has been discovered since the protocol was last published.

RECOMMENDED FOODS

John: The foods on Dr. Bernardo's recommended list, "DO EAT" is an absolutely superb array of cancer-fighting sustenance from God's garden. Most of it is self-explanatory—however, here are a few questions:

WATER: Distilled or Spring Water with freshly squeeze lemon and stevia to taste.

RM: Lemon juice is great prior to eating to help aid in digestion. Yes, the lemon juice will cause an alkaline tide to help bring the PH to a normal level. Baking soda can do the same, but most people don't like the taste of baking soda.

MILK: Almond and Goat Milk are listed. What about Rice or Soy milk?

Rice Milk for some would be ok but the content may have more sugar content and they should not have sugar while they are on the protocol. Soy milk, since soy now has been chemically changed here in the US, it is not recommended. Also, soy can change the hormonal levels and since cancers can increase with the increase of hormones it is not recommended.

SOUPS:

John: What are your favorite cancer-fighting soups?

RM: A good vegetable soup is my favorite. A lot of different vegetables with a little bit of barley.

TEAS:

John: In terms of teas, Dr. Bernardo's protocol mentions Essiac, Sierra Madre, Purple La Pacho (Pau D' Arco), and Green Gunpowder. What is the nutritional value of the teas, and why is it better to drink tea with meals than water?

Dr. Kotsanis: All the teas have phytonutrients that promote health. The teas Bernardo was recommending also have anti-cancer properties. My favorite tea is Essiac; it seems to help most, if not all, people.

When eating, one should not drink water with meals because it dilutes the activity of the enzymes. If one wants to drink water, one should drink all the water one wants 20-30 minutes before meals and two hours after meals.

SEA PLANTS:

John: These are great, and easy to find in Whole Foods or Asian markets. What are the main anti-cancer active ingredients found in sea plants?

Some patients have asked how to incorporate sea plants into recipes. Any ideas? Great in soups and salads…

Dr. Kotsanis: It's best to visit the Chinese and Korean markets. All seaweeds can be incorporated into soups and salads. They are very rich in minerals and especially magnesium. Most if not all Americans have magnesium deficiencies.

Personally, when I cook vegetables or soups, I cook with color. Take a pinch of 40-50 veggies and herbs and make a healthy soup!

JUICES:

John: Patients absolutely love Dr. Bernardo's juicing protocol! The only question is, must one do the whole regime twice a day?

RM: Depends on the individual and what they are experiencing.
Preparing the daily juices is time and labor intensive, so was wondering if there was a time when these could be scaled back a bit?

RM: Yes! As the markers come down you can slowly scale back on the juicing.
Anything new you've learned about juicing in the last few years?

RM: The importance of using asparagus in some of the juices. Dr. Bernardo's juicing protocol calls for separate asparagus juice, but also the Enzyme Juice calls for asparagus.

John: How important is it to do asparagus juice as a standalone juice?

Dr. Kotsanis: Asparagus is a great anti-cancer vegetable! One can make soups, salads, or even eat it out of a can if fresh is not available. Patients with cancer should incorporate asparagus daily.
Also- everyone seems to want to know- Why is it important to drink the juice through a straw?

RM: It's important for your foods to mix with your saliva prior to swallowing. Sipping through a straw helps to slow down the process and collect enough saliva prior to swallowing.

John: Would a glass straw be even better than a plastic one?

RM: Yes, Glass would be better if it is available to you.

POTATOES:

John: The only potatoes allowed are redskins and Yams. What about Sweet Potatoes?

RM: NO sugar content is high…

John: Are Sweet Potato French fries OK?

RM: NO. Why would you want to eat anything fried?

CHEESE:

John: The protocol states that Brie and Havarti made from Goat Milk are OK. Does any cheese consumed by a cancer patient have to be made from goat milk?

RM: It is best if you can use the cheeses made from Goat milk.

MEAT:

John: Why would red meats like Buffalo and Lamb be allowed, but not beef? Would the answer still be no even if it was grass fed, hormone and antibiotic-free beef?

RM: Yes! Do you know for sure the Beef hasn't had hormones or antibiotics; did the parents or grandparents to that cow have no hormones and antibiotics?? To be safe stay away from beef while doing the protocol for the best benefits.

NUTS:

John: Why are peanuts not allowed?

RM: When peanuts go rancid they give off aflatoxin. If a patient wants peanut butter, make sure it is fresh all natural and to add a ¼ teaspoon of vitamin C powder to help remove the aflatoxin.

RECIPES:

John: Do you have a favorite recipe book that sticks to approved ingredients from Dr. Bernardo's protocol?

RM: Yes, I put together a cookbook for Dr. Bernardo's patients. But it is important for the patients to take their favorite recipes and convert them. That way they will enjoy the foods they eat.

Dr. Kotsanis: Our cookbook **"Food for Thought"** can be ordered on Amazon; or call our office at 817-481-6342.

John: Recently, "I Cure Cancer.com" documentary filmmaker Ian Jacklin commented on Facebook that Dr. Bernardo had approved buckwheat pancakes. Is that true? But what would you put on them, as surely butter and maple syrup are prohibited foods?

RM: For those whose cancer markers have dropped an occasional Buckwheat pancake can be done. Butter is OK, yummy if you can find butter from goat and a little pure maple syrup. Yes! The maple syrup you are to avoid that is why it is NOT recommended to have, on a daily basis. Only as a treat once a month or less.

NOT RECOMMENDED FOODS - "DO NOT EAT"
BREAD
John: Are other types of Sprouted Grain bread acceptable, or just the Ezekiel brand?

RM: Sprouted breads are great but watch for the sugar content and soy or soy by-products in them.

CHOCOLATE
John: What about raw organic cacao without sugar? Could one healthfully make chocolate or chocolate smoothies with cacao and Stevia?

RM: As a chocolate lover I would hate to give up my chocolate. But, during the protocol, it is important to stay away. What is important is that you receive the nutrients you need for your body to heal itself. By adding extras that may compromise your healing process and it may take you longer to heal.

VINEGAR:
John: Almost all salad dressing you buy from markets are loaded with sugar. Vinegar and Oil seem like the only alternative if you want to avoid sugar. Is vinegar in this context OK?

RM: Why not try Lemon juice and Oil? Extra Virgin Olive Oil is great. Why not mix up some of your favorite herbs and spices to make your own special salad dressing. You never know what you might come up with. It may be the next best thing in salad dressings.

DAIRY PRODUCTS:

John: Is Insulin-Like Growth Factor, IGF-1- the main reason to avoid dairy products?

RM: One of many…

Is ghee an acceptable substitute for butter?

Dr. Kotsanis: Organic ghee is an excellent fat. Ghee is clarified butter and it can be used for any chronic illness.

John: Would the only other exception to the diary rule be Dr. Bernardo's wonderful weight-gain formula of heavy whipping cream, blended with berries of your choice and Stevia?

Dr. Kotsanis: The number one problem is late-stage cancer is muscle wasting. The cancer eats up the patient's muscles. One can control or delay cancer by keeping an optimal weight. The best weight gain formula according to Bernardo is "heavy whipped cream, berries, protein powder and stevia." This works brilliantly, by the way, for all patients who need to gain weight.

DRINKS:

John: Why are iced drinks prohibited? Even something like iced green tea with no sugar not allowed.

Dr. Kotsanis: Cold drinks upset digestion and the autonomic nervous system (causes the imbalance of sympathetic-parasympathetic axis).

John: Some alternative practitioners suggest that the benefits of drinking grape juice or wine, for example, due to the resveratrol, make up for undesired sugar content. Would you agree or disagree?

Dr. Kotsanis: If one were to use the entire organic grape (seeds and skin included), it would have great benefit. Dr. Petron, a Greek physician, used to reverse cancer with grape therapy. (Between 1976 to 1979, he had great success using organic grapes, clean water, and emotional healing).

MEAT

John: What about turkey bacon?

Dr. Kotsanis: No processed meats. All processed meats are potentially carcinogenic.
If a patient were doing well- would it be possible to add any meat- if it was free-range, grass fed, hormone, antibiotic free, etc.?

Dr. Kotsanis: Till the cancer is under complete control, one should minimize animal products. One can return to a controlled animal diet, this is organic after cancer is in remission or stable.

POULTRY:

John: A little free-range chicken is OK. One Thanksgiving, I asked Rhonda Majalca if it would be OK to have a little turkey. My parents always buy Amish turkeys and she said that hormones were the main thing to avoid. So, a little hormone-free turkey OK once in a while?

Dr. Kotsanis: Three to four times a year one can enjoy the spirit of the Holidays and eat organic, hormone free, animal products.

FRUIT

John: Some holistic practitioners have recently suggested that the benefits of fruit outweigh the negatives of the sugar for the cancer patient. How do you feel about loosening up the fruit restrictions?

Dr. Kotsanis: I am working on a phyto-chemotherapy regiment that includes fruits and vegetables. However, this should be done under medical supervision by a trained practitioner.

EGGS:

John: What about eggs? They don't appear on either the Recommended List or the Foods to Avoid List. Are Eggs OK?

Dr. Kotsanis: Organic free-range eggs can be used once a week.

SUPPLEMENTS:

John: Supplements can be a bit tricky since everyone is biochemically different, with a different set of deficiencies—but I think we can all agree that supplements are vitally necessary.

Beyond our biological differences—there are many different forms of cancer- requiring different approaches to supplements. Dr. Bernardo was a master at prescribing herbs and supplements according to the needs of his individual patients. It says in the protocol, "All of our supplements have been tested for electrical energy. Many similar brands are toxic with traces of benzene or other elements which will deplete the body of its electrical energy, therefore making you feel weaker."

Do you still create supplement programs for patients?

RM: Yes! If they are my client, I am happy to help them with a protocol. But, at this time my time is limited and I'm not taking on a lot of clients.

John: If not, who can patients turn to now, to help them design a plan of just the right supplements according to their individual needs?

Patients can call Dr. Kotsanis in Grapevine Texas. He was working with Dr. Bernardo prior to his death.

John: Is there a way, patients can test supplements for electrical energy themselves?

RM: If they are into muscle testing that is great. Dr. Bernardo did a lot of muscle testing with patients. He was very observant when looking at a patient and his years of study taught him what a patient needed.

John: What are the basic supplements that should be the standard of care for every cancer patient? [See Chapter 7]

MUSCLE TESTING:

John: How important is muscle testing of supplements?

RM: This can be very important. We naturally know when food is good for us. Our bodies tell us every time we eat. Listen to your body and it will guide you.

John: The muscle testing procedure is described on Page 20 of Dr. Bernardo's patient guide, [See Chapter 7]. However, if one lives alone, is there a way to muscle test food or supplements on your own?

RM: Yes! In fact, this is what I have always done with my muscles testing. Hold the item you want to muscle test up to your chest. Close your eyes for a moment. Say, "Is this product good for me?" Which way does your body sway?? If your body sways forward it is good for you. If it sways backward it's NOT good for you.

DETOXIFICATION:

John: Dr. Bernardo discusses the benefits of taking a daily hot salt bath in the evening to increase circulation and encourage the discharge of toxins. He is emphatic NOT to use Epsom Salt. Could you please explain why no Epsom salt?

RM: Regular salt is what the body recognizes. Keep to what is natural to the body.

John: Dr. Bernardo also mentions saunas and sweat therapy as helpful in the detox process. Any other favorite detox remedies you'd like to share?

RM: There are so many, this would be an individual recommendation. Some cannot afford saunas; it may not be available to cost-effective for them. A good sweat in a hot bath is great for all of us.

John: Is there any particular type of coffee one should use in a coffee enema? Is it possible to over-do them?

Dr. Kotsanis: Only organic coffee. Cancer patients are instructed to use coffee enemas in the AM. Like anything else, one can overdo it. Patient needs supervision by a trained practitioner. Careful with electrolyte imbalance!

ADDITIONAL THERAPIES:

John: Other substances commonly administered in the alternative world include; Poly MVA, DMSO, Cesium, Cannabis Oil, Sodium Bicarbonate, Vitamin C IV. What is your opinion on the efficacy of these treatments? How and when should these treatments (or others) be used in conjunction with Dr. Bernardo's protocol?

RM: Dr. Bernardo did not use Poly MVA with what he saw, it did not work. DMSO is great especially if patients are doing multivitamin IV. Cesium, Cannabis Oil, sodium Bicarbonate all work well with his protocol. Again, this also depends on the individual.

BIOLOGICAL DENTISTRY:

John: Dr. Bernardo discusses in the book the dangers of mercury poisoning. "In 60 years of treating so-called "terminal cancer patients," we have never seen a case where patients are not contaminated with mercury. "How do you test for Mercury poisoning? How do you detoxify from Mercury poisoning?

Dr. Kotsanis: This must be done by a licensed physician. This is the most intense procedure in Alternative Medicine. One should use DMPS or DMSA. One must keep track of kidney function. We prefer the "urine challenge test" to verify toxicity.

John: Where are the best places to have Mercury amalgam fillings removed?

Dr. Kotsanis: Always use "functional Dentists". They are few and far between, but one can find them on the Internet. Many alternative practitioners have made a link between improperly extracted teeth, root canals, "cavitations" and cancer. Some even claim that when these problems are corrected, cancer goes away.

John: Did you detect such a strong link with your patients? Any particular Bio-dentists you recommend?

Dr. Kotsanis: They are in every major city. In Texas: Dr. Evans, Dr. Glaros, Dr. Nunnlee, Dr. Cole and Dr. Petre.

[Editors note: For more resources, please see: International Academy of Biological Dentistry & Medicine: https://iabdm.org also see Holistic Dental Association: http://holisticdental.org/find-a-holistic-dentist]

ESSENTIAL OILS:

John: What is your feeling about Essential Oils? Sacred Frankincense, for example—has been scientifically proven to have significant anti-tumor properties.

EMOTIONAL REALM:

John: One of my favorite quotes by Dr. Bernardo is on the cover, it says: "Cancer is not a Death Sentence, It's a Major Inconvenience." One of the major things that Dr. Bernardo did for me was instilling confidence; that I could actually beat this. That I could actually reverse this cancer and be well again. And that made all the difference in the world to me. How important is a positive attitude, a belief in one's own innate healing ability?

Dr. Kotsanis: Extremely important. A positive attitude is critical in healing.

It has been said, "Cancer is a disease of the body, mind, and spirit." The physical realm, diet, juicing, exercise, lowering stress, etc. seem easier for many patients to deal with than calming the mind, or improving our unseen spiritual side. Anger, resentment, unforgiveness, even guilt, for example, are acidifying emotions known to increase cancer markers.

John: What are some of the best techniques you are aware of for resolving emotional issues, which may be contributing to cancer problems?

Dr. Kotsanis: Re-call healing, mindless meditation, positive affirmations.

[Dr. Kotsanis: Dr. Piefer, DeWitt, and Dr. Lee Cowden are among the best.]

ENERGY MEDICINE:

John: What is the role of energy medicine in healing? Things like Qi Gong, acupuncture, reiki, quantum physics, rife machines, etc.?

Dr. Kotsanis: Energy Medicine is the missing link in Western Medicine healing. Here we use biophysics to treat and heal people.

INTEGRATION WITH ALLOPATHIC MEDICINE:

John: Sometimes there is no choice for patients other than to do some conventional therapy. For example- if a patient discovers their cancer in a very advanced or aggressive state- and it is administered. (Which is actually how a lot of people discover they have cancer, unfortunately.) We all know the toxicity of the treatment is very damaging to the immune system- and that has to be weighed against a benefit short term of regressing cancer cells. Can one still make a full recovery even after conventional therapy?

RM: This is always a good question; this depends on the individual and how their body responds. Also, how they adhere to the recommendations. When it comes down to it is all up to our Lord and savior. Treat each day as a gift, live each day without regret. Tell the people you love that you love them, and those things in the past let them go move on. The people in our past have let it go, why hold on to it; it is only making you sick.

ARE ALL CANCER PATIENTS TOO ACIDIC?

John: Dr. Bernardo had tremendous success alkalizing his patients; however- are there exceptions to the rule? The highly regarded and recently departed Dr. Nick Gonzalez MD,.. for example, has stated that his mentor Dr. Kelly realized that those who run too alkaline are prone to immune cancers like leukemia, lymphoma, myeloma, and connective tissue cancers, and the various sarcomas. Are there cancers for which the alkalizing protocol is not suitable?

RM: Like in all things we need to find balance not too acid not too alkaline. Smack dab in the middle is what you want.

TO VISIT A CLINIC OR NOT TO VISIT A CLINIC:

John: Many patients seek out alternative clinics in Mexico or in Germany for holistic or CAM treatments. These clinics are typically very expensive, and rarely covered by insurance. In your experience, are these clinics necessary? Assuming one could afford a visit, when and where should one go?

RM: This depends on the individual and their needs and also their finances.

FINAL THOUGHTS:

John: What new discoveries have you made in the field of alternative cancer research and reversal in the years since Dr. Bernardo has died? Any final thoughts you'd like to share?

RM: I have discovered that my husband in all he did loved his patients. He was passionate about people and their welfare. He was always right in the conclusions he came up with. Most of all, finding true balance in life is important for all of us

John: Is there anything in the protocol that you would now amend, strike or add due to new information?

RM: I would keep the protocol as is and only add to it if the individual needs something specific.

John: What are your "must read" books and "must see" documentaries for cancer patients?

RM: Dr. Bernardo's patient guide. Ian Jacklin's documentaries and dish network also have a documentary; "The Incurables" I believe it is on Veria.

RM: To everyone out there that is dealing with a health issue, I pray all of you to find the protocol that is best for you. Take time out to listen to your body, you are the expert. You are a precious gift. Tell the people you love, you love them. Wake up each morning knowing that the day is a gift. Live the rest of your life in love and without any regrets. Everything else is not important.

ABOUT RHONDA MAJALCA

Rhonda Majalca has practiced Classical homeopathy since 2005. She has been involved in the medical community for over ten years. She started her journey into alternative/complementary health as a Bio-Energetic Technician in 2000. During that time, she has worked with renowned doctors and their patients both in traditional and alternative medicine. Her interest in investigating the causal factors of the disease led her to her attainment and proficiency in Homotoxicology. It is here that Ms. Majalca has become a beacon to those seeking superior health.

Rhonda is a member of (NCH) National Center for Homeopathy, (NASH) North American Society of Homeopaths, Georgetown Chamber of Commerce, Biltmore& Stanford

Learn more: IntegrativeHealthResearch.com

ABOUT CONSTANTINE KOTSANIS MD

Since the age of three, Constantine (Gus) Kotsanis knew he wanted to be a doctor. He loved the smell of ether at his uncle's surgical clinic in Athens. He was hooked on the mystique of medicine. Little did he know then that in November 2014 he would be kicking off his second thirty years of practice in Grapevine, TX.

He moved to the states as a teenager – eager to experience the American dream. His family settled in Chicago, where he attended Austin High School and went to Northern Illinois University. He then returned to Greece for medical school at the University of Athens. After finishing medical school, he continued his specialty training in otolaryngology, head and neck surgery at the Loyola University of Chicago which is when he met and married his wife and business partner, Beverly.

Beverly, the practice CEO, a Loyola graduate with an extensive business background, worked in government, insurance, and education before tackling the business of medicine. Both Gus and Beverly are outside-the-box thinkers. They attribute this to being of Greek descent.

After moving to Texas in 1983, Kotsanis began the practice of medicine quite conventionally, doing surgery and allergy treatments. Several years later he began to experience health problems. After extensive testing, he was told nothing was wrong with him. But he was in pain, fatigued and experiencing severe gastrointestinal issues. So, he began to look for answers in less conventional places. This was before Google and the Internet. He had to find answers the old-fashioned way – books, journals, and other sick people. His answer came in the form of animal stem cells in Mexico. At the same time, they realized that patients coming to them were more challenging. Treatments that worked before were no longer as effective. What was happening? This is when they widened their horizons and turned to other disciplines for answers. Gus first explored the world of nutritional treatments for digestive disorders. It made sense that if digestion breaks down, nutrients can't get where they're needed, and a cascade of deterioration begins.

Lyn Dart, a dietician, and nutritionist who was then a master's candidate at Texas Women's University worked in Kotsanis' office and needed a project for her master's thesis. They had already begun using nutritional interventions to affect behavior changes in children with attention and behavior disorders, so they agreed to study the effects of diet and allergy in a group of autistic individuals. Diets were designed for each child based on test results. These individualized nutrition and allergy treatments proved to be highly beneficial and the results were presented at the annual meeting of the American Academy of Otolaryngic Allergy. This research laid the foundation for the biomedical treatment of autism. Lyn went on to get her Ph.D. and is now teaching nutrition science at Texas Christian University.

Thus, began a long Kotsanis tradition of translational medicine (evidence-based research that is translated into practice). Kotsanis Institute has done several studies in autism and currently has an active study on low dose chemotherapy and insulin for cancer. They offer many different types of treatments for a wide array of conditions including hormone balancing, autologous stem cells, pain management, detoxification and oxidative therapies to name a few. Gus has edited a book in which he authored a chapter on Insulin Potentiation Low Dose Cancer Treatment. (The Kinder, Gentler Cancer Treatment) and they co-authored allergen-free nutrition and recipe book (Food for Thought – The Free Food Cookbook).

Together they created a medical practice that delivers health care that is customized to each person. Their method in a nutshell is:

1. Listen to the patient's goals
2. Draw them a roadmap and give them options on how to get there
3. Partner with them to help them stay focused

Now in the legacy phase of their careers, they are focused on educating people to take charge of their health. This is why in 2011 they expanded their physical facility to accommodate the educational part of their mission. Kotsanis Institute's monthly educational series, "Digging Deeper" offers subject experts sharing their knowledge during a one-hour gluten-free lunch. Afterward, attendees can ask questions and even get a tour of the facility.

Kotsanis Institute would not be who they are today without the people that bring it to life. The staff gives the institute a relaxed family feel. Beverly Kotsanis says that the staff is her family and credits staff longevity and responsiveness with the fact that patients stay with the practice. Eighty percent of Kotsanis Institute patients are word-of-mouth referrals.

In addition to the Kotsanis commitment to education, Gus and Beverly have served on the Board of Directors and Medical Advisory Board of the Best Answer for Cancer Foundation. They also reach out to the Grapevine, Colleyville and Southlake chambers and actively participate in the Leadership Colleyville program by sending key staff members for leadership training. Another key activity for the couple is educating elected officials on the emerging technologies that will influence the future of medicine. Sometimes this involves testifying in Austin before legislative committees or visiting legislators personally.

While there is not a lot of downtime at Kotsanis Institute or household, favorite pastimes include creating new recipes, traveling, reading, and catching up with family. The couple has two grown children, Andrew 29 and Katerina 22.
http://www.kotsanisinstitute.com

CHAPTER 9:

INTERVIEW WITH PROFESSOR BRIAN PESKIN

(EFA's Essential Fatty Acid's for Cancer!)

"After Prof. Peskin saw my movie, he contacted Dr. Bernardo and they had a superb professional collaboration until Dr. Bernardo's tragic, accidental death in 2010. Dr. Bernardo implemented the Peskin Protocol EFAs for all of his cancer patients, stating in a medical journal article appearing in 2007 in Townsend Letter for Physicians that, 'The Hidden Story of Cancer [Peskin's book] has provided a great breakthrough in the treatment of our cancer patients. The addition of 5-725 mg Peskin Protocol EFA capsules t.i.d. along with our protocol has brought a dramatic difference; unbelievable and rapid improvement [4 of Dr. Bernardo's remarkable cancer patient success stories follow]. In ten days' time, one can see a physical improvement in patient condition. We believe Peskin Protocol EFAs are the 'missing link' in cancer therapy. The cost of treating our patients has dropped from $20,000 (US) per month to $1,500 per month by eliminating the use of eight IVs daily. We saw no side effects. Within two weeks, patients typically see great physical and mental improvement.'"

Ian: I am so lucky to get Brian Peskin on the show tonight. He was my mentor's guy that he went to, to learn about how to cure cancer. Otto Warburg figured all this out back in the early 1900s, and Brian wrote a book about it called, "The Hidden Story of Cancer." You're not going to believe it. It's amazing. There are so many things here. Right now, the big thing about cancer cures is cannabis oil. Don't forget about Peskin's book folks. I was helping people cure cancer for 17 years thanks to this kind of science—way before the cannabis-hemp oil. So, that just another weapon to your arsenal. This (book) is the key – diet, and nutrition. Brian Scott Peskin, welcome my friend!

Brian P: My pleasure!

Ian: Good. Good. Man, you have the nicest office there and more books than I have of VHS tapes!

Brian P: Why . . . I have a new one too, it's called, PEO Solution – for Pure Essential Oils solutions with Dr. Robert Rowen. He's raw food vegan, and the editor-in-chief of Second Opinion

Newsletter; a very big medical journal. So, he's vetted my work for five years, and now he's on board.

Ian: Yeah. This is huge, huge news. Where should we start? Should we break it down from your first book, and then come into this new stuff?

Brian P: Sure. It's the same stuff with a different format. This one is focusing exclusively on cancer and the story of cancer and it's very important to you and your followers. PEO Solutions takes it even a step further and applies it to everything; from sports medicine to martial arts, to beauty, almost everything because it's fundamental. So, what very few people talk about is what causes cancer. This is what got me. "Hundreds of causes" – they'll say, and "blah, blah, blah, blah, blah war on cancer", has basically gotten nowhere. In Houston, Texas, we have the world's largest cancer center. It's right in my back yard. Some of the hospitals there have an abysmal success rate. Absolutely abysmal. Many oncologists there do not know the name Otto Warburg, and, this is why none of their new drugs work! (Ian hides his face with his hands.) The latest one I was in Germany with a lecture and a doctor was over there, and he goes, "I was just at the national cancer thing in America and the big hoopla was "an extra week of life" if you had cancer with the drug. And it was unbelievable. If this is, the best you guys can do…"—and it is because they're not using Warburg's discovery. **So, IN A NUTSHELL, THERE'S ONE PRIME CAUSE OF CANCER: LACK OF CELLULAR OXYGEN.** Not oxygen in the bloodstream, cellular oxygen. Now, there are hundreds of secondary causes, but they all have to impact cellular oxygen.

Now, there are hundreds of secondary causes, but they all have to impact cellular oxygen. So, Warburg knew this. It was proven in America in 1953 and 1955 by medical scientists—MDs and PhDs here. They deprived heart cells of oxygen over a two-year period, even intermittently, and they became cancerous. The same cells that were not oxygen-deprived never turned cancerous.

Then they proved that with the low oxygen in a brilliant experiment with mice in 1955. So, they absolutely proved it, but back then no one knew how to oxygenate a cell, and that was my discovery. The parent Omega-6 — cannabis-hemp oil has that in it—is the cell membrane's oxygenator. So, the cell gets oxygen two ways: 1) oxygen transfers from the bloodstream into the cell, but, and everyone has enough oxygen in the bloodstream unless they're diseased. So, you can get a pulse oximeter, this is what you get in your surgeon's office or during surgery, which puts some infrared light into there and it's about 90 – 98% oxygen saturation, you're fine. That's everybody unless you have a disease as I said. The question is why is the cell not getting the oxygen?

The parent Omega-6 in that cell membrane can dis-associate, meaning the oxygen can come out of the Omega-6 oil. Now every cell membrane is 50% fat and 50% protein. There's almost no carbohydrate in there. Out of the 50% fat about half the saturated fat and about 25 – 33% is unsaturated fat. That is the parent essential oils: Parent omega-6 and Parent omega-3. Those are the only two essential fats your body can't make. So, fish oil—anybody listening—throw that in the trash. That is a derivative, it is not essential, your body makes it as needed, I'll talk about that later. I've published journal articles about that in 2013 destroying it. And, this is why it fails. So, when you have the right Omega-6—Omega-3 combination in the cell membrane, it is fully oxygenated, you're not going to get cancer.

Now the big thing: and this is what changed everything in 2009 – is INFLAMMATION. Everything is inflammation (i.e., that is disease-related). Inflammation is a cause of cancer. Dr. Weinburg, a professor at MIT got (discovered) this, and he was the originator of the oncogene. It's not genetic. There is no oncogene giving you cancer. That's garbage. That has been changed but the average person hasn't heard it. The average physician hasn't heard it. It's all inflammation, and the omega-6 oils allow what's called PEG-1, and that's the ultimate anti-inflammatory. Now the reason we're deficient in it — and, you have to ask yourself 'why the heck am I deficient in this stuff?' — is because of the food processing that has taken over the food industry. So, all the commercial stuff you get at your supermarket, Safeway, Kroger, Food City, Walmart whatever you have, ANY COMMERCIAL SUPERMARKET – the food is all processed. Why? So, it doesn't go bad. So that Canola oil can sit on the shelf for years, and that's a good thing except that we need the oxygen transfer in the cell. And the oxygen transfer is the reason the (good) oil is going bad. So, if you put margarine out, for example, in your garage, come back a year later there'll be no fungus, no mold, no bacteria, no animal or bug will have touched it. It's called plastic food. And if we get this in the cell membrane from eating processed oils, as all the processed food has it, it goes into your tissue as a percentage of what you eat. So, if I'm eating 20% adulterated oils, I have 20% screwed up in the cell membrane. You get to 30% - 35% oxygen deficit. Intermittently, over a long period of time, this will give you cancer because it's cumulative. And it can be in any tissue in any cell membrane anywhere in the body. So, everybody, even in the finest restaurants, Ian, are using adulterated oils.

Unless it's organic it is adulterated. And all of them are using this stuff. First of all, it's cheap, then they use extenders, anything to keep using the same oil. It's in all baked goods, it's in all fried goods, it's in all cooked goods, it's just ubiquitous (everywhere)! You need to get organic oils. I like a blend of about 2:1 parent omega-6 and parent omega-3 with some GLA in it. GLA is the direct precursor of this anti-inflammatory I said has PEG-1. That's what makes it so efficient. That is what I spend 90% of my waking time day in and day out looking at and now, it's absolutely provable. Everything is tied to the adulterated oils. The hidden story of cancer has all this and now the PEO solution I've added right up to 2013 with the journal articles like "Fish Oil Fails" and they can't figure out why it's because there's no parent omega-6 and no parent omega-3 in it. It's all derivatives, and your body makes very, very, very little. So, I look at physiology.

People want to know what my background is: I'm an electrical engineer from MIT. You go, 'what the heck does electrical engineering have to do with medicine?' Well, to start with, everything is electrical in your body. Everything goes by this. So, it does a lot. But, I brought the concepts; the input of what you're eating, the system is your body, and the output is your disease/state of health, how fat you are or how thin you are. So, I look at it as an engineer looks at it and I'm all about a cause-effect. Associations mean absolutely nothing to me. They may get my interest and my attention, but if I do this, it has to give me that output. If I design a TV to work on 120 volts AC, it can't blow up in my face every 5th time.

Now in the medical profession that would bring great results. Every 5th time – that's not bad, because that's 80% working okay, and that's only blowing up 20%, you'd be a trillionaire. That's when I quit statins. They have a one percent success rate. To me that's a 99% failure rate; and yet they're a 15 billion dollar-a-year industry! I'm for natural foods, just like you said in the beginning. And oils are key. That is number one by a factor of a thousand compared to anything else you're doing.

Ian: Thank you. That's what Dr. Bernardo always said. He really harped on that: No fish oil, it has to be vegan sourced. And he always offered a brand called "YES". Neither of us makes money on it. It's just that that's one of the better ones. But stick to the vegan source for the oils, right?

Brian P: I like a blend of four or five oils. So that minimizes the sensitivity issue anybody can have. A lot of people are sensitive to one specific oil, so if you have four or five in there it minimizes any sensitivity issue and you need a GLA-containing oil. I like evening primrose, that's what I recommend to people who want to follow my advice.

I like it better than hemp. The problem that I have with the hemp is that it doesn't have a culinary history anywhere in the world, anywhere. There are isolated uses of it, but I have to recommend things that have been around for hundreds of years. So, Evening-primrose oil is edible. Flax oil is edible; Sunflower oil, Safflower oil, Pumpkin oil, Coconut oil.

Those are all edible with hundreds of years' history. If you want to try something else, I don't know. As long as it has the right ratio. Cannabis is a little high in the Omega-6. I like 2 or 2.5 to 1, that's more like 3 or 3.3 to 1. So, it's a little too heavy is my opinion on it. But it's a good step in the right direction. So, if people look at my web site they can see what's needed with the oils and the ratios.

Ian: Yeah. Exactly, and the Cannabis-hemp oil is sort of a thing on its own. It's the THC does its own thing. It's magic. It's like frankincense oil. It's another oil that is so magical that they don't even know what it does yet. They just know that it's good for you. The formulation that you're talking about… is probably the best, and to anybody with cancer, if you're taking chemo or cannabis, I would also be taking these EFAs wouldn't you?

Brian P: Yes. They are the ultimate thing to take with conjunctive therapy, with chemotherapy, or radiation. Whatever. The radiation causes more cancer! The radiation typically kills 90% good cells to 95-99%. There is a big journal article that just came out this year as a matter of fact that you increase the cancer stem cell by a factor of 30 after radiation! So, what you've done is you've wiped out the good cells, the ones that are not a solid cancer. Solid cancer means it's 100% malignant. Typically, cells until the later stages or a certain amount of them are combinations. There are highly malignant cells, and medium. Now, what the heck does that even mean? A typical cell breathes oxygen. It's called cellular respiration; just like we do. There are two ways the body can get energy. It can get it using oxygen that is in the mitochondria, it can get it in the cytoplasm which is the inside of the cell from glucose, from sugar. That is getting energy as yeast does. So, it can get energy very inefficiently, it's about 1/20th as efficient, but it's quick, it's easy and there's no intelligence, so this is why cancer cells just keep growing. That's what they'll always say is the defining aspect of a cancer cell. They're wrong. It's not that it just grows uncontrollably. That's a result of its lack of intelligence. The defining issue of a cancer cell is its respiration is highly impacted, so it can't use oxygen, it has to run on sugar. So, it's inefficient and it becomes "dumb." And what cancer really is, Ian is a short-term time frame so you don't die. Remember it's cellular lack of oxygen. So, what can happen?

Well, if I smothered you, you're dead. So, the body has two things it can do. It can kill the cell, it can kill the tissue right away: stop your heart, stop your kidneys, stop your lungs immediately so that you're dead. Or, it can allow it, to revert back to just existing, and hope you fix the problem. The problem is that nature never intended that humans would be so stupid as to be adulterating the one thing in every one of your hundred-trillion cells which have these oils. A hundred-trillion cells a minimum of a quarter to a third is made of these oils and we're screwing them all up. So, cancer is created. The amount of pro-genetic cancer would be 0.0001% which is next to nobody (nothing), it's the one in a million literally or one in a hundred thousand. Everybody else: you created it unknowingly, it's not your fault, but the solution is here, and that's the new book "PEO Solution" and that's these parent essential oils.

So, I term parent omega6 and parent omega3 the only two essential oils that your body can't make. PEOs. So that is what everybody needs to remember. PEOs . . . they use the term wrong because they call fish oil DHA-EPA EFAs, and that is wrong, so I'm one of the biggest proponents of fixing the terminology in the journal articles with Parent Essential Oils so that it's 100% clear.   And the results are absolutely incredible! From oncology surgeons to heart surgeons . . . what a lot of cancer victims need to know is that heart disease is right around the corner. It kills about 20% of the people that have cancer because it impacts the whole system: your blood flow, your vascular system gets highly impacted too with the lack of cellular oxygen. That's the same reason you get a heart attack. So, cancer and heart disease are tied together, and the cholesterol is the common link and that transports the PEOs. So, the cholesterol is magnetized, picture a magnet, two of them one of them is the PEO and the other cholesterol. So, cholesterol is moving the PEOs into the tissue. Statins came along going "ah we're going to minimize cholesterol." What happens when you minimize cholesterol? You minimize the PEOs. Now the good thing is that you minimize the adulterated ones, but you've also minimized the good ones and that's why people taking statins have a higher rate of heart disease actually, and a higher rate of cancer. And this gets hushed up.

Ian: Yeah, I know, those statins are just horrible. I can't believe they're even still around let alone the chemo and everything else. The thing that I like about this book and when I was reading it . . . I've always been a bodybuilder, kick-boxer kind-a-guy, so every now and again I'd give myself a rest and I'd take a whole month and not work out. So that means that the next two weeks of training – like any other professional athletes, or even weekend warriors know what I'm talking about – after that first day of training, you can't move the next day! You're so tight, you're full of lactic acid and you feel like you're going to die. I did this for decades, and then finally I read your book and I went on EFAs a week or so before I started lifting, lifted, lifted – no pain at all; no stiffness at all! Unbelievable. You wrote about that experiment in your book, I did it and it's right!

Brian P: …. Had video talks about it with his athletes. He's in Italy, and he's the team sports physician. And your threshold of the acid burn goes way, way up. So, you can do the hardcore lifting, your muscle just fails, you don't get the burn. You have 25% more endurance you have 25% faster recuperation. It is unbelievable. So, in PEO Solution – the new one, there's a whole chapter on sports medicine.

Ian: Wow. That whole little scenario I just described, that's also how you explain how the cells become cancerous. Right? Isn't there some process?

Brian P: The oxygen deprivation. You have cells that – it's called fermentation like a yeast – when you give it heat give it sugar, the output is lactic acid. So that's a by-product called glycolysis. It's not respiration. Respiration doesn't have that when you're using the oxygen. But if you're using the dumb way, because the cell can't do it, and bodybuilding and under intense physical endurance your muscles initially use glucose because it's fast. This turns over to respiration after a couple of minutes, but initially, it's that. That's why you get that lactic acid burn. And, this is why the worse the cancer level is, the lower the PH of the blood and the saliva is. And that is the measure of how aggressive the cancer is.

Dr. Bernardo would always do that. So, there are always a few things you can do to impede that. Lemon juice (organic fresh raw) is one thing you can take. Now even though that's acidic there are other components so that once you ingest it, it becomes alkaline. That always bugged me until I got a Ph.D. in chemistry and said, 'how the heck can this be, it's an acid?' There's something else, I forget what it is because I'm not a chemist, but that makes it alkaline in the body. So, if you can alkalize your body, you can make the cancer reaction much harder to proceed. Now, you're not going to change your PH by what you eat. I want to make that very clear to everybody because there are all kinds of diets and stuff. Your blood stays PH 7.35 to 7.45 regardless of what you do. It's called the bicarbonate system. It's the acid-base system. Nature would never be so stupid to allow us to control that. Doesn't matter what you eat, your kidneys can take care of maintaining the acid base. The only time you have to watch that is if you have cancer. And if you take these oils, I don't know how you'd get it.

People ask me, "is there anything else I can do?" There is also another product I like called Essiac. Now that is an old one, and it is the best blood purifier I've ever seen. It's another anti-inflammatory. It soothes everything. And I added cats claw to it so there are formulations with companies that I work with that have cats claw. It's the best upper-respiratory conditioner you've ever seen.

So, Essiac is a phenomenal daily detoxifier. I take it every day myself. Because unless you're a raw-food vegan, you are eating some junk. This is like a chelator, I take on a daily basis. It is unbelievable; non-stimulating, non-irritating. I would always go to the health stores in Houston early on, like twenty years ago and I'd always see people from MD Anderson with their drip bags from chemo. And I'd play dumb. They'd be buying that I had consulted for and I'd go, "why are you getting that?" They'd go, "Because I'm taking chemo and radiation and I don't have any of the side-effects. My hair is still here, my energy is still here." I'd say, "Really!?" And I'd see another one and another one. It was very, very rewarding. And it's one heck-of-a product. But if you're doing the detoxifier with an Essiac-concept formulation and the PEOs, I do not know how you could get cancer unless you walked through a radiation field, or, poison yourself or ate something radio-active.

I mean, there's no causal mechanism of getting the oxygen deprivation or getting the inflammation. And if you take away oxygen deprivation and inflammation, you're not getting a heart attack, you're not getting cancer. So, the two top killers in America – it's over! And the beauty effects are unbelievable. Your skin becomes soft like you wouldn't believe. Your fingernails become like a mirror-glass because there's no omega3 in the skin, it's all parent omega6.

Ian: Well, I have to tell you . . . Do you remember my call to Cynthia Brooks? She loves you bro. I mean she's so disappointed that she couldn't come on tonight . . . but I'm probably going to beg that you come to our telephone show again soon because she wants to talk to you. She's got the Essiac phase and she's showing off her nails to me, and her hair and she's so happy with it.

Brian P: It's a dilator, so it opens up the arteries naturally. There's nothing forced here. This is what your body does on its own. And when things work, nature is pretty damn good! My thing is, I am amazed how long and how healthy people are given that we're doing everything wrong. Now, it's unknowingly, and the problem is the "health solutions" for our health problems are typically the cause of the problem. This is how backward we are. It's a very unfortunate state of affairs today! And, this is why the bulk of my time is spent with physicians, MDs, really giving them state-of-the-art science, and they just love it because they really want to do the right thing. Most of them are misled themselves. So, it's the blind leading the blind honestly.

Ian: Really? You've gotten MDs to listen to you? Because I find that any time I give them any truth they're like "I don't want to know because then that means I am a murderer!"

Brian P: They come to me. I do a lot of journal articles. I don't go to anybody. I don't try to convert anybody. So, the physicians I get say, "I read your article, fish oil or whatever I was doing didn't work; you've answered every question, every metabolic pathway, and physiology. It's bulletproof. So, I understand why my method didn't work, and why this does work." And then they're onboard. So, the answer is yes, in the PEO solution the dedication is for American's physicians. And every chapter has a dedication by how important it is, for a particular physician. There are about 25 accolades and 98% are physicians.

There are two DC (chiropractors) which are very good, but the rest are MD or Ph.D. There's never been this kind of book with this kind of accolades. Yeah, I have a very big following of physicians around the world because what I tell is based on medical science, and it's the science, Ian, that they haven't seen. So, the mandate of PEO Solution is giving physicians the 21st-century medical science they haven't seen elsewhere. And it's not their fault if they haven't seen it, for example with fish oil: it doesn't work. Yet it's still the number 1 supplement in America.

The first question you would ask is, "How much DHA and EPA do the brain use?" Because the brain is the number 1 depository along with the eyes and nervous system. Most other tissues have none of it. Nobody's ever asked that. The answer is about seven milligrams (7mg). So, if anybody out there is taking fish oil, look and see the dosage you're taking of the DHA plus EPA and compare that to seven milligrams (7mg); you're getting overdosed by a factor of 20 to 500! This is the overdose, on a daily basis of fish oil. 20 to 500 times overdose!

Now if you want to know what that does, imagine—and don't do it!...taking 500 aspirin! Take two and you'll be okay. Take twenty—you are dead. This is what they're doing with fish oil on a daily basis in America! So, this is why I give the physicians the 21st-century science. When they see this, they get sick because they don't want to hurt people.

I've got one doctor, he wrote a four-page dedication, and it starts, "I have a confession to make…" He had been recommending fish oil, massive doses and thought he was doing good. So, he wrote a four-page – and basically an apology which is unbelievable.

So, this is the book of the 21st century. I hope people will look at my web site. It's www.BrianPeskin.com There are all kinds of papers there. There's a coast-to-coast radio interview that has a good summary of this. And they'll see about PEO Solution too. But you don't have to spend a penny. You can read, and get all of these papers for nothing. But you owe it to yourself if you really care about health and if you don't look at what I have on this site you're in the dark.

Ian: Yeah, and I can a witness to, like I said, Dr. Bernardo who cured more people than anybody I know just followed your science basically.

Brian P: The PEO really increased his effectiveness a lot. (Ian: Yes!) He had his own protocol, but then he added the oils and the results were phenomenal.

Ian: I want to add to that because you said something earlier and I don't want to confuse my people because I'm one of the guys saying, "Hey, you've got to get on an alkaline diet and get your PH up" because that's what Bernardo said. If you have cancer, your PH is probably 5 or 5½ and you want to bring it up to 7.2 to 7.4 where cancer can't.

Brian P: Absolutely right! if you have cancer. If you don't have cancer there's nothing to worry about. If you do have cancer you want to be on a very low glycemic carbohydrate meaning it raises blood sugar. Some carbs don't raise blood sugar much. And Dr. Bernardo was very good with that, so a lot of the vegetables don't raise it at all. So, whatever Dr. Bernardo told you was right.

Ian: Yeah and I've thought that exactly, diet and protocols from the different patients that were his. So, I'm going to come back with that to my own book because he/I took from everybody and will hand that to people and let them use what resonates with them. Because, I've learned that the person has to be spiritually connected, mind, body, soul for healing. It's really nice when you get what's like the third eye, they're more open and more awake because they can really pick it up quickly. What you're saying though for Dr. Bernardo's diet, because you're saying food doesn't change things so much, you're saying that it's the oils, the EFAs.

Brian P: For cancer prevention and the ultimate cure of the disease you should never get it (cancer). I mean, polio, you don't get it. They don't have a cure once you get it to reverse it. The ultimate cure is prevention, and these oils are the ultimate prevention both for heart disease and cancer. And I have journal articles, peer-reviewed journal articles that, . . . you've got to understand, I encountered every physician typically unless they've seen my work when it comes to fish oil. So, you can imagine what it gets. The reviewers typically are PhDs in biochemistry. When they see this, they go nuts. And the stuff they come back with I have to do a rebuttal of it and one of them: The Journal of American Physicians and Surgeons was ten pages! And I won. They published the article. I destroyed everything they said and showed them to be wrong, which took a while – a few months of course. Ten pages. So, it's very, very, difficult to get published when you're going against the mainstream. And just this year I've had two journal articles come out. 1) "Why fish oil doesn't prevent heart disease", and 2) "Fish oil can give you cancer." Gives it to you! The journal article came out in the journal of the National Cancer Society or Association and the people taking fish got the most prostate cancer. And they're going, "what the heck is this?!" So, I gave the first explanation in the world why I would expect that. So, stop the fish oil, the PEOs are the answer for about a buck-a-day. If your life not getting cancer not getting a heart attack isn't worth a buck-a-day there's nothing more for me to say. Have a nice life. But don't say you weren't warned especially with Obamacare coming in. You'd better be concerned.

Ian: Yeah right! Dr. Joel Wallach who has the Youngevity Product Line, but he was also a veterinarian before he became a physician.

Brian P: I saw him a month or two ago in Brazil!

Ian: Right on, he's a good guy. Yeah, he was in my movie "I Cure Cancer – one". He tells everybody you need 93 essential nutrients, I think is his number. He's got a multi-vitamin that you can take and take EFAs because your body can't make them. And that's what you're saying the best EFAs are not fish oils, they've got to be vegan sourced, folks.

Brian P: Yes, plant-based, plant-based. They have to be organic! If they go to my website they can go to my papers and see what the ratios need to be. Because you can't just take Flax oil, for example, which was a big deal a few years ago with the Budwig diet. Years ago there was not the adulteration of the parent omega6. They didn't have the adulteration of the cooking oils. It was lack of the omega3 series. Today the problem is 99% adulterated omega-6, and remember it goes in the tissue and each cell as a percentage of what you consume. So, if you're at 30%, 40% adulterated oils, then, it's really easy to get there.

I did some calculations: just a half a percent of adulterated oils over-powers every cell in your body by a factor of like 3,000. So, imagine trying to fight 3,000 people. That's the trauma every cell in your body has with a half a gram of adulterated oil, and that's only one percent adulteration. It's unbelievable the damage that's getting done! So, any kinds of margarine, any of these products you are getting adulterated oils. Unless you're raw-food vegan, you need to be taking a supplement to guarantee you don't get the problem.

Ian: Absolutely, Yeah. That should be in every cancer protocol, and the only one I know of offhand is "YES". Do you have a name brand?

Brian P: I consult with different companies on the air because it's disease prevention, I can't recommend any specific one. So, what I tell people is: It has to meet the requirements of multiple oils, 2:1 or 2½:1 in favor of parent omega6, no fish oil! What they've done now is, they've changed the strains now on a lot of the seeds, for frying. So, it's a lot of what's called oleic acid which is omega-9, like olive oil – that's a non-essential. So, they have oils that they use that are high oleic. You want high linoleic which is the omega-6. (laughter) Not good at pronouncing this stuff. But you want high parent omega-6 so there's enough magnitude, enough amount of the active ingredient. Because if you get say a gram of a high oleic one, it'll be 90% ineffective. So, you want high omega-6 content, and, it has to be organic, of course. And, it has to have, GLA! So, there are a few specs. And if people have questions they can go to my web site and pop an email and somebody will answer it for them.

As I said, it's critical, and just how good you feel people don't have a clue. Remember you've got to oxygenate it. So, you're not exhausted all the time even if you're doing nothing. Most people are exhausted doing day-to-day stuff. That changes. Now you're not hyper. It's just if you got tired at 10 o'clock, all of a sudden, you're tired at 11 or 11:30 at night. And then you wake up . . . you know, I get up at 4:30 and start working and then go to bed at midnight. It's unbelievable. We even have surgeons taking these oils for more focus, more attention. Kids: there is no ADD, ADHD. There's none of that garbage. Lack of these oils is the cause for virtually everything: Alzheimer's . . .. like I said the new book PEO Solution hits all this and why these are titled. But if you think about it, a few fundamental things, have to be at the root of everything. Have a strong foundation, and the house never falls down. Have a weak foundation, I don't care what the paint color is, or what the body looks like, it's the engine. If I have a strong engine the car is going to run. It doesn't matter what that body looks like. Have a Ferrari engine in there, I could put it in a Toyota and if it has the Ferrari engine, it's going to run. And I concentrate on the fundamentals.

Ian: [chuckling] Speaking of Ferraris, we had one young lady there that has a Ferrari and had her headlights cut off – speaking about Angelina Jolie; she had her breasts cut off just because she had that gene that may mean that she is genetically more closely susceptible to cancer. Yet from my research, there's no such thing as genetic cancer. There are habits from your parents…you may be doing, but I don't know if there are any genes that are connected. A lot of people ask me about that and say, 'what would you have said to her?' And I said "I would see what your PH is, and if it's just average say around 6.3, maybe even 7, you're good. But if it ever drops below 6, gets down to 5.5 that's when you can decide whether you want to either cut them off or maybe just go on an alkaline diet and bring your PH back up to 7 and you get to keep your breasts." That was my opinion. Do you have any thoughts on that whole scenario?

Brian P: Oh yeah, I have, because I got barraged too. But it's tragic. The biggest problem is these physicians saying this garbage—and it is garbage—actually, think they're right!
There's no way on earth with the BRCA (called Braka) gene and whatever else should possibly have had that there was an 87% chance that she'd get cancer. I mean that is nonsense. The average person with this braka genes …that's all been discounted, I told you the genetic theory the oncogene thing, I don't know why these physicians are still grabbing on to that. It's just tragic.

The average person with these genes does not get cancer. They don't! This is like smoking. Here are the statistics, this is an interesting one because it's called a 'conditional probability'. And I'm trained in this stuff, so I understand. You smoke two packs of cigarettes a day for 28 years. That's two packs of cigarettes a day for 28 years. Out of 100 people doing that, how many of those do you think would get lung cancer? I would say 100%. Two packs a day . . . that's 40 cigarettes a day for 28 years, of course, I'm going to get lung cancer. But the answer is 16%! That means 84% of people living on cigarettes are not getting lung cancer. (Ian looks to the sky with his hands spread open.) Therefore, the first thing is: smoking cannot be the damn cause of lung cancer. However, and this is where they get you if you look at the people that have lung cancer, 85% of them smoke. Okay, but you just said it was 16%. No that was a different question. The first one is: What is the probability that you get lung cancer by smoking two packs of cigarettes every day for 28 years? The answer to that is 16%! But of those who do get lung cancer, 85% of them smoke. So that's what these doctors are looking at with Jolie. And it's just exactly what you just said if she got the oils if she was taking the Essiac concept tea and looked at what her PH was, [shaking head 'no'] absolutely insane! And these poor women doing this. It's like what, to stop brain cancer lop off my head? I mean this is where we are in the 21st century with oncology? (incredulous tone) If I was one of them, I'd be walking with my head bowed on the floor in shame. That's what I tell these doctors. I'd be looking on the floor in utter embarrassment. Because coming from an engineering level, this is beyond pathetic! So, they don't even understand statistics, and as I said, I'm sure they think it's an 85% chance she really would when it's 15%! And that's doing nothing. With the oils and the Essiac concept tea, it's a non-issue. It's tragic.

Ian: It's unbelievable what's going on with our world. I'm finally coming into a potential way of dealing with this, and I've been hearing it from Gary Knoll – talks about it a lot and certain gurus. We have to go to grassroots! We have to be neighbourhoody… because right now, judges, oncologists [Ian is animated with his hands as he lists] lawyers, all the people that are in charge, not all of them are as good as the guys you talked to who are coming to you and realizing "Oh shit I was doing it wrong." Most of them don't give a damn.

Brian P: You're absolutely correct! They never admit they're wrong. And they'll never admit that they don't know anything. It's the rare one that comes to me. And that's all I can work with. I can't give you a solution if you don't think there's a problem. It's like, "who the hell do you think you are?" So, they have to come to me admitting, "Brian, I've got a problem" to give the answer why. And that's what I get. But if they don't have a problem I can't do anything with them.
Same thing with people. If you want to listen to your doctor you're probably going to die. And it always comes back after 5 years. Remember the radiation makes the inherent cells that can run on fermentation much more virulent, and it takes decades to develop cancer. This is why they put it out five years so when they kill a lot of the stuff the ones that are the strongest or very small, five, ten years later now they're dominant. And you're dead. That's why it's so bad when it comes back. If it comes back a second time you're dead. Maybe it'll postpone it a little bit, but you're dead.

Ian: It goes back to those stem cells that you were talking about, just to clarify for people. Stem cell cancer cells are the ones that kill you. Regular cancer cells – that why tumors shrink drastically when you do the chemo and radiation because it's killing all those cancer cells. But cancer cells don't hurt you like the cancer stem cells.

Brian P: A cancer stem cell is a full-blown cell that can only run on glycolysis. It can't use respiration at all with oxygen. So, what's the difference between malignant cancer and benign cancer? I can never get the answer out of any physiologist over at the cancer hospitals. And I'm going, 'you guys don't understand this!' It's the degree of the impact of cellular respiration. So, it starts at 100%, or 98% is normal because any cell especially muscles can run on glucose short-term. So, there's always the potential, but it's little. So, n when you have a cancer cell that's only 98% and can only run on sugar, where it should be 98% and running on oxygen, that's what they call a cancer stem cell. They don't even know what-the-heck it means. But that's what it is; its metabolism has changed and it's irreversible. This is why you cannot reverse a malignant cancer cell back. You have people saying they do, Harvard did a paper saying they could, I wrote a rebuttal to it and of course, I never hear an answer to it from the MD that wrote the paper because they're on to the next thing. It's impossible.

You have to cut it out or kill it, or don't get it! So, a full-blown cancer cell is irreversible, and Warburg said that. It's in the book and he's never been shown wrong in anything. What they did is they gave chemicals, made the respiration go up, but that's like putting a gun to a handy-capped kid's head and saying "move or I'm going to kill ya!" He could be probably fully paralyzed and with that kind of stress – that's the kind of experiment they did. Not fair at all; not normal conditions and they just give wrong answers, so they mislead every physician that looks at it: "How I can make a cancer cell normal again". No, you can't. If it's fully malignant – no you can't. The key is, if it's benign you can make it normal again. It'll never turn cancerous. And even if it is cancerous, Ian, as you learned from the book, if it doesn't metastasize you're not going to die. Unless it is on the brainstem where it's shutting down vital functions because it swells if that puppy doesn't metastasize even Weinberg at MIT said: "95% chance you don't die." There's no issue if it stays localized. So, these oils and the Essiac tea – worst case you're going to keep that puppy localized.

Ian: That Essiac tea, people, if you don't know a Canadian nurse named Rene Caisse got that from the American Indians. What's ironic is that I went and interviewed the Hopi Indians recently, and they didn't even know or have heard of that! They no longer know tribal medicine that I know came from them! So, I'm hoping to go back there and bring it all back to them because they're getting cancer on their own reservations since the government came in and dug it all up with the plutonium, or whatever the radiation stuff is, and instead of cleaning up properly they just sprayed it with sprinklers to keep the dust down. So, they're getting cancer. And I'm like, well why don't you use Essiac tea? And they're like, "I don't know what that is." I'm like, "Oh man! We gotta hang. We gotta hang out." Cause they (the government) they're on their land poisoning them and then giving them their white-man poison to them which is killing them right off. Whereas if they were to go back to their own ways (the Indians), they'd probably be healing better. Plus, with all this new stuff I know about – forget it. We'll have 'em on EFAs pretty soon. Okay, so we have 15 minutes, so let's think. Are we missing anything? What do you want to get into here?

Brian P: Suggest/ask something and I'll give an answer if I can. I mean there's just so much. In the past year, I've just been working on the PEO Solution. But every journal article, 2013, is confirming. There was just another one came out two weeks ago; a doctor actually from California sent it to me. Women eating the most peanut butter had the least breast cancer. And, of course, the people writing this, the doctors, they have no idea why. Well, what must be in peanut butter? PEOs! And there is the parent omega-6. So, I can explain almost any result they get, and their hands are going up. They tell you to eat nuts, for example, because of the omega-3. There's almost no omega-3 in any nut. One has omega-3 in it. I forget which one it is. But it has five times more parent omega-6! All the other nuts have no omega-3.

So, everybody keeps getting this led (to them) because the medical community just doesn't know what-the-heck they're doing. It is a tragedy. It is really a tragedy. This is one of my charges: to educate the physicians, and start with them. Most of everything we're told is wrong. High carbohydrate diet – that's the cause of diabetes. Two things: high carbs, meaning glycemic carbs which put the blood sugar through the roof – your pancreas is not designed to deal with this – and lack of the oils in the cell membranes so the insulin can't work. Well if the insulin can't work, what is that called? Insulin resistance. Gee! That's type 2. Pre-1940 there were no Type-2s. Zero. Type-2 Diabetes is a created disease by the person unknowingly. And now it's rampant in the world. China now has a higher percentage of diabetes growth now than in America. They're following our nutritional recommendations! All the countries do. Italy has a diabetes epidemic.

Ian: Yeah, I heard Brazil kinda went downhill too. I was there in the early 90s and everybody was healthy, and I was told if I go there now, twenty years later, it's not quite the same because all the American diet came in. It's a sad man. I just got out of that. I just went on a blend fast. Look! [Ian pulls up his shirt and shows his sculpted abs and chest – with a satisfied grunt ☺ then laughter] I had to do that [laughing] and I didn't work out or nothin'! All I did was blend. Take all these vegetables and stuff and the only thing I was missing was the EFAs – the essential fatty acids.

Brian P: And they fulfilled your appetite; not quench it, not curb it, they fulfill it so you're not a human billy goat. That's another thing I talk about: because that's another side effect of the oils. But here's why it does that. Because these oils are so critical because they're so adulterated if you don't get 'em, what can nature do? I gotta make the guy hungry. Now eat another batch of food and you (still) don't get'em. Well, what else can I do? Make you hungry again and hope you get these things. So, eat-crave, eat-crave, eat-crave . . . I call that the human billy goat syndrome, then your little nutritionist goes, "Oh yeah you're supposed to eat six times a day." She/he doesn't know any physiology, doesn't understand the pancreas produces insulin in very small amounts twice a day. You start eating four to six times a day, you're overstressing the pancreas. You're going to blow it out. It doesn't store it the way people think. You look at curves: two times, you eat more than three times a day; get a picture of yourself; get a bullseye; on a dart board and put that picture there and write "DIABETIC TIME BOMB" because you're going to become diabetic. I get this all the time. A lot of athletes become diabetic. High carb diet and they start dropping the exercise. Exercise burns sugar. So, if you're exercising a lot you can eat those carbs 'cause you're going to burn them up. But my comment is, "I don't want to live in the gym seven days a week." Then don't eat the damn carbs. And that's the trick. If you want to work out that's great. I used to do weight lifting. I trained with Lee Labrada.

Ian: Really?!

Brian P: He came in second in the Olympics. [Ian's jaw drops.] Samir Banout, I trained with him a few times too.

Ian: Wow!

Brian P: He won just before Schwarzenegger. (Ian clearly impressed) He won it. So, I was doing a very hard-core reverse pyramid. You start with the highest weight and go down, and the difference was incredible. They didn't know about these oils. So, even sports nutrition people don't know about this, that's why PEO Solutions is going to hit this market too. It's incredible. And it also dispels the myths. Like what do they tell you in America? 60% carbohydrate diet. What does that translate to? Well, 2,000 calories a day — 60% — that's 1,200. Okay, big deal. Yeah, it is a big deal. How many calories per teaspoon of sugar? 20. 1200 divided by 20 is 60. That means, Ian, our government the brilliant nutritionists, and your doctor is telling you to eat 60 teaspoons of sugar a day. [Ian shakes his head'] You go, yeah that doesn't sound too swift but tell me more. I'll give you the last thing: How much sugar is in the bloodstream? Less than one teaspoon. So, you're overdosing your bloodstream by a factor of 60 to 100! Where the hell does it go? Insulin is a fat-storage hormone – this is physiology — right to body fat. So, I've created all this body fat and that's where you've got to live in the gym now or do aerobics or you've got to run, or you've got to exercise six days a week because I just told you to make yourself a fat pig.

Ian: Right!

Brian P: This is why I get so irate with this whole nutritional field. I can't stand it. I don't like it. I'm not in the nutritional field. My joke is "nutritionists aren't qualified to talk about nutrition". They don't know anything. They don't know any physiology I don't even know if they can spell it. Unless they're a Ph.D. in it, and even then, it's iffy. Even then it's iffy to get one that understands this and physiology. But again, with my systems engineering, I put things together, I connect the dots perfectly. So, I can explain the diabetes epidemic in a nutshell and nobody else can. It's very obvious and simple as heck as to how to get rid of it. Protein. Huh! "Protein is bad for the kidneys." No, it isn't. Your kidneys have the capability to get rid of the hydrogen ions from the protein. There's no issue at all. (verbiage I couldn't understand – the name of some proteins is my guess) spits it out all day. And your urine PH varies all over the place to keep your blood PH constant. If something has to be constant something else has to be able to vary. So, urine PH is completely irrelevant. That's why you go with saliva as Dr. Bernardo would tell you.

Ian: Right.

Brian P: So it's incredible. Saturated fat. There's no saturated fat in a clogged artery. Every cardiologist I've ever asked – one knew it---probably from my work somewhere. The rest, they think there's saturated fat in a clogged artery. This was known in 2001. 1997 high-resolution chromatography was published in Lancet, it's been published, it's been duplicated. You can measure what-the-heck is in there. There's no saturated fat. So, America has got everybody petrified about eating cheese, butter, eggs, all saturated fat – is no issue at all. What is in the clog? Answer: adulterated omega-6. That's 85% of the clog. Case closed.

Ian: Wow!

Brian P: So, everything everybody is taught about this stuff is wrong! "Protein causes osteoporosis that leaches the calcium out of the bones." Absolutely insane. The calcium is transported via protein and it's going into the bone. These guys measured it once and were backward. They didn't even understand that calcium was going in, not out! It's just unbelievable, and what gives you a strong bone is protein collagen and the oils. They make the bone matrix itself. The minerals are dumped on it. So, if you picture a screen, the screen is the bone structure. That's made of protein and oils. The holes in the screen are where you slop on the minerals. Like when you put some mud on. That doesn't give the screen any integrity. That makes it where the bone fractures. That why the women taking the most calcium have the most bone fractures. The opposite of what these guys say. "But my bone density went up." That's because the x-ray measures bone density any way you can get it. So, it's like they're putting concrete on what is supposed to be a flexible bone. It gives you a better bone density and it's the exact opposite of what you want.

[throws his hands up in the air] Every time you turn around, you're told one thing and the medical science is the opposite. It is tragic, and why I deal with physicians, because it's complicated, and I don't have the time to talk with individual people is why I write so well. I spend a lot of time on the articles, on the reports, and this is all on my web site. You can get these reports for nothing. So, I hope people will take the time: www.BrianPeskin.com and it's all there. And it's current as of 2013 [when this interview took place]. I am one of the few that continue to do very relevant journal articles, lectures, and everything I've said only shows itself more important as I write as time goes on. I've never been reversed in fifteen years of leading the field in what's right. And usually, it's contrary to what everybody says. I told people not to take calcium supplements 20 years ago. And now with just this year – calcium supplements – the most heart attacks in women. Why? The last stage of heart disease is calcified plaque which precipitates from the calcium supplements you're taking. Nobody needs more calcium. That's not the cause of osteoporosis by the way. And that's in the Textbook of Medical Physiology. That's lack of vitamin D. It's a different term. It's a different condition. It is not osteoporosis. Osteoporosis is the bone matrix, it has nothing to do with calcium. We just keep getting misled. And it's one thing after another.

Salt. We're told to be on a salt restricted diet. Just came out this year again: people on the least amount of salt have the most heart attacks. What do you need salt for? No. 1 – it's the most critical amount of extra-cellular nutrient. Meaning if you're looking at anything, what's floating around? There's more salt than anything. You need it. No.2 – You can have ten times the amount of salt that they say is good for you or that you normally eat in a day. Your kidneys produce something called anti-diuretic hormone to stabilize it. So, it's no problem . . . [Ian interrupts…]

Ian: Aren't you supposed to eat pink Himalayan salt... .you don't want white table salt, right?

Brian P: No. White table salt is awful. It's 99% sodium chloride. What's better than even the pink Himalayan salt is "Flower of the Ocean" brand. That is sea salt from France. And it flows to the top. That is the best. The physicians have said the land-based salts have given them problems. But I've never heard anybody say they had any problem with the sea salt. The other thing is if you put an elderly person on a salt-restricted diet, you've just given them digestive problems. Why? Because they can't produce the hydrochloric acid from the salt! Where do you think you get the chlorine to make the hydrochloric acid? It's from the salt and you've just put them on a salt-restricted diet that's why all the elderly can't digest anything. It goes on and on and on. We're our own worst enemy. So, I hope people check out the web site and learn some of this stuff.

Ian: www.BrianPeskin.com & www.yes-supplements.com correct?

Brian P: Yes sir!

Ian: Okay well Brian, thank you so much, my friend, for coming back on. I still gotta get in front of you with my actual camera (Brian grinning broadly) so I can put you in my film "ICureCancer-2".
Brian P: Beginning of next year I should be coming down to California your way.
Ian: Oh perfect, perfect, sounds good. Okay, thank you, Brian Peskin. I appreciate you very much. Have a good night everybody. Peace.

CHAPTER 10:

INTERVIEW WITH BURTON GOLDBERG

Palm Springs 2008 I was lucky to fly Burton in to speak at an event in Palm Springs. I caught him before our dinner party in the hotel room. It would be the last time I saw him. RIP Burton.

[See Pic 10.1]

Ian: How are you tonight?

Burton: I am perfect, thank you, look at me. (smile)

Ian: Yeah, right on man, you're looking great. (broad smile)

Burton: 87 and I'm going strong and getting' younger.

Ian: Oh, wow man! When I first interviewed you, I think you were just 82 at the Cancer Control Society for my "ICureCancer" film.

Burton: You interviewed me when I was a younger man.

Ian: Yeah! (laughter) You still look, great man. You're obviously staying in shape. . . . Well, we spoke about . . . I was in, where was I?... I was in a magical place. I was in Arizona. Where the energy is, the vortex. Anyway, I did a show with you then and that we probably three, four or five months ago. So, what's new? Is there anything new and exciting that we want to get into? Or shall I just start from the beginning?

Burton: We can start from the beginning.

Ian: Okay. So, you basically – I've always looked up to you. I've studied your book. I still have it right here (reaching for it from a nearby shelf). This is one of my favorite books, folks (The word CANCER figures prominently in the title – nothing else could be discerned on the video). Back in the day, man, this is what Suzanne Somers read to learn how to write her book. And if it wasn't for Burton we wouldn't be where we are today. So that's why I always love having him on my show. And he had a follow up to this book as well. What was the other big one that came out after this?

Burton: Well before that came Alternative Medicine – the definitive guide which covered all health conditions. (Ian holds up book …) That's Cancer. And then subsequent to that, I did a documentary that one can see on the internet called Cancer Conquest which updates that book. Because at the time I did that book, took me from 1995 to 1997 to do Alternative Medicine – the definitive guide to Cancer. In 2002 the genome project came into being. And when that happened one of my mentors in Germany went to a laboratory and they created a test in Germany on circulating tumor cells so that the doctor knows which chemotherapeutic agent will target the circulating tumor cells. You know, whenever a physician puts a needle in to do a biopsy or a knife in to do surgery he spreads the cancer. (like bursting a balloon full of water) Conventional medicine tells you "no" but that's not true. It does. And even if the knife or needle doesn't go in the cancer cells mutate and that's why after doing conventional cancer treatment from two days to ten years later, it comes back with a vengeance. And it's the circulating tumor cells; whatever works on the primary will not work on it because it mutates. And it goes into other forms. So, you may need two or three different chemotherapeutic agents. Now, I am not against chemotherapy. But I am against chemotherapy the way conventional medicine uses it. They use it medievally.

Can you imagine treating cancer where you vomit and lose your hair? Nothing could be further from the truth. The way to use it is to know in advance which chemotherapeutic agent will target that patient's primary, and what will target their circulating tumor cells. And that can be done with a company that I put into my DVD called Bio-focus. And you can read about bio-focus testing on my web site www.BurtonGoldberg.com. You're sent over to the German site in English. And you can learn all about it. And there's another way of knowing, and it's by using quantum physics devices known as electro-dermal screening. The ability to tap into the body non-evasively, and see what's going on; to see what organs and systems are malfunctioning; what poisons and toxins allow you to come down with cancer in the first place. Always drain the swamp. Detoxify. That's essential. That's number one. Always find out what the cause of the cancer is. You ask conventional medicine what causes cancer and they say, "Cigarette smoking, the sun, and we don't know." Well, we do know. We need to know, in order to put it into remission. Our doctors never use the term "cure". It's a "remission". And once you have cancer you must be vigilant by doing the various tests that are available to see it in its early stages and in its regression to come back, or, to clean up the body so it won't come back. And that's really, truly our goal.

Ian: Now how did you get into this Burton? When and how did you get into helping people with cancer?

Burton: Well it all started with the publication of my book, Alternative Medicine – the definitive guide. I had to do a chapter on cancer. And a Texas doctor, Rosco Vansant, called me from Arlington, Texas and said, "Goldberg, do you know what causes cancer?" and I said, "No. What?" This was back in the early 90s. It took me four years to do that book. So, it was somewhere around '92. He said, "call this number." And he gave me the number of Hildegard Staninger a toxicologist who now resides in L.A. And she was my mentor in what causes cancer. It's poisons. We're being poisoned to death and we're being starved to death in the land of plenty.

Ian: Right.

Burton: And it is not a question of 'will I have cancer'? It's a question of when.
When my daddy was born in 1900, one in 33 Americans had cancer of any kind, shape or form. When I was born cancer was the tenth cause of death in children. Today, cancer is the first cause of death in children. Accidents are second. Today, every other man and every other woman will have cancer in their life and climbing!

Ian: And wait until the Fukushima adds up, and we start seeing what happens after that.

Burton: It is not only Fukushima which is a total disaster. It's all nuclear power plants in the United States. All nuclear power plants cause cancer. The strontium-ninety which never existed on earth goes up in the sky the winds push it down, the rains bring it to the ground, it falls on the grasses, the cows eat the grass, and strontium-ninety gets into the children and adults and people. How do we know this? Because the U.S. government who knows this, who did the study, and everyone can look up that study by looking up the Tooth Fairy Project on the internet. Google it! We have charts on the internet that show that there are higher rates of cancer down from every nuclear power plant in the world. Not only Fukushima. Fukushima is a disaster, and yet they're still building nuclear power plants, and the government lies about it. They don't tell the truth. It's really sad!

Ian: Before your book, what got you interested at all in health and helping people with their cancers? Cause were you a restauranteur or a businessman?

Burton: Yeah. I have been a restauranteur. I have been a builder, developer, a publisher. I sold door-to-door. About 45 years ago my girl friend's daughter at the age of 19 slit her wrists. She was depressed, anxiety, panicked, and her psychiatrist said to the mother, "I give up." "Did you ever hear of vitamin therapy?" The mother came to me. I never heard of vitamin therapy. And I had a psychic and her name was Iris Saltzman from Miami, Florida. And I asked Iris about vitamin therapy and she said, "Yeah, my son practices it in California." So, we flew to California with the young girl who slit her wrists. And lo-and-behold she was hypoglycemic. Simply a blood sugar imbalance. And when treated with diet and nutrition, she got well from mental illness; and ended up with ten children training horses in Florida.

Ian: Wow. I heard the same thing with people who have schizophrenia. I heard that they use high-dose vitamin C and some other things, and they've been able to bring people out of the schizophrenia.

Burton: I happen to be very aware of mental health, addiction. I've done documentaries on addiction. All of this is on my web site. And nutrition is extremely important. Of course, some schizophrenia can be caused by food. The best book I've ever read or seen on that is by William Walsh, called Nutrient Power. He covers everything from autism to mental health, depression, anxiety, panic and all those. Wonderful book. Nutrient Health by William Walsh. And I belong to an organization called "The Alliance for Addiction Solutions". I'm on the board. And there we use amino acids and fatty acids, and important is 1) eating properly, 2) not being a vegetarian – very important. 3) and feeding the body with the body it is screaming for – which is nutrients, amino acids and fatty acids that produce serotonin and whatever is deficient in the body.

Ian: That's right. You've done a number of films. You came down and blessed us with your presence and film that was talking about GMOs, and it had three things in it. Do you remember that time you came down to Palm Springs and you screened your film? Which one was that? That was
Burton: That film was called Greed. I never did get it out. Greed is about cancer, autism and mad-cow disease.

Ian: Oh, okay. I remember that. So that never went anywhere? Oh my god, it was such a great film too!

Burton: It was a great film and if you want to, take a look at it, let me give you codes to see it. Let me see, it's called Greed, g r e e d, that's the passcode to see it too, go to Vimeo. Write it down: www.Vimeo.com/65614716 and you'll be able to see this film.

I'm trying to raise money to pay for the B role, but it's very important. The bottom line to the film is until we take back our government from the corporation's nothing will change. We are dead ducks. As Leonard Cohen says in one of his songs: "I see the future, and the future is murder."

Ian: Ah. It's a sad state of affairs… what's been going on I'll tell you that. I'm glad you're on my team too man. We need some young guys to start coming in there and help out, which is starting to happen. I'm starting to meet a lot of people that are really, man, those young people have got a different way of thinking of things. I still think there is hope for us. All right, so let's see, you've got . . . tell me about the whole Suzanne Somers experience. What was that like? Did she just contact you out of the blue and say, "I've been using your book . . . do you want to work together?" Or, how did it happen?

Burton: How it happened is, I had a magazine and I knew her because I did an article on her and her health years before. But she went on Larry King because one of the scheduled sheets had squealed on her that had had liposuction. So, Larry asked her why she had liposuction. And she said, "I had cancer and I wanted to even out my breasts." So, he said, "I didn't know you had cancer! What are you doing for it?" She says, "Alternative medicine." He said, "Alternative medicine?! How'd you get into that?" And she said, there's another nice Jewish boy by the name of Burton Goldberg who wrote a book." Every book in the country sold out. That was the book you held up which is now ancient history. But my DVD is really important! It's called Cancer Conquest and it takes place in Mexico, Germany, and the United States. And it tells how we go about putting cancer in remission in stage four!

Ian: (nods) Okay. Good. So, you're a cancer coach basically. You help people if they're in need.

Let's just say I've got a buddy right now that's got testicular cancer and he's taking the cannabis oil; he's juicing and doing the whole alternative stuff. Have you got any tricks of the trade for testicular cancer?

Burton: All cancers are about the same. Diet is extremely important. You must get him on an alkaline diet. Because when the body, the sweet spot is 7.4 saliva before you brush your teeth in the morning and it's difficult to get there alone with diet. And I recommend a diet of some juices, organic, and believe it or not, in the diet that Dr. Bernardo – you remember him – I give that to the patients. Dr. Bernardo allows certain meats. You can have buffalo and deer, goat and lamb, and some fish and some potatoes and some rice but you've got to be very careful. And lots of juices. So, diet is extremely important.

Ian: Yeah, I had a wonderful time when you came down to visit a few years ago to show us the movie and we started talking about Dr. Bernardo (smiling) because he was in I Cure Cancer as well. You two were basically the stars of that film so it was cool to continue our relationship. I really miss Dr. Bernardo man. He was a good guy to have around you know. You agree with his alkaline diet and so do I. I mean... and, also Dr. Gonzales from New York City has helped me realize that some people with blood cancers, that maybe they're too alkaline and may need to be more acidic. And, they actually need some of the meats too.

Ian: How do you get an honorary degree?

Burton: Well, I was in WW2 in the Navy. After the Navy, I went to work. I never went to college. I improved my vocabulary by using the dictionary and reading and writing down words and looking them up and so forth. Anyway, I was very successful in business. And I started the book Alternative Medicine, the Definitive Guide. Muffie Fanning, a woman who lived in Philadelphia, (her husband at that time was a retired Rear-Admiral), she ended up with lymphedema, a swollen leg. And they couldn't find out what caused it. He went to every doctor she could find. He (her husband) bought my book and read about a physician in Oregon. He traveled from Philadelphia to Oregon with Muffie Fanning because she was dying. The leg was like a balloon. And what happened is this woman put her to sleep. And then woke her up two hours later, pricked her finger, looked at her blood and there was a parasite which turned out to be elephantiasis.

And God in His wisdom seals off the body so that the parasite stays within the area and the leg blew up. So, um, they used conventional medicine out of England, which was flown over, a vaccine, and Muffie ended up killing off the elephantiasis parasite. And they used many of the aspects of the light beam generator to fracture the molecules and open-up the blockage. And her leg went down, she lived and Timothy Fanning, Admiral Fanning, decided to join Capital University in Washington D.C. as a board member in honor of what alternative medicine did.

It was a college of physicians for physicians to teach other physicians . . . like Robert Atkins would teach there. He got no money; he'd just go down from New York to Washington – all over the United States. And they, because of my work and the "definitive guide" put the school together of alternative medicine for the various therapies and the 360 health conditions, including cancer. And they gave me an honorary doctorate in Humanity. So, when people call me "Dr. Goldberg" I answer. (smile)

Ian: (laughter) That's awesome. Yeah and so you should. We're finding out that people are actually following the law and getting a marijuana license for their cancer and it's taking away their tumors, it's taking away their cancers. They're losing weight. I mean it's just amazing what it's doing. Yet, some states are still throwing people in jail regardless of having the card. And it like what we've always been fighting against with just alternative medicine in general. You can't say "cure" you can't say this you can't do that. Is there anything we can do legally these days? I mean I talked to Dr. Coleb recently, and he's talking about some sovereign law. Have you thought about what we can do? Like children's rights. My movie I Cure Cancer – 2 is about how if I have a child I can't treat them holistically. I have to get chemo, radiation or surgery (or all three) or I go to jail. Let's talk about this for a bit Burton. Where do you feel this is going? Is there any hope for us?

Burton: Well there's no question that medical marijuana has a place. San Jay Gupta, the doctor of CNN just converted. His mind was opened-up. He had been brainwashed. So, he now is in favor of medical marijuana. And I just think the only thing you can do is become politically active in your state.

We live in California which is a legal state. I have a license for marijuana, and I use marijuana. It's my drug of choice. I find it to be very healthy, also for cancer. You have to know what you're doing. I don't believe it's a panacea. The object is to take the marijuana without the hallucinogenic aspect because a lot of people are disturbed by how stoned they can get from this oil that's consumed. But there are people making marijuana oils that remove the hallucinogenic aspect of it. It's good medicine.

Ian: Yeah. I'm learning about all this now. Fortunately, the THC is really good for cancer, so, people who have cancer I say, 'you want to go high THC.' From what I understand if you have seizures high CBDs which is not the psychoactive ingredient is better. So, it kinda depends on what you have. And I think we're all just learning as we go. I'm talking with growers and people making the medicine. I'm kind of learning as I go to figure out the best way – what cannabinoids I need and how much THC and you know, it's science that we have to figure out on the street because our government won't do it for us I guess.

Yeah, I'm recalling a couple of horror stories that are going on there. Have you heard of anybody ever beating anything legally using "sovereign"? That's what I'm looking at, like "sovereign" the law that our constitutional rights upheld. Do you know if this stuff is going somewhere where it may work? Cause' I don't know anybody that's had it work.

Burton: You're talking about the legal aspect of using marijuana?
Ian: Yeah, like, when if they get busted . . .
Burton: I'm not up on that.

Ian: Okay. Okay. Just checking. All right, um, let's see . . . you're the publisher . . . you've written books, too right? Have you written any, or are you just publishing?

Burton: No. It's neither. I hire writers. I have the knowledge and I guide them where to start. And then from one doctor, we go to the next doctor and I create the voice and edit and then I publish. I no longer do that. I've been making some films. I did a film on depression, anxiety, panic. Another one on addiction. Another one on cancer.

Cancer Conquest, which is what is the latest in the remission of cancer. And I do guide people from all over the world thanks to Suzanne Somers who has done more for alternative and integrative cancer than any person ever because of her celebrity status and her brilliance. She's quite an extraordinary woman.

Ian: Yeah, she's a hard gal to track down. I tried to get her for my first film, I tried to get her in the second one. I've gotten close to her through her secretary, but I'm not quite there yet. It may happen. I got Muriel Hemingway. She's told her story. She helped cure her husband of "terminal cancer" years ago. So, you never know. We're getting some people in this film. It should be done by the end of the year, Burton, I hope. I may want to shoot you again too, so if you're ever in L.A. make sure you know, uh, let me know so that we can hook up. Um … . . okay . . . What, what else is going on? So, what happened new since um, um, the last time we spoke? Are you traveling anymore? Do you still go to Europe?

Burton: Yeah. As a matter of fact, I was in Europe recently. I'm very much into stem cells. And I have a product that I'm on which regenerates the body. So, I'm a year older than the pope that retired. And when he retired, I was skiing in Switzerland with friends. And I ski in Aspen. So, at 87 I'm doing amazingly well. And I'm younger now than when you interviewed me because of the stem cells that I'm on. It's orally delivered, the sheep placenta and it's absolutely amazing!

Ian: I remember you starting to speak about that, yeah. Okay. So, if somebody …. What do you use it for? Is it just for general wealth, uh health and wellbeing? Is it, uh, specific to anything?

Burton: No. It goes where necessary. It goes into the body and regenerates and the first thing you think about is energy, the second thing is clarity, and your skin looks younger, fewer wrinkles.
Ian: And what is this called – the product?

Burton: The product is called "Swiss-cell". And I handle it, so if anyone wants it they have to get a hold of me on the internet.

Ian: Okay so we get . . . and that's … uh … BurtonGoldberg.com right?
Burton: Yes sir.

Ian: Okay Swiss . . . I still couldn't get that right . . . Swiss…?

Burton: Swiss-cell. I don't have a web site, although there is one in Europe. And I don't want a web site because I don't want publicity. It's by invitation only.

Ian: Yeah, yeah, they're lucking to hear. So, if anybody . . . when you hear that folks and you need to call me, or Burton and we'll take care o' ya' on that one. You look good, you look the same as you did ten years ago or whenever that was. Unbelievable.

Burton: That is unbelievable and, um, I'm the same age as the Queen of England and she walks like an old lady. Before I went on these cells, I couldn't bend without aches and pains. Today I fold into a car like a youngster. And sexually, it's amazing. I'm like 35. (Ian laughing)

Ian: You go, Boy! (laughing clapping hands)

Burton: Very important. You have to be healthy, to have sex.

Ian: Right. Yah. Well, I've started blending lately. I've dropped 30lbs myself and I've gotten my PH up to 7.4, cause, it was five for six months. See, in a way, it's the best thing that could have happened to me, if for no other reason that I tell people and teach by example. I put a video up, today actually, where I'm showing how to blend, you take one of those 3-horsepower blenders and just pack it full of all the organic stuff – dark cruciferous vegetables and everything and wow, in three months man I feel like 20 years ago. Do you know? It's amazing. (Goldberg smiling) I'm ready to make a comeback (putting up his fists and laughing).

Okay, so let's go with, I have another friend that has, needs to get a kidney replaced. Because he got it replaced when he was young, and he went through it and now got to do another one. Have you heard of any . . . do you know anybody getting-off of transplant lists but finding something that rejuvenated their liver like . . . does hemp oil do anything for the liver? Have you ever heard that or kidneys?

Burton: Uh. Stem cells would be the way to go. Stem cells are really important! They can regenerate organs. As a matter of fact, one of my doctors in Pennsylvania gave this woman who had multiple sclerosis. And he treated her for a year and a half. He put her on Swiss-cells for about three months and several of her lesions disappeared on a PET scan. So, stem cells are definitely helpful in regenerating. Again, I recommend anyone who goes to a doctor to look for a physician who does electro-dermal screening; the quantum physics to tap into the body non-evasively and look for trouble. By the way, by the time you've been diagnosed with cancer you've had that cancer eight, nine or ten years.

Ian: Right, right.

Burton: It takes that long to double and double and double. So, you look for trouble. You look for heart disease. You look for diabetes. And you can nip it in the bud if you catch it early. That's the game. And yet in conventional medicine and alternative medicine, we're not looking for it early. So as a matter of fact, I send all my clients a medical detective. I wanna know what caused the cancer and have them remove it and I send them to physicians who can help them. Because I'm not a medical doctor. I am a knowledgeable man who knows and studies who knows and I'm able to send people to physicians. I don't practice medicine.

Ian: Right. You and I are both kinda the same. I'm just kinda following your footsteps, I kinda just learn from you and uh, many other people and, and, peep…. I didn't plan on this being my gig man. I was an actor and kickboxing champion. You know I stumbled across it and I learned it well and I seem to relay it well to people. So, I got no problem helping out with this, you know. I'm trying to learn how to monetize so, uh, until one of my movies makes some money you know, then I'll just make movies for free for people. But I'm trying to learn how to monetize and up some things. Well, let's see, is there anything on your mind that you haven't talked about tonight?

Burton: I think the best way for you to monetize is to charge people for your direction because you've studied it. You know rightly how to put it in remission. And you should be a consultant as I am. I make a living that way. It's very difficult to do it on movies. Very, very tough.

Ian: Yeah, I know. I keep thinking that just one is going to do it. You're right. Um . . . the key is again, I never thought of charging. Really, I mean I asked for money for my video and if they want, but I'll look into that. Ah, what else is new? There's got to be something new man, (leaning back looking into the air) we've been talking about the cannabis oil, what about Moringa trees and Soursop. Have you heard much about these things?

Burton: No. No, I'm not eh". I'm basically um, into what caused the cancer and into how to remove it. And I'm not into specifics. Because when it comes to specifics I want to know scientifically what that patient can use. Will this be effective? Will this be tolerated? Or, am I wasting my time? And that's why I am into quantum physics or electro-dermal screening. Your audience can look that up. And these devices are now amazing. They're computer operated. You hold two electrodes and they spit out what's going on in your body. Which organs and systems malfunction. And then you can find out which product. So rather than ask somebody about it, or you can use a pendulum. I love pendulums.

Ian: (enthusiastically) Yes! yes!

Burton: I use pendulums. And uh, what is a pendulum? You're talking to God. It's quantum physics. You're in the field. And they've been using for thousands of years to find geopathic. And that's something that most people pay no attention to in cancer. Geopathic stress. Google it! These are noxious rays from the outer sphere down to the ground. I learned this in Germany years ago. And every one of the patients I have, shield their house by putting steel rebars in the ground: one foot in length, and surround the house every four feet, drive a one-foot iron stake, iron rebars, in the flower beds outside the house every four feet and that will acupuncture the earth and stop it. But, google "geopathic stress" and make your clients aware of it.

Ian: Yeah, this is new.

Burton: It is one of the aspects of getting cancer. And I don't know of one doctor (medical doctor) in the world that pays attention to it. But I learned this by going to school in Germany back in the 80s. I went to Lake Starnberg working with doctors and learned how, what causes cancer and how to avoid it and overcome it.

Ian: Okay. Geopathic stress; so that's got to do with mother earth basically?

Burton: Exactly. It's the ionosphere down to the ground. And it goes up, it'll go up the Empire State building. But you can put a simple iron rod and that will acupuncture the earth. And uh, there are certain houses that are cancer houses. And that's what they found in Germany. There is lots of research. There are movies and lots to read. Geopathic stress. Google it! So that's something I pay a lot of attention to with patients.

Ian: You brought up a very important thing at the very beginning of the interview that I want to reiterate for our folks: Never get biopsies folks! If you're my fans you've probably seen my video with Dr. Bernardo? If you think you have cancer? No biopsies. Once you cut into that the cells get into the bloodstream and spread throughout the body. I just met a great guy down in Mexico and I should tell you about it sometime. Basically, they're MDs that do holistic first. Everything you believe in (Burton), everything I believe in, they do it all, I mean, it's just unbelievable … and, if they have to use some chemotherapy they will.
They use stem cells too. They're in Mexico https://americanbiodental.com/. So they can do that. Somehow, they're using certain stem cells even with some kinds of chemo I think. So, they're not against chemoeither. If you need it, they're going to give it to you. But nine times out of ten they're not going to use it. But it's Alessandro Porcella's clinic in TJ.

Burton: I want to tell you, you must use targeted chemo in low dose. And low dose is something like 10%. That's why I'm not against chemo, but I'm against the way conventional medicine uses chemo. And it's never the cookbook. For instance, you may use an ovarian drug for prostate. You may use a colon-rectal cancer drug (chemotherapy) for breast cancer. You never know. But when you use low dose, with insulin potentiated and full-body hyperthermia it is 14 times more effective. And then there are vaccines that build the immune system. There are vaccines that take away the shield on the immune system.

You know, cancer uses the same mechanism that God uses to shield the baby in a pregnant woman. In other words, when a woman becomes pregnant that baby is a foreign element. And yet the immune system would wipe it out had God not developed nagalase, an enzyme, that shields the immune system. Cancer uses that shield. They use nagalase to shield, and they have a CG-math vaccine that wipes away that shield so that when you do dendritic-cell therapy you take out the blood and train the person's immune system to attack their cancers. This is the latest.

This is unheard of by conventional medicine. Conventional oncologists are butchers. Period. Let me show you the disconnect. When you do a PET scan, the oncologist, in order to get the radiologic molecule into the tumor,—the cancer cell—so it shows up on X-ray, gives the patient sugar! And yet they tell the patient they can eat anything they want. And the oncologists give them candy, cookies, and cake in the chemo room! That's like putting gasoline on a fire. That's the disconnect. Which means you don't have to be smart to be a doctor, you have to have a memory. If you have a good memory you can become a Ph.D., a psychiatrist, a medical doctor you can be anything you want. Remember; take the test, and they give you a license. But the oncologists in this country are mad (i.e., senseless crazy). They don't understand cancer. They truly don't understand cancer. And that's why they have such failures. And that's why it comes back.

Do you ever hear an oncologist yell, "What causing cancer? Why don't we find out?" They don't want to find out. They want to keep this whole thing running because it's a money train. And until we take back our government from the corporations (and rich elite), nothing is going to change.
As Leonard Cohen says in one of his songs: "I see the future, and the future is murder." And let me give you an example. Autism. Autism is bankrupting this country. It's on its way. Autism alone. The official rate of Autism today is 1 in 88. That's what my movie is about. The one I told you. Greed. One in eighty-eight. That's the "official" rate. My doctors who treat Autism say it's now 1 in 55. In 1970 it was 1 in 10,000 (one in ten thousand). And in 1950 it was unheard of. Because of vaccines, because of mercury, mercury in the fish. I mean there are kids who have become Autistic who have never had a vaccine. Because if you want to detoxify become pregnant. It goes right into the umbilical cord right into the embryo. This is a holocaust! Autism. And Autism is reversible. That's the good news. And I have helped a lot of families with Autism.

Ian: What's the key? The gut bacteria? With cleansing, are people getting well?

Burton: Yeah. You just said the word. Drain the swamp. Detoxify. Get rid of what poisons are in there. Diet is very very important! It's many, many, many things and this program isn't about Autism. But Autism – and the government knows this – anyone listening out there that thinks I don't know what I'm talking about Google: "Simpsonwood CDC Autism". That is a study that was put out——Google it——by the CDC and achieved by the Freedom of Information Act where the scientists of the CDC know that the vaccines a problem. And although they've taken mercury out of some they haven't taken it out of the flu vaccine, the Marisol, but they have aluminum in them which is equally as bad; and excitotoxins. So, we are poisoning ourselves and because we have a crooked government that pays attention to corporations rather than humanity. And until we take back our government, and this president (Obama) is no different than the two that preceded him.

Ian: I know man! It's so sad. How are we going to do it? Do we do what Iceland did, or . . . do we pull off a revolution do you think, or are they just going to kill us all?

Burton: What you have to do is educate yourself. Tune into Ian Jacklin shows and educate yourself. You have to take charge! You mother. You father. You have to take charge of your health! You cannot allow your doctors. You think your doctors know it all. "Oh yeah, if it was any good my doctor would know about it." Your doctor has become a conventional doctor; a legalized drug pusher. He spends five or ten minutes and he gives you drugs not to cure the situation but to mask the symptoms.

Ian: Isn't it funny and the stuff the people used to smoke on the streets, instead of having a beer, smoke some weed – and that's supposed to be the illegal one. Even though it's becoming legal, they're still making it difficult. Yeah. I don't know what to do Burton, man, I just keep talking. Keep asking, keep educating.

Burton: Well you're educating, and that's what you do. So, you're doing the best you can. And you the listener (reader) have to educate yourself because the government won't do it.

Ian: That's right. So, the bottom line is . . . cause' I have some friends with cancer right now ... get alkaline, right!? Cannabis oil is good, right? Anything else you want to throw ideas you have for people who are working on their own and they don't have anyone to teach them.

Burton: Ninety-five percent of females with breast cancer have dental involvement. The oral cavity is as important as anything else. As much as 50% in the remission of cancer can be in the oral cavity. But 95% of females with cancer at a German University study had dental involvement. So, if you have cancer and if you need help give me a ring (phone call) I'm here to help you.

Ian: That's right that BurtonGoldberg.com. Do you have any other sites that we should bring up?

Burton: No.

Ian: That's the main one.

Burton: Yeah, and if you have mental problems, emotional addiction: The Alliance for Addiction Solutions. That a very good web site. It's a non-profit for people who use nutrition to deal with all that. Mental health is a huge problem because our food supply is denuded. As much as 30% to 70% less nutrition in certain vegetables than in the 1970s because we're not reinvesting the nutrients back into the soil. So, consequently, our food is not as nutritious as it should be. These are (seen on) government charts.

Ian: Right. Yeah, not like the carrots my grandpa used to pull up out of the ground in his garden 40 years ago.

Burton: That's why it's so important to go organic.

Ian: (nodding) Yeah. I don't even mess around anymore. Just straight up organic and blending most of it you know. I'm starting to eat vegan too, not vegan, but more vegetarian which I've never done. I'm a proud meat eater, but still instead of three times a day

Burton: Let me say this: I don't believe in most Americans who will come from Europe – you know two or three or four generations back, it takes many, many years, and the China studies about Chinese people; they haven't had very much meat. But we've had meat and we've had dairy and so forth…but we adulterate our food with pesticides and herbicides, the antibiotic in the food supply. They use more for animals than they do for humans. And it goes in and it destroys our gut. So, we depreciate our own immune system. And then we go into the emotional aspect. The psychological. The immunological aspect of the disease. All of these things, when you've seen one cancer patient you've seen one cancer patient. You treat the individual who has cancer. Because we're all different, we all come from different backgrounds, we all have different poisons.

Ian: Very true, very true. Have you experienced any, sort of, magical healing where somebody got blessed by a priest or you know, you know what I'm talking about like spontaneous remission . . . anything like that?

Burton: Yeah. It does happen. I've heard of it.
Ian: John of God in Brazil.

Burton: Well that's for using his psychic powers. And then there's Lourdes and so forth. Um. There are spontaneous remissions but that's extremely rare. I wouldn't depend on that and I wouldn't look to that. No. 1 drain the swamp. Find out what caused your cancer in the first place. That's what my clients have to do because I don't want it coming back. When they hire me, they hire me to keep them alive. And non-compliance is for a lot of people who don't want to live.

Ian: Right.
Burton: You've got to recognize it and lay off because you can't beat them. No. 2 But diet is extremely important.
Ian: Well, I guess that's a good way of wrapping it up folks. It's an alkaline diet, very important. Let food be thy medicine. Cannabis oil is working great for many things: seizures, weight loss, cancer, mental issues, M.S... I mean it's . .. look into it folks. I'm not saying you should take my word for it. Just look into it. Burton and I both agree on it. So, it's worth looking into it.

So, again: www.BurtonGoldberg.com and this is www.ICureCancer.com. Burton, it's a pleasure as always having you man. You're one of my old buddies now. I can't believe we've known each other for like 20 years! (laughter) But thank you so much sir, and I will be in touch, okay? (Burton blows Ian a kiss) All right, thank you, Burton. See you in New York. Peace. Bye, everybody.

FYI: Burton Goldberg passed away before this book was released. The world lost another good man. I really enjoyed being mentored by him and Dr. Bernardo. I hope you guys are both sitting up there in heaven watching over me and I'm making you proud.

[See Pic 10.2 and 10.3]

CHAPTER 11:

RONNIE SMITH ON CANNABIS OIL

Ronnie: That's what killed my mom, was chemotherapy. If it wasn't for chemotherapy, I think she'd have lived a lot longer! Yeah… My name is Ronnie Lee Smith. I do stand-up comedy under the name Roland A. Duby.   Roland A. Duby opens for Doug Stanhope in Cincinnati 2005 And I was the editor for Jack Herer's, The Emperor Wears No Clothes.

Now before I went to see Jack I'd lost my mother, my father, my brother, and a sister and many cousins and uncles to cancer. And I had lumps all growing in my hands… and one between each knuckle [rubbing hands] and I had a thing in my rear end that was bothering me real bad! And I assumed I probably did have cancer. You know, I was never diagnosed, but I was feeling very bad. And luck would have it, I went out to see Jack Herer… ended up getting my medical marijuana card here in California, started growing pot with Jack and his wife. And when we harvested it, it was my job to make the oil… I mean to make the hash.

So, I was making cold water bubble bag hash and I would make my little pallets of hash with a tablespoon, I would eat a spoonful, every four or five pallets, I would eat some. Did that for a couple of months and all the lumps [rubbing hands] disappear out of my hands?

Well, that got us to searching the internet for marijuana and cancer which led to discovering Rick Simpson and what he was doing. And Jack Herer was doing a thing called [picture of Jack Herer on High Times] Jack Herer TV at the time. So, we started putting Rick Simpson on Jack Herer TV and getting the message out there.

And then Jack got Steve Hager to write a story about Rick Simpson's oil and that was the thing that really skyrocketed! Because up until then, people, it was hard to get anybody to believe that marijuana cured cancer. You know, people would say, even potheads would say, "Oh yeah sure, it's good for the symptoms," you know, "It'll give you the munchies and make you want to eat and it'll help relieve the chemotherapy stuff," but they won't believe that it's the cure, you know.

And here it is! The most simple thing in the world, soak some pot in alcohol, cook the alcohol away and you got oil. And all you gotta do is eat it and it's the cure for pfft almost everything. Not just cancer, so many things, diabetes, Parkinson's… maybe not a cure for Parkinson's, but it relieves the symptoms enough to where people with Parkinson's can function on a normal basis every day, you know, everything like that, glaucoma.

People with cancer who also had glaucoma, they would say, "Oh wow, my glaucoma is gone!" Just out of the blue, you know, "Oh, Wow! It's gone." Who'd a figured? Things like that, you know. Somebody has a pain in their back, all the time, and then they get cancer and they start taking the oil. Well, the pain in their back goes away too! You know, cause the inflammation, marijuana is the most wonderful anti-inflammatory that there is. So, it gets rid of all the inflamed arthritis, you know, the sore fingers when old people wake up in the morning. That stuff all goes away when you're taking oil every day. It's like a miracle!

You know in the 1800s, they had these guys, they called them snake oil salesmen, and they would go around selling their bottle of Dr. Feel Good's Miracle whatever… well if it had cannabis Indica in it, I believe it was the cure to just about all your ills. - Outdoors - Ronnie shows Ian how to make oil… [Shot of blue bucket] And you can see the red in it.

Ian: Oh yeah!
Ronnie: Can you see the red?
Ian: So that way you know it's …

Ronnie: You know there's THC in there when it's red because the crystals are amber. Well, we're just making this oil, my friend had a lot of trim and stuff that was donated to him and he wanted to make it into the oil. So, he invited me out to make the oil for him and we're going to split it. So, then I can give mine away and he's going to give his to his friends that have cancer.

Ian: So it just goes to show that you don't necessarily have to get kind Indica buds.

Ronnie: Oh no. Man, I've cured cancer with Mexican brick weed, you know. When I lived in Atlanta that's almost all there was, Mexican brick weed, sometimes I'd get good mid-grade from Arizona. But people would come to me, and say, "Oh, my mom has cancer," bring me a brick of weed, and say, "Can you make oil out of it?" Well, "Yeah." Three weeks later they're saying, "My Mom is doing much better." And two months later, "Mom's cured of cancer!" It happens, all of the time!

Ian: Wow.

Ronnie: But online you never hear anybody talking about all that, you know. If I said online, that I'd made marijuana oil out of Mexican brick weed, I would get called so many names. And I will, once this is out there, but I don't care because it's curing people, you know.

Ian: It sure is.

Ronnie: Yeah, it's helping people; saving lives!

(Ronnie only uses top grade Indica buds for the oil he sells for $2000. He makes oil out of shake and gives for free to those that can't afford it.)

Ronnie: Ideally, you wanna use a good strong Indica, you know, so that the person who has cancer can sleep. Usually, like if you're using Mexican or something like that it's going to be a Sativa. So, you don't really wanna use that for somebody who's really, really, sick and they need to rest. You don't want them cleaning the house while they're dying of cancer. Right.
[See Pic 11.2]

Ronnie: [High Times pic with Jack Herer on it.] Oh, you know, it's hard for me to even imagine people don't know who Jack Herer is. [Chuckling] Jack wrote a wonderful book called, The Emperor Wears No Clothes. [See Pic 11.1]
And it is the end all, be all of the hemp and American history. And Jack's book taught me so much. If it wasn't for his book, I would have never known that our country was founded on marijuana.

It was because of Rick Simpson that I started doing this. [Pic of Rick holding up oil tube.] I mean, people have known that cannabis is a medicine for years because before 1937 it was in almost every medicine. But Rick brought it back to the forefront and said, "Look, it's a fucking cure for cancer," you know! [Chuckling] If he hadn't done that, I wouldn't have known... Jack wouldn't know. If Jack hadn't known, the rest of the world probably wouldn't know. Because it was Jack who really spread the word. You know the sad thing is there's a lot of people who are so lazy they take the oil for a couple of weeks, they feel better, and they stop. You know, and then they start getting sicker again, so they'll take the oil until they feel better and then they'll stop. And it's just SILLY. Note: Ronnie passed away a few years ago of Leukemia. He stopped taking his cannabis oil. Was just smoking it and went off his diet. Boom, dead. Oh, the irony! RIP buddy.

Ian: Right.

Ronnie: You know, it's just lazy.

Ian: What do you recommend?

Ronnie: Just do it until... Yeah, 60 grams, eat it every day until it's all gone. And then eat a drop a day, every day, for the rest of your life. We have an internal cannabinoid system, the endocannabinoid system, without a drop of oil every day, all of our organs, are going to go right back into that state of dysfunction without the cannabinoids because they need them to properly function.

Ian: Wow.

Ronnie: Ronnie: Doctors don't tell people this. And Why? Doctors gotta know about the endocannabinoid system! If they don't; they have to learn. It can't be stopped. No way. You know I was in a... I was in a warehouse with some friends of mine, years ago, before I went out to even be with Jack Herer and to grow pot. And at a time, we were all on this holy anointing oil kick. Have you heard about the holy anointing oil?

Well in Exodus 30:23 in the Bible, there's an oil; Moses' holy anointing oil. And the first ingredient, in the English version of the Bible is, Calamus, but if you read the Hebrew, it's cannabis.

So, the holy oil, that Jesus was anointed with, and all the priests were anointed with, was about 80 percent hash oil.

And, so, we were making this stuff up and using it for all kinds of things. I was brushing my teeth with it. I would put it on my head when I went to Hemp Fest, and I wouldn't get sunburned. Incredible stuff!

So, when I went out to be with Jack and told him about what I was doing with it and come to find out, he already had a guy who was helping him with the holy anointing oil, named Tom Brown, who would rub it on his legs and got rid of his diabetic ulcers and stuff on his legs. So, we knew then that is was curing diabetic ulcers and all this other stuff.

Yeah, yeah… it does, it makes you better. Our organs need it. We have an internal system called the endocannabinoid system. Every organ in our body has a receptor site for cannabinoids, CB1 and CB2 receptors. And they're all over, in our brain, in our liver, everywhere.

I think that's why the cannabis oil works so well on liver cancer, because when you look at the… they have these ways that they can video, or take pictures of the organs and see where the receptor sites are, by putting some kind of chemical in you. And they're focused on the internal organs and on the brain, and all of the cannabinoid receptors.

So, every organ in our body needs it, and without it the organs… they fail after a while. I think that's what causes long term sickness, you get… your organs just fail, because they don't have the CB receptors activated.

It's what helps diabetes because of the… if you watch the video of that guy on YouTube, he talks about the scientific reasons that he tried to use the oil for his diabetes because it said the cannabinoids cause your pancreas to do its job correctly. [Chuckling] So… [Hands spread palms up] Oh I know I've done cured well over 350, terminal, stage IV, and that's not counting stage I, stage II, stage III, glaucoma, Parkinson's, diabetes, hundreds of people I know have wiped out diabetes, wiped it out, and diabetes. Yeah. Any diabetes. There's a great video online, I don't know if you've seen it… the big guy?

Ian: Yeah.

Ronnie: Yeah. He was in… he was in bad shape, you know.

Now, I think I had it too, cause, I had a… I would get sores on my legs and they wouldn't go away for a long time; my legs would swell up over my socks. That doesn't happen anymore, you know. I'm still fat. I was 340 pounds [chuckling] now I'm down to like 280. So that's pretty good.

Ian: You didn't do anything differently?

Ronnie: Uh huh, no. Yeah, a lot of people having good success with that.
– I've had four brain cancer patients, [holding up four fingers] that don't have brain cancer anymore, yeah. Most of the people that call me are liver, pancreas, stomach cancer and breast cancer; that's most of the people that call me. If I had… I would say that of the people who got to me in time, it's about 75 to 80 percent success. Yeah!

Unfortunately, most of the people that contact me are at the end of the… you know, because most of their organs have been cut up and pieces of their liver cut off and their… I can't remember… [Gesturing to arm pit] lymph nodes have all been cut out. You know, when your body has been chopped up like that and mutilated like that, it's not going to function correctly no matter what you do to it.

And that's a drag, because if these people would take the oil, first; if you take the oil [banging hands together] FIRST, you don't have to cut those organs away. They go back to the way that they were. You could have your liver, half of it, cancer cells and eat hemp oil and the cancer will go away and your liver will still be there just the way it was before. But doctors go in there and cut it away. So, you've got half of a liver. It makes no sense, you know. You'd think that we've got past that freakin' bloodletting, cut it off crap. [Shaking head]

Hell, I'd send it to anybody in America. Anybody in America that needs it, if they're dying and they need oil and they contact me I'll make sure they get it. Yeah. I have no problem with that. I've been doing it now… as soon as I found out that it was the cure for cancer, I said to myself, "This has gotta be spread far and wide."

And then, talking with Rick one day, he was telling me that they needed somebody in America to make oil because he gets all these phone calls. So, I said, "Well, I'm your Huckleberry, [hand up], right here. I'll do that!" It's easy to make.

So, I was getting referrals from Rick for two years before he went to Europe and got stuck out there, you know. So… and I still get calls from people who were originally referred from Rick, even though Rick doesn't do any more referrals. I still get calls from people who were referred from Rick saying, "Hey can you help my friend? You mind if I give him your number?" Well, it's just… it's snowballing like that, you know.

Which… and that's a good thing for me because that means people who I helped six years ago, five years ago, are still alive, and still helping other people.

Ian: YOU AREN'T WORRIED ABOUT THE POLICE?

Ronnie: "Come and bust me," is what I say. I beat Marijuana charges in my county of Kentucky 9 times because of religious reasons and they quit bothering me about marijuana. That's why I've got these felonies on me because they had to find something that they could do to get me out of the way. My plan I was running for Sheriff… [chuckling]… this is a "wild dream" okay. I wanted the farmers in my county to grow the Marijuana; the Sheriff's Department would process it into oil and distribute it to the people in our county that had cancer. Because our county had the highest cancer rate of any county in Kentucky, Gallatin County Kentucky, the highest cancer rate of any county in Kentucky.

There was a billboard on Highway 42 that said, "Gallatin County Highest Cancer Rate" yadda yadda yadda. So, I put my billboard for Sheriff up right up above it, "Marijuana is the Cure for Cancer!" [Laughing] You know, [chuckling], "Vote for Me, and we'll make sure everybody has access to cancer medicine!" So, they wanted to get rid of me. Oh, I've been doing this for six years, vacuum sealing the oil and sending it out to people in the United States.

Well, I grow my own pot and I charge $2,000 for oil, made out of buds. And I buy lots and lots of extra trim and sugar leaf and I make stuff out of that and I give it away for free. Right now, I've got 75 people that I'm giving oil to every month, 2 grams a month.

THC causes cancer to go into... I don't know if you've heard of this, a state of autophagy where it eats itself. That's what THC DOES to cancer. It makes it eat itself away. So, any pot has THC in it, unless it's really old, then it's degraded. So, if you can get a pound of cheap Mexican weed or get ya a couple of pounds of the trim leaf that somebody has sitting around, make your oil out of that if you're poor, and you're going to cure your cancer or whatever disease you have is going to be taken care of.

For other diseases, Sativa is good, you know, because if you wanna go to work. You got diabetes and you still wanna go to work, take a drop of Indica in the morning for your diabetes [head hung back] there ya are, the rest of the day. [Head still hung back]
[Laughing]

But you take a good hit of Indica... I mean of Sativa and you can go to work, you can do... you can drive your car; you can do whatever you want. And it still cures your diabetes.

Ian: HOW DO WE FIX THE WORLD?

Ronnie: How to fix it? Oh, God! I don't know. I know that there are certain people who are the controlling factors, and these are the upper echelon royal families; relatives of Dick Cheney's and George Bush's, these people are all related. The bloodlines go way back. And if we could take our world back away from those people, whether they're lizard alien families or whatever they are. The people have to take that back away from 'em.

It's like here in America, we had a great thing going on, individual sovereignty, everyone in America is a King. We are all Kings and we don't even know it. We don't even exercise our kingship.
What they're really trying to do to me is... is... what is the word when they try to make you look bad?

Ian: Discredit you?

Ronnie: Discredit me, make me look like a fool or make me look like somebody who is out there trying to hurt people.

And there's like two profiles on Facebook that harass me all the time. There's 2. But I think they're both the same guy and they go around Facebook telling people that I make oil out of crap weed and it's killing people. Ask 'em to show you somebody who's died because of it, [chuckling] you know.

Ian: Yeah… yeah…

Ronnie: It's the front, the front line of the war.

Ian: Yeah.

Ronnie: You're right. Yeah, it is… it is. I am quite certain that they want me gone.

I mean, I was threatened with death, by the Deputy Sheriff who arrested me. He told me, he says, "Yeah we're going to put you in jail and you ain't coming back out!" That's what he said. [Chuckling] Was just a local county sheriff in the county where I was running for Sheriff, you know. A Deputy Sheriff where I'm running for Sheriff and I'm going to be his boss. Hey, they hated me. Pot leaves on billboards with a Sheriff's badge on it. [Chuckling] They hated me. There are only two cops came to me and shook my hand and said, "I hope you win."

Of course, then we gotta fix our election system. Because [chuckling] you know, I ran for Sheriff and it was definitely rigged. I've had over 500 people that came to me and say, "Hey, man, I voted for ya. I'm sorry you didn't win!" [Slaps hands together] I got 25 votes on the ballot. [Laughing]

Ian: Whoa.

Ronnie: You know, like if you voted for me, how come it didn't work? I mean, I know why. I know how they rigged it. They had the ballots all rigged. What a lot of people don't know, in the Bible, in Ezekiel, I don't know which chapter or verse. But in Ezekiel, it talks about the plant of renown, that the leaves of this plant are for the healing of the nations and the people who use the plant will no longer be called a heathen.

You think that when you go to some other country and you say, "Marijuana." They know exactly what you're talking about. Or even like Yugoslavia, you can tell 'em, "Do you know what cannabis is?" And they won't know what you're talking about, but if you say Marijuana, they'll just go, "Ahhhh, Marijuana! Yes, yes yes!"

But, that is the plant of renown in the Bible. I think it is… It's the key to everything.. the healing of the Nations. The leaves of that tree are for the healing of the Nations.
If it was me, and they were forcing my child to take chemo.

Ian: Yeah.

Ronnie: As soon as I had my hands on my child and I was in a car, we'd be gone. We'd be gone. And as soon as we were gone and somewhere safe and had my child on hemp oil. Then I would sue the bastards that stole him, that kidnapped him and tortured him and forced poison into his body. That's poison. Chemo is nothing but poison. Doctors take a freakin' Hippocratic Oath that says, "I shall not administer POISON." [Giggling]
And they're all doing it. [Hands spread wide] AND NONE OF THEM WILL DENY THAT IT'S POISON, right? They're fucking administering poison. Did they take the oath? Do the doctors still take the Hippocratic Oath? Kidnapping your own children, crazy isn't it?

Ian: Yeah.

Ronnie: Crazy. How do you stand up against a corrupt system like that? I wish the aliens would just come and change everything, you know. The galactic federation would come down and say, "Uh, we're taking this government out and we're going to put in these people until you guys can figure out who you want in their place," you know. That would be awesome.

Camera Man: I wish they'd freakin' hurry up.
Ronnie: Right.

[See Pic 11.3]

CHAPTER 12:

INTERVIEW WITH RICK SIMPSON

[See Pic 12.1]

Ian: Okay are we live? Are we live yet?

Frank: Yes.

Ian: That you Anthony?

Frank: Yes, Ian this is Frank from New York and you are live.

Ian: Hey Frankie.

Frank: It's all you man, it's all you. We're strapped and on behalf of the whole network, welcome and we can't wait to work on this show with you.

Ian: Right on. Well, it's my pleasure man. Thank you for the opportunity. This is a good venue, to actually get some truth out there because there's… well first of all everybody, this is Ian Jacklin. This show is going to be called I Cure Cancer for any of you who don't know I made a film called I Cure Cancer.com back in 2006 because about… I was just reminded that it was almost 19 years ago my girlfriend at the time, J. Cynthia Brooks had cured herself of terminal cervical cancer and we were doing a play together at the time and I basically overheard her tell her friends she cured herself of cancer. I just couldn't believe it. I've never heard of anybody curing themselves of cancer, so she explained it to me over many months and years, actually. So that put me on a path to make this film I Cure Cancer because you have to cure your own cancer you can't expect your doctor, so the "I" is not me it's you, you have to cure your cancer. So, you have to say "I" Cure Cancer, not your doctor, not your oncologist, probably not your oncologist.

So, basically, I set out to make a film to prove her wrong that she was just a fluke because we didn't want this kind of information screwing people up and from getting proper treatments. But as I found out it's true, alternative cancer healing is the only way to go. In general, for most tumor type cancers, chemo only has a three percent success rate. It's up to 40 percent with some of the blood cancers and testicular cancers, but you're still getting hit by 60 bullets out of a hundred and that's not good. Because what I did find out about holistic healing is it's more of a 75-85 percent success rate, especially if you haven't done any of the chemo or radiation or the surgeries.

I mean, there's, sometimes surgery is necessary if you're getting something cut off or whatever, one of your arteries is being pinched. But in general, holistic methods can reverse cancer and make it… die and it'll never come back. That's the difference between, you know, curing your cancer holistically other than with western medicine is that it doesn't come back, cause you fix the problem and that's what you have to do, you have to fix the cause.

So, I basically spent the last, man, I guess it's almost 17-18 years interviewing people that have cured themselves of cancer. Because I used to be a kickboxing champion and that's how I became champion, I studied the best. I studied all the best kickboxers, the best boxers. I got to box at the Lennox Lewis stable for a while in England when he first turned pro. So, I just did the same thing, I wanted to find the world champions in the cancer world and to me, that would be the ones that are basically cured now that weren't supposed to, they were given, you know, a year to live. Like Cynthia was given a year to live and she cured herself in 8 months.

So, I made the show… the film, and since then I've also been shooting part II. Because I found out after I made that film, that, okay, great I know how to cure cancer, so I'm set, I can help my family friends or whatever. But then I found out if I had a child that was not 18 yet, under 18, they're forced chemotherapy, surgery, and radiation. It's a standard of care is what it's called. If you do anything different, they arrest you and take your children and give them to child protective services which I just… is horrific, I mean, what are we… is this… are they Nazi's? Is that what… and as I found out, as I was making my film, the FDA and the AMA they are Nazi's. It's hysterical what's going on.

And that actually… boy, my eyes have been so opened-up as to what's really going on in the world, we ain't in Kansas anymore, Toto. Because unfortunately, our leaders are no longer, you know… we're not the United States of America, we're U.S., Inc. So, the corporations run everything.

So, we have to be, our own best advocates and be our own healers. So that's why I made the film to show you that basically cancer is curable my good friend Dr. Bernardo, may he rest in peace, starred in my film, he used to say, "You don't die of cancer, you die of acidosis!" Your PH level drops down to about 5 where you're too acidic and people that get their average, so you know it's 6.3 and if you get it up to 7, 7.2 cancer can't live. And most cancers are acidic, some of the blood cancers, I've learned from my good friend, Dr. Gonzales, who I should have on the show next week or the following. He explained to me, some of them, some of the cancers, the blood cancers can be because you're too alkaline.

So... and then PH isn't the end all be all, it's just a good... it's a good sort of once over, see where you're at. So, the average is 6.3... cancer is 5... you want 7.2 – 7.4 and cancer can't live. And that's... you can just google alkaline diet and figure that out. And then hopefully you learn a lot more from this show and many others what other things that you can do since you're just not going to get this information from your oncologist. They're taught one way.

Oh, and real quick, before we get to my guest, I just want to say just so you understand this, cause I had to figure it out myself, like how could our medical system be so screwed up? Well, Rockefeller who's, you know, one of the elite. Back in the early 1900s owned the pharmaceutical companies, him and Carnegie. And they realized if they could get control of the medical schools then they could, you know, basically, boost their pharmaceutical business and that's what they did.

So that's why we have a pharmaceutical-based run medical business today and that's what it is, unfortunately, it's a business. So, you have to be your own person and that's why I'm coming out to the people the best I can to try and explain to you, be your own doctor, be your own researcher. You can use them for their tests, I would definitely use them for the tests, but I wouldn't use their treatments. Because'... and what I found out recently... I mean I've been helping people cure themselves of cancer, geez, like Cynthia said, I think almost 19 years. And I didn't even know about cannabis hemp oil yet. [Chuckling] I mean you... it's... you can cure yourself of cancer if you get alkaline and you detox, and you boost up your immune system and use things like the Rife machine and there are many ways. But now, we've got the closest thing to a silver bullet we've ever had and that is in cannabis hemp oil.

And I am so honored tonight to have Rick Simpson on my show. He is the godfather of cannabis. I think it was Jack Herer that was the main cannabis guy back in the day, but since he is passed on, he sort of passed the torch over to Rick Simpson. Are you here with me tonight, Rick? Is Rick here?

Frank: Ian, I was actually just going to say, do you want to go on a quick one to two minutes break just so we can get Rick on the phone for you?

Ian: Oh yeah… sorry… start first…

Frank: Cause' I didn't know if you wanted to… if he was going to call us or we're going to call him. But…

Ian: Yeah… yeah… give him a call for me, would ya? And…

Frank: Alright.

Ian: And we don't need a break or anything, just go ahead, I'll keep talking I got plenty to say [chuckling].

Frank: Alright, cool, so Anthony why don't… you'll switch between some… okay… cool… do your thing.

Ian: Okay. Cool. Yeah and this is our first show folks, so we're kind of figuring it out as we go. But this is really cool; because Anthony and Frank they're back at… in New York City at the studio and they're actually able to handle all of this for me. So, unlike any of you that may have heard my last radio show on Saturday, if anything goes wrong they can fix it, which is nice cause I don't know all that technical stuff. But yeah, Rick Simpson is going to be on in a minute and he brought cannabis hemp oil or simply Rick Simpson Oil aka RSO to the world.

Basically, if you take a pound of marijuana, mix it with high grade, 195 proof vodka, alcohol, boil it down, distill it basically and get it down to two ounces of the oil, it cures cancer. Not only cancer but like almost everything. People… people have a bad back and they get rid of their cancer using the hemp oil and they realize they don't have a bad back anymore.

Crohn's disease is helped with it. Diabetes... you can take a maintenance of the hemp oil and it erases diabetes. I mean, just get on YouTube. Get on YouTube and google cannabis hemp oil cures, hemp oil cures, marijuana cures and you'll see. The proof is in the pudding folks. That's... that's what sold me on it. I'd heard about the cannabis hemp oil, I watched Rick Simpson's movie Run from the Cure and I just had to... I had to have more proof, cause it just sounded too easy. Like God gave us the plant that cures cancer? What?

After all these years of research and they ... humans couldn't get it right. And, sure enough, I... YouTube video, after YouTube video and then I started calling the people and I hung out with some people that make it and I got... I just... the proof is there, man. So, this is... I would say... but do not just do the cannabis hemp oil. That... you should get on an alkaline diet. You gotta boost your... do everything, I mean, you're fighting cancer. You're going to... if you lose you die. It's not a Jenny Craig diet; where you're just going to stay fat. No, you're going to die. So, you have-to-do everything, alkaline diet, essential fatty acids are very important. EFAs, get your oxygen to your blood. Again, cause it's that whole alkaline thing. Otto Warburg figured that out, you know, in the early 20s. I think I got Rick coming in right now.

Rick: Oh.

Ian: Rick, are you there?

Rick: Yes. [Laughing]

Ian: Hey, we did it. Right on, man.

Rick: Okay.

Ian: How are you? Can you turn on your camera?

Rick: Oh, I'm sorry. Just one second. The camera is on, okay, can you see me alright?

Ian: Yeah.

Frank: Yes, and gentlemen, we're screen capturing your feeds right now, just keep talking, everybody hears you, but we're getting your video set up right now.

Ian: Okay so...

Rick: Good.

Ian: Yeah, they're handling it man, we don't have to worry about that stuff this time.

Rick: [Laughing] Had me wondering there a little bit brother. I was waiting and waiting [laughing]

Ian: Oh I know, I know and then when you have that extra hour. I thought you were like New York time but you're even further than that.

Rick: Yeah, we're way out in the Atlantic here I guess. [Laughing] Four… four hours difference between here and California.

Ian: Well, I'm glad you hung in there, man, I hope you're not too tired. So, I was basically explaining to everybody, you're the guy. I mean, you're the Godfather. You brought cannabis oil to the world. If it wasn't for you… cause' this is what kills me, and we'll get into this in a little bit, but sometimes… I belong to a lot of cannabis groups; you know, online to learn when I started researching this. And a lot of people will start yapping about, "Ah, well he uses naphtha and that…" and I'm like, "Excuse me, do you know how many people got cured by that Naphtha?"
Okay. I mean, sure now we can talk about it in a bit but there's. There's better… there are new ways of doing it, but back then that's what he had, that's what he used and who knows how many thousands of people have been cured. And now the word has spread, has evolved. It's on the internet everywhere, people know about hemp oil thanks to this man.
So, it's an honor, man, thanks for… thanks for being here.

Rick: I'm happy to be with you, Ian. But, actually, you know, the Naphtha, I know it's a real problem in the U.S. because they add… they put a lot of additives and things like that to different solvents down there. But you know, here in Canada you can buy 45-gallon drums of pure Naphtha right from the fuel suppliers and they get it from the refinery. But, actually; the oils that we produced using Naphtha, you know, we've had them tested and as far as I know, nobody has ever produced oils that tested that high in cannabinoid content. You know, very often we're getting up around 99 percent pure cannabinoids, and that's pretty hard to beat.

Ian: Yeah, that is. And… and my friend, Ronnie Smith, who I think you crossed paths with before. He was teaching me… or showing me how he makes his oil and stuff. And he explained to me Naphtha's different in Canada. In Canada it's pure, it's clean. In America, you can't use the Naphtha down here. But I mean…
Rick: Yes.

Ian: all that aside, cause really, I hear… Everclear is good. Basically, a good potent, a pure alcohol 190 proof vodka will work, you know. But the point is, we have it. We now have this… some… the closest thing to a silver bullet we're ever going to get. Can you tell my listeners, who are new to hearing about you a little bit about your situation, how you got cancer and figured out the hemp oil thing? And then we'll go from there.

Rick: Well about 16 years ago I suffered a severe head injury and that left me with a condition called post-concussion syndrome. And I went through the medical system and of course, they never did anything for me. Just everything… every pill they gave me just made me worse and worse. And then about a year after I was injured I watched an episode of The Nature of Things with Dr. David Suzuki and the episode was called Reefer Madness II and it showed all these different people, you know, on this show smoking cannabis and it was helping with their medical problems.
So, I went out and I got some cannabis and I had smoked cannabis in the past, but I didn't look at it as medicine, you know. So, I went out and I bought some and smoked it and sure enough, it worked better than anything the medical system had given me. But the problem was they wouldn't give me, you know, a prescription so I could use this substance legally.

And then in 2001 the medical system finally cut me loose, they said that they had tried everything they knew, and nothing was helping me, so I was on my own [chuckling]. And again, I asked for another prescription for cannabis, but no way, they wouldn't allow it. So, I mean I was left to my own devices. So, I actually… I turned to the oil. You know the smoking aspect of hemp did help me some, but it didn't… still didn't have the knockdown power that I needed. Because… see my head rings 24 hours a day from the injury. And if I don't have… like something that's very sedative to knock me out then, you know, then I just don't get any sleep.

But man, when I started producing this oil [chuckling] talk about knocking you out [chuckling]. You know, 8, ten, twelve hours of sleep at a time and it made a dramatic difference in my health. But then in late 2002, I went in to see my doctor about three areas, you know, that I had that concerned me. There was one close to my right eye and one on my left cheek and one on my chest.

And I'd had these lesions for quite a few years and I strongly suspected they were skin cancer. But you know I don't think I really wanted to admit it to myself. But, anyway, when the doctor saw them, they sent them in to have the one next to my eye removed because it was so close to the eye. And then they said, they'd take care of the other two; at a later date.

So, I went in and had the operation. But about a week after the operation a report I'd heard back in the 1970s, it was from the Medical School of Virginia Study. And I'd heard this announcement back in around '74 or '75 on the radio. And it just popped back into my mind, you know, THC, the active ingredient in cannabis has been found to kill cancer cells.

So, I knew the oil I was producing was full, you know, of THC, it had to be. So, I'm ashamed to say it, but I almost didn't try to, because where I was ingesting the oil at the time, I really thought, that, you know, well, if this actually worked, then my cancer should be gone. But you know like the skin of our body is… it's the largest organ on our body and you know, it takes a lot of oil to reach out to the surface of the skin. But just for the hell of it, I went into the bathroom and I took a little bit of oil and I put it on the other two areas on my chest and on my cheek and put a bandage on them. And, I have to admit I didn't feel a thing, you know.

So, I left the bandages in place for about four days and then when I went down to the bathroom I removed them, and I was just shocked. They were all healed up. There was nothing but pink skin. But when I started telling my friends about what I had done, they all just laughed at me, you know, "Yeah, sure Rick, marijuana cures cancer!" Well, guess what, it does! [Laughing]

Ian: [Laugh]

Rick: And then about seven, about 7 weeks later, the one they had surgically removed by my eye, it came roaring right back, you know, the same splinters in the face feeling. You know, it puffed up and it was bleeding. So, I watched it develop for about four or five days and then I just went in and I put the oil, a little bit of oil on that, put a bandage on and that's been well over ten years ago. And it's never returned.

Ian: That's amazing. And I'm so glad you brought that up. Ladies and gentlemen, I hope you heard that. Skin cancer – okay – and I can say this as a filmmaker, 100 percent curable. And there's a couple of ways… there are a few ways using holistic and thank God for cannabis oil coming along, cause the other way wasn't pretty. It was called bloodroot. The American Indians used to use it back in the day. And it's… you can still use it.

If for some reason you can't get cannabis oil, you can get bloodroot, but it HURTS… I mean it hurts like childbirth, from what I hear. You put it on… if you have… wherever you have it. It is unbelievably painful. And you'll know it's cancer right away. If you put it on there, you will feel the pain. One lady, she told me, she had it here and it gets… the reason why blood root works is, cause it gets the roots, cause she could feel the roots all the way to the back of her head. And it was just agonizing pain for weeks. So, I mean, it's better than nothing. But since cannabis oil doesn't hurt. Pffffffttt I'd wait till I found some.

Rick: [Laughing]

Ian: You know.

Rick: And it works on all types of cancers, let alone skin cancers.

Ian: Yeah, let's get into that. Cause I got a friend right now that… oh, my God. This is Rick, I told you when we were on the radio last week, whenever that was, about my friend, Eric, who, actually got child services to side with him and let him, you know, get off the chemo and try all the natural stuff. And this guy is a smart man, he had her… his daughter for leukemia, on everything you could think of, did everything perfectly. And I told you, you know, it was a victory, cause' we beat it. Well, unfortunately, we just found out like last night I think it was, I found out that it's back. So, she's going to… she's forced the chemo now. Unfortunately…

Rick: Wow.

Ian: Ya but it is leukemia… it is leukemia, right. Now, and I've found two or three parents right now doing this because… if you have a child… as I explained earlier, that's not 18, you have to do chemo, radiation, surgery. That's just the law or you go to jail. Well… so, they're doing the chemo and the radiation, whatever they gotta do, but they're also sneaking in the cannabis oil in the feeding tubes. And apparently, it's working. Did it not cure that one that you know of, so far?

Rick: Oh yes. I mean, the oil definitely works, but it should be the first line of defense, you know, against cancer, not the last. And… I mean, I think, you know, giving any child or giving anybody chemo or radiation, I think that's just absurd. Because these are cancer-causing treatments for God's sakes. You know, to me, it's just insanity what the medical system is doing to us, Ian. And I just can't believe that it's, you know, that it's going on like this, because, you know, all of the experts, are all agreeing, to you know, now about what cannabis can do. Harvard University agreed back in 2007, even the American Cancer Institute, is singing a different song about cannabis these days.

But still it's not out there for people, you know. And people are dying left and right. And there's no damn reason for it. It's just all this corruption over a God-given plant that never harmed anyone.

Ian: Oh I know… I know… it was Michaela… Baby Michaela that you…

Rick: Yeah, Michaela, yeah, she's doing well.

Ian: Yeah. Here ya go folks. Okay. Doing the chemo wasn't doing anything. They started giving her cannabis oil. All-of-a-sudden, no cancer. What are they doing? They're making her go two full more years of chemo anyway. Cause they think that's what's doing it. Ridiculous. The… oh, my God… and now, unfortunately, my friend Eric, is going to have to go through the same thing. Thank God, at least he's got the cannabis oil to treat her as well. But, I mean, cause if he didn't, it's death. Cause, it's leukemia, basically, they've got a month to bring her numbers down and if they don't come down, it's bone marrow transplant time. And I just learned, from again, my friend, Dr. Gonzales, in New York City who was being trained to do this and he quit because of it. He said, 30 percent of the people die immediately and the rest usually die fairly soon after.

Because what bone marrow transplant is… is basically they just blast you with the regular amount of chemo until you're almost dead. Then they keep you alive, they give you that bone marrow and they can give you more chemo and radiation. So, she's not going to be able to have children now if she does all that. So, we're just hoping and praying and everybody out there that believes in the power of prayer, pray for… pray for my friend, Eric's daughter. Sorry her name escapes me right now, but pray for her because we need her… we need this oil to work in the next 30 days, or it's going to be really bad.

Rick: Well brother, I mean, [chucking] if you've got good oil there… I mean, I hate to see anyone taking chemo because, you know, if you're taking chemo you do have a better chance of surviving if you're on the oil, there's no question. But you still have… you still run a great risk of dying. Because I mean they're literally poisoning… you know, poisoning you. And this case with Michaela in the United States, I mean, this young 7-year-old. I mean, she is cancer-free today. But there's the madness of our system. You know, they're going to continue to give that child chemotherapy for the next two years. In other words, they're going to kill the child.

Ian: I know. And while I'm going to have it all on tape, so what… you know, we're… that's the only thing I've learned that I can do, cause, I can't pick up a gun and go shoot oncologists. I mean, I could, but then I'm done. I'm not going to do any more good for the world. So, all I can do is shoot my camera and I want the pictures and the faces and the names of these people because I think… you know, it's just… it's a travesty what's going on. And hopefully, my… but for you, that know me or if you're just joining, I'm making a film called I Cure Cancer Part II and it's going to address this main issue. It's going to show you that cancer is curable and it's going to say, "By the way, you can't use it on your children."

And I am a starving artist, so if anybody wants to go to ICureCancer.com, we do have a donate button there. I'm just doing it on blood, sweat, and tears. I'm not getting any Hollywood money for this, cause, they don't support anything that doesn't support big pharma. So, it's just We the People doing this one. So, real quick, Rick, just… I want to clear this one up so I can explain to people in all these chat rooms I go to about what… how would you make oil today? What kind of solvent would you use? Cause I know when… when you brought out your movie, your Run from the Cure which everybody should watch, by the way, it's free on the internet, Run from the Cure. He showed everybody how to do it with a rice cooker, just in case that's all you can get. But there's newer and better ways, cause, that was what, eight years ago, 7, 10 years ago?

Rick: Well actually, I showed people that method out of desperation. You know, years ago, I used to have a five-gallon stainless steel still that was properly designed to boil off solvents. And I used that for the first four…four years or so, but then the police took that.

And so, I was in a real panic then because I had all these people coming to me and all looking for medicine. So, one day I was in the local Canadian tire store in Amherst and I got looking at the rice cookers. So, you know, the rice cookers had two heat settings on them, high and low. So, when the temperature in the rice cooker gets up the cooker will automatically kick itself onto low heat.

So, I thought that you know, that might work. But so that's the… you know, I took, I went and bought one and I brought it home and sure enough, it worked like a charm. And that's the method I showed people how to use because a lot of people already have a rice cooker. It's very simple. If you follow the safety instructions, like… you know, that we put up on the site and in the movie, I don't think anybody will have any problems because I've done it that way thousands of times and never a problem.

But to this day, I would still prefer to use, oh, either Naphtha or Ether. I've used Ether too. And Ether is a wonderful solvent. Very volatile. But it does… it makes a wonderful oil. And, so does the Naphtha. I mean, I don't really have anything against alcohol, but the only problem I find with alcohol is that it dissolves more of the chlorophyll from the plant material.

So normally an oil that's produced with alcohol is generally darker. But some strains will just produce the dark oil anyway. But I mean, the main thing is, as long as the cannabinoids are in there because I used alcohol too and I cured a lot of people, you know, that had cancer using that method. So, it's definitely viable, but just as you say there are so many new methods now coming out. You know, I'm in favor of anything new and safer. But as far as I know to this time, our methods have proved… produced the most medicinal oils.

Ian: Yeah… you know what, darn you, Rick, you've made a couple of confusing things [chuckle] because you made this famous. [Chuckling].

Rick: [Laughing]

Ian: Cause down here in the states, they… we don't have the good Naphtha. So that's what the talk is always in the chat rooms, "Oh, you can't use Naphtha, that's horrible!" I'm like, "It's not the same as Canada. No, don't use Naphtha down here, get Ever-clear, or something better," you know.

And the other thing [chuckles], everybody… I've had people come up to me with a bottle of salad dressing, hemp oil and say, "Is this the hemp oil." [Chuckles]

Rick: [Laughing]

Ian: I'm like, "No… no, no, no!" [Laughing]

Rick: [Chuckling] Well and something I would strongly recommend, Ian, to anyone, you know. I mean, the Naphtha I was using here in Canada is called Lite Naphtha and it's boiling vigorously at about 150 degrees Fahrenheit. But if you're going into any store to get a solvent, the best bet is to simply take the lid off, stick your finger in it, and you know, and just watch your finger. And if it's a good solvent, it should evaporate off your finger within 30 to 40 seconds and leaving no residue. But if there's an oily residue or anything left behind or if it takes two minutes to evaporate away, that's a solvent that I wouldn't use.

Ian: Oh, okay. And then just to clarify that thing about the hemp oil. Rick just called it hemp oil when he first started it because it became famous at that point, that's what we all call it, hemp oil, at least the ones that have done the research. But there are so many people out there that think it's hemp seed oil that you put on your salads and it's not. That is good for you too, very, you should be eating that anyway. But it's different.

Rick: Oh, yes. [Laughing]

Ian: Yeah, it's very… marijuana is what makes the oil for them… cause' it's got the THC and the Cannabinoids, that's… so it's gotta be a dark black thick oil and it tastes like marijuana, basically. So just so everybody knows, but [chuckles] those are the two things that I'm always getting, "What about the Naphtha?" Oh, and what about, "Is it hemp seed oil or hemp?" But, anyway… the point is the proper name is Cannabis oil.

Rick: There's been… there's been a real foul-up over that over the last few years. But, you know, I mean, you know, farmers everywhere that grew this plant for thousands of years, they always called it hemp. So that when I produced the essential oil from that plant, I called it hemp oil.

Ian: Yeah.

Rick: And then the… the hemp seed oil companies, they got… they got mad at me, you know, there was no reason to get mad at me. It was simply… the problem is… is that they're mislabeling their product.

Ian: Right.

Rick: If they would, you know because on the back of the label it says cold pressed hemp seed oil.

Ian: Right.

Rick: Well why doesn't it say that on the front? You know,[Chuckling] So this is the kind of thing you run into. But I know it has caused a lot of confusion and I do apologize for that. But this is… you know, the essential oil, off of this plant, is truly the most medicinal substance on earth and I really don't know of any medical situation where it can't be used. As a matter of fact, I don't know of any pharmaceutical that's nearly as effective for any condition.

If you have properly made oil; it's the best you can get!

Ian: Yeah, I was telling everybody at the beginning there about them… it's good for diabetes, it's good Crohn's… really good for brain injuries! I mean, I was a kickboxer…

Rick: Oh, yeah.

Ian: I was a kickboxing champion. And even though I won most of my fights I took a few shots. So… I… and I… you know, I've tested this. I don't want to just talk about things that I don't know about. And I swear, when I was on it, I almost felt the re-circuiting going on up there, could be psychological. But… so, anybody, that has kind of… you know, what I was wondering, what about schizophrenia. I heard… is that possible?

Rick: Yes, that's another disease that it works very well on. You see when you take the oil, what happens is… you know, when it enters your endocannabinoid system it gets up into your pineal gland and it decalcifies your pineal gland. And your pineal gland basically controls your perception of reality. So, you know, and like I said your melatonin levels, actually also go out there. The pineal gland also produces the melatonin; the greatest antioxidant on earth and it travels to every cell in your body. And your melatonin levels go up thousands and thousands of times once you get on this oil. But I literally, I've seen schizophrenics get on this oil; get off their medications in no time they're back to work and they're back to normal.

Ian: Wow, that's good for me to know. Because one of my best friends EVER, you know, disappeared basically about 10 years ago because of that. So; I'm going to look into that one. And how about leukemia? You heard a lot… much about that?

Rick: Oh, yes, very positive. Leukemia, actually… leukemia and lung cancers are two of my favorites to treat, because of you… you know, generally, you see results very quickly with this medicine. You know, with lung cancers, they're walking further every day, they're breathing easier. And with leukemia, well a lot of leukemia patients, their white blood cell count is right through the roof.

Ian: Yeah.

Rick: Now I've seen people that were dying, or they are on their death beds with leukemia and in two days their white blood cell count comes down by half, as soon as they get on the oil.

Ian: Yes, you hear that Eric? Right on! This is what I needed to hear. Good. Good, good, good. Yeah [chuckling]. I got… I got a really interesting story, you're going to have to wait for the movie on that one, to hear this good one…but [chuckling] Okay, let's see… What else should we hit? What else for the oil, would you say? I know diabetes, it kicks that pretty good.

Rick: Well there's just no, it's like I said, there's no disease that I know of that you can't use this for. You know, and I don't call it a cure-all for no good reason, because it literally is, one medicine, that you can use in any situation. You know, I mean, you can take it in suppository form. You can take it orally. You can use it topically or you can vaporize it. You know, mix it with skin creams. Whatever you wanna do. And you know, the results are just phenomenal.

Ian: Yeah… yeah, you're looking a little young there, have you been putting a little on your…

Rick: [Laughing]

Ian: [Chuckling]

Rick: [Chuckling] No, it's… it's also anti-aging, there's no question about that. I mean I've seen animals… like we had a dog that was about 18 or 19 years old and she was really slowing down. You know, animals have this same endocannabinoid system we have. So, one day, my son mentioned it to me. So, I started giving the dog, like two doses of oil a day, one in the morning and one in the evening. And I was giving her… you know, she was a big dog, (about 130 pounds). So, I was giving her about a ¼ of a gram each dose and it was just knocking her to down. You know, it was funny watching her because she'd be laying there panting, you know, on her side.

Ian: [Chuckling]

Rick: And I thought the first dose, I thought it might scare her. But as soon as she got back up that evening when I put another dose on my finger she came right over and licked it off. Because in reality… here's… you know, like… dogs have… they're more sensitive, much more sensitive than humans, you know. [Chuckling]

You know, I wish… I wish humans would behave like dogs and then there'd be so little trouble taking this medicine. But you know, within five days, that dog was running back and forth to the road. And, it's over 100 yards from my house out to the street. That dog was running back and forth like it was a two-year-old. And I firmly believe that even animals, like, you know, an old dog would be 20 years old, but if you started giving an animal small doses of this oil on a regular basis I honestly think you might even see their life expectancy double. And that goes for humans too!

Ian: Right. Well, this is… this is good news, because another one of my Facebook friends, Jore, I think his name is, his dog has a lump on his leg and I told him, you know if you can't afford… cause cannabis oil is expensive, folks. I mean, you're looking… if you're lucky you can get it for two grand, like three months' worth of oil. Down here in the states because it's legal in a lot of… like California is. I mean, for me to get a pound of weed from the dispensary it's $3,550. So, nobody is going to make the oil for cheaper than that. Although I have found a couple of places and I know guys on the street and stuff. So… but, yeah, it's expensive. So, I told him about the bloodroot. But that's good to know for… he's got like a lump… in his… insides… you would recommend probably orally and maybe topically?

Rick: Yes. And I often treat like… if you have a big tumor that's sticking right out, you can treat it both ways. But… I mean, ingesting the oil is by far the most important. But I've had wonderful results topically too. But, you know, what's going on in the U.S. with the prices and everything, this is all caused by your corrupted government, same thing here in Canada. I mean… if this… if this plant was grown properly, the same as we grow any other farm crop, I mean, what's a pound of corn worth? Well, a pound of hemp wouldn't be worth any more than a pound of corn.

So, in reality; if it wasn't for all these… all this corruption… and all these idiotic laws which, in truth, are not even real. If these weren't in place, you'd be able to buy a pound of good hemp bud for five bucks.

Ian: Right. You know, it's hysterical. I just thought of that the other day, cause street value, we were always paying sixty bucks an eighth, down here, for the chronic, for the kind buds. Okay.

Rick: Right.

Ian: So… it now becomes legal, right. So, we're thinking, "Great, price control, it's going to come down." It's not, it's the same. It's the same price today, as it was when it was illegal. So, who's making the money now? You know.

Rick: Well this is what scares me too Ian, I mean, you know, people are out there running around and most of… you know, most of the dealers and growers, they won't take a pound of good cannabis bud and melt it down, you know, cause, they can make more money selling it the other way. And that's… that's the horror story because they're so many people running around trying to make it out of clippings and leaves and you just don't get the same quality.

You know, I've had people send me test results that showed like 30 percent THC. Well to me, I mean, I might use that on a skin condition, but I certainly would not even consider giving it to someone with, you know, with a serious internal medical condition like terminal cancer. You know, only the best will do for those people.

Ian: Well… is it about… what do you want? Obviously, you want the most powerful, like 95 percent would be best. Which, you know, if you make it from a good kind Indica strain you can get that. But some people, you know, like Ronnie, for instance, told me one day, he goes, "You know, when I used to live in New Mexico, or whatever, somebody would bring me a pound of Mexican brick weed and it would… that's all we could get… so we had to use it… and it worked."
So, do you what the… is it 40, 50, 60… how high do we want it in THC to know it's good?

Rick: Well I always went for the highest THC levels possible. Because I mean, when I started producing this oil I didn't have any test facilities here in [chuckles] Nova Scotia.
So, I mean, I just note and look for the strongest most sedative cannabis I could find. You know, I would just sit there and smoke a half a joint, if it made me want to go lay down on the Chesterfield, well, then, that's what I made the medicine from.

Ian: Right.

Rick: But today, I mean, people are screaming so loudly about, you know, CBDs and all these other cannabinoids and you know, I think all cannabinoids, actually play a role. But right now, they are putting so much emphasis on CBDs; but in reality, I think the THC content is the most important.

Ian: Yeah… yeah… you wouldn't want to lose that, cause' it makes the cancer cells eat themselves from what I understand, there's a lot more science behind it… but, yeah, you definitely want to get that kind. And some… you know, here's a little warning for somebody out there [chuckling] cause this happened to my friend. He smokes pot so he's a little cocky, and he took the first rice grain size, you know, that's all you need is a little pea size.

Rick: [Laughing] Yeah, even less.

Ian: Yeah, and he's like, "Ah, that's nothing." So, he upped it a little bit, he ended up in the ER having panic attacks. [Laughing]

Rick: [Laughing]

Ian: And let me… let me tell ya folks, nobody has ever died from an overdose. As a matter… again, my buddy, Ronnie, I keep bringing up, he was… he used to have to fly to… cause his mom died of chemo. So, he's been on a mission for this, you know. And he flew to Jamaica, cause you can get the weed cheap and he'd swallow a couple of balloons and come back and make it, you know, here. Or sell it here…. or give it… he gives it away a lot of the time. Anyway… they burst in his stomach, so he had three full grams of cannabis oil burst in his stomach and he's on a plane from Jamaica. [Laughing] And nothing happened to him. I mean, he slept for about three days… but, you know.

Rick: [Laughing]

Ian: And if…

Rick: Well that happens quite often. I mean, I've had… oh, three or four people over the years, that actually took too much. I mean, you gotta have a lot of respect for this stuff. As you said, it won't kill you or harm you. But if you… you know, if you start with a… like I had one woman… and, actually, she took… the first dose, she took one gram of high-grade oil. One Gram.

Ian: Ohhh.

Rick: It knocked her… it knocked her down for three days.

Ian: [Laughing]

Rick: And then she calls me on the phone screaming at me. And I mean, I told her… I had talked to her son and I had told him, you know, how to make the oil and I told him how to give her the dosages. But, you know, when she called, she… I asked what happened and she said, you know, "I took a dose of that three days ago and I'm just coming down now!" And I said, "Well how much did you take?" And when she told me the amount, I said, "Why would you take so much?"

So, like… it was about… I told her, you know, the proper way to ingest it. And about six weeks later she called me back on the phone and she told me, she said, "I've increased my dosage, you know, just like you said." And she said, "You know what Mr. Simpson, I enjoy taking this stuff!" [Chuckling]

Ian: [Chuckling] Oh, I know… I know. That's what I tell… like some of the people are kind of square, you know, straight-laced and they're like… I'm like, "Don't worry about it, okay."

Cause I've had to talk… I… you know, I messed around with everything when I was a kid. I was in Hollywood in my twenties, you know, and I know how to talk people down. That's all you gotta remind yourself is, you're on a drug, okay, and thank God, it's not LSD, you're just on weed and you're not going to freak out. You don't need to go to the hospital. Just get a hold of your breath, relax, calm yourself down and know it will pass, that's all you gotta do.

Rick: Well I like the definition, you know, years ago, Nixon had, he had formed The Safer Commission to study this… this plant. And, The Safer Commission come right back and told him, "Legalize it." And they also stated that they did not feel that this plant was a narcotic. They felt that the cannabis plant should be put in a category by itself because it wasn't harmful like all the rest of the narcotics or anything like that. So, they felt it should be in its own category.

But unfortunately, instead of Mr. Nixon legalizing it as he should, he started the War on Drugs. Good for you tricky Dicky, look how many people you killed.

Ian: [Laughing] Oh, I know.

Rick: There's a name that'll live down in history now isn't it.

Ian: Yeah, yeah. It's… it's just horrendous what's going on. And I was listening to that show that I called… remember when you were on the radio and I called in, I'm like, "Hey Rick how's it going!" They played that today earlier, so I was listening to it and you brought up some interesting points, you and I are on the same page exactly and I want to bring it up tonight on my show because most of my friends will probably agree. What is wrong with… why is it, the way it is, it's because we're not run by the good people anymore, we're run by the evil elite. The Rockefeller's, the Rothschild's, whoever… the Illuminati, the one percent, whatever words you want to use, you explained it quite well too. Don't you agree, that's why our country is going to hell?

Rick: Oh, God yes. That's… that's the entire reason, you know, the rich elite are really running the planet. I mean, they own the oil companies, the pharmaceutical companies or they own the major stock, you know, so they control things. And this is going on all over the damn world. So, what, you know all the governments… they've got all the governments corrupted everywhere it seems. And then, in turn, the governments control the legal system and the medical system in each different country, and they've got that all corrupted. And this is what we're fighting against.

I mean the corruption is on such an enormous level. I don't know why people put up with it, I honestly don't, you know. We should… today, I mean, you know, with the internet and the world is becoming enlightened. You know, I think it's just about the time we know the truth, you know.
But for these people to run around and hide everything and give us all these lies and propaganda, so they can fulfill their own agendas. I mean that's truly what's been going on. And; I mean, I have to admit completely, I cannot name a politician that I trust. Not one.

Ian: Yeah, yeah… we need a whole new system. It kills me when people start to talk politics about the left and the right and the democrats, republicans… whatever. I mean, I'm like; they're two heads of the same snake.

You know that right! But half the people out there don't even know 911 was an inside job. They think I'm a nut case, cause I say, "Well the Building 7 didn't get hit by a plane and it fell. Did you not notice that? Did you not notice there's not one suitcase, not one body part, not one seat of a plane or engine in the two other crash locations?" I mean hello people. You know, I understand people don't wanna know, they're busy enough with their own lives. And that's… the elite knows that. They know that they are keeping 'em busy with Dancing with the Stars and the football and their hockey. And that's all people… we just need to wake people up, man. Because one percent and then there's this, there's the 95… all we gotta do is like… we just gotta blow on 'em.

And we don't even have to… and I like what you were saying too, you were saying, "We don't have to kill 'em, we don't have to take their money, their riches. Let's just make it so they don't tell us what to do anymore."

Rick: Well I'm in favor of that. But, in reality, Ian, I'm in favor of taking their riches.
Ian: [Chuckling]

Rick: Cause' I mean, what these people have been doing. I mean, all they talk about now is, you know, let's legalize cannabis and let's tax it. So, they want the cannabis plant to pay for it all.
You know, but I mean, the simple truth is, the rich elite, you know, all of these… of the resources and the money that these people have, they're the proceeds of crimes. Crimes they committed against us.

Ian: Yeah.
Rick: Now if you or I committed a crime, they take the proceeds away, don't they? And I think that's exactly what should be done. I think you should take the rich into a common law court, make them admit their guilt, take their resources away, leave them enough. I'm not saying to lock them up.
Ian: Right.

Rick: Just, you know, leave them enough so they can live out their lives, but take the money and power away from them. Because of they… you know, these people are destroyed. And they've done so much harm to our earth already the only way to put a stop to it is to take the power away from them.

Ian: Absolutely, absolutely. And that's probably better… yeah, we definitely need to take everything back that they took. I mean, look at the Fed, the Fed's not even legal [chuckling].

Rick: Ahh' yeah, I mean, the banking system, that's so ridiculous, you know, paying all of this interest. And… I mean, it just seems that no matter where you turn these days somebody's reaching into your pocket. And it's usually something to do with the government.

Ian: Yeah, yeah. That's the truth. Well again, that's why I'm not afraid to speak the way I speak because… I already know if they want… for example, Jason Vale, a good friend of mine, he's in my film. He was selling apricot seeds, to help cure cancer.

Rick: Oh, yeah.
Ian: Cause' they do.
Rick: Laetrile. [Chuckling]
Ian: Laetrile.
Rick: B17. Yes.
Ian: Exactly.
Rick: [Laughing]
Ian: And he… they went after him and put him in prison for five years and he had to do every day, nothing off for good behavior or nothing. But… cause' they say you can… you can talk about a cancer healing modalities, but you can't sell anything on the same site. He didn't even do that. He did everything legally to the T. It turns out the Judge… he told me himself, the Judge lied on the stand about what had happened. So, what I'm learning is it doesn't matter when they want you, they get you, you know. Whether… whether it be to put you in the jail or they off you, you know.
And so that's why I personally don't care about any… what I say and getting in trouble. Because, first of all, I'm a filmmaker and I'm just saying, this is what I've seen. This is what, so and so did to cure their cancer. But I mean, if they want me gone. I'm gone. What are you going to do? You know. So, I'm… there are no rules. So that's why I'm not afraid to bring this to the public.
Rick: Well actually I'm surprised they didn't put a bullet in me a long time ago because if they had a done it back in 2004, 2005 that would have been it! Nobody would have paid any attention.

Ian: Yeah.

Rick: But I think they honestly, Ian, I don't think they took me seriously. You know, I figured, they just figured, "Well we'll put him in court and we'll make sure he is found guilty." And, they actually tampered with the jury to do that. And I guess they thought that I would just go away but I didn't go away, I just kept going with this. And I have no regrets… and you know, about it in any way because… you know, I was left back in 2003, when I realized what this substance could do. To me it was just a simple matter of right and wrong, you know. And I contacted the government and I thought within six months or a year that the medicine would be available to the people.

Ian: Yeah.

Rick: And that's when I started finding out just how corrupted these governments are, and I also found out that… you know, cancer societies, United Nations, none of them… none of them, want a cure.

Ian: [Chuckles]

Rick: You know, it's just a sad joke on the public. So, I think what happened… what has to happen, is we all have to get together and we have to stand up and take our freedoms and our rights back.

You know, especially our natural rights, you know, the right to grow this plant and use it as a medicine. I mean, that's a God-given right. And they had no… well, they had… they never had any reason, other than greed, to put these laws in place in the first place.

So… I… you know, I'm hoping to see this happen, in the near future. And I would love to see America become the country it used to be. You know, when I was a child America was the greatest country in the world and today, it's a fascist state.

Ian: Yeah.

Rick: There's no other word for it. And it's the same thing here in Canada. It's all fascism.

Ian: Yeah. Iceland is the new heavyweight champion, by the way, folks. Iceland. If we did what they did… they didn't kick the homeowners out onto the street, they… they… not only…

Rick: Kicked the bankers out [chuckles]. [Laughing]

Ian: Yeah, they kicked the bankers out. They kicked the politicians out and arrested some of them. Go Iceland!

Rick: Right.

Ian: See that's the new America, is Iceland. And we need to get that back, but we just gotta get the word out on the street for this, cause' Americans wouldn't put up with it, the Canadians wouldn't put up with it. But they just don't know yet.

Rick: Yeah, well it just seems that they're all living in fear of something, Ian. Because, I mean, around here, practically everybody knows. But nobody is doing anything about it. You know. So many of them, they get cancer, they're still running… taking the chemo and of course, the doctors are still passing it out like popcorn. You know… and… I… although there is, all kinds of evidence, you know, about… millions worldwide now have used this medication and they know what it can do. So, there's no stopping it now. And then when we put all the information right up on the website how anybody can produce their own because there is nothing to it.

I mean, just… if you have a bit of a green thumb, grow your own plants, produce your own medicine. There's nothing to it. It's no harder than making a cup of coffee.

Ian: Yeah… and word on the street is everybody should be taking it as a maintenance dose. Take two or three little… like one at a time, little rice size.

Rick: Yep.

Ian: couple times a week at night before you go to bed or… you know what, if you don't wanna drink and get drunk, take a nice little size… it'll make you feel good like you had a couple of glasses of wine and that kicks in your cannabinoid system. So, you don't have to just take it when you're sick, you get those cannabinoids kicking; running the way they're supposed to, you don't ever get sick. So that's… that's another thing.

I mean, and you're right about… I… my own dispensary here… I'm like, "Why don't you guys got hemp oil here?" "Ahh, cause' we make too much money selling it for people who smoke!" I'm like, "Well, you know, have a heart!" Have a little side … for… you know, for people that need it, you know. Cause… and that really had shot the prices up. Cause people wanna get the oil, but again, it's $3,550 for a pound of chronic here in America, to buy it legally. And, I mean, how can you afford that, you know?

Rick: Well I mean, I certainly have nothing against people smoking cannabis, I smoke it myself.

Ian: Yeah.

Rick: You know, and I don't see a problem with it. It actually, it's just another form of preventative medicine. Because it's already… it's a proven fact that people that smoke cannabis, on average, lives about six years longer than people that don't.

So that's preventative medicine, as far as I'm concerned. It just happens to be a medicine that you can use recreationally [chuckling] you know, without harm.

Ian: Yeah.

Rick: So I think it's a helluva good idea. But if you have a serious illness don't expect smoking pot to, you know, to take care of your problems, you have to get, the raw unburned cannabinoids right into your system, that's when you see the magic.

Ian: Exactly. And the reason why even smoking it is better than nothing is you…I hear you can still get … oh, is it 16 percent, maybe even higher of the THC just from the smoking it. But you'll get 95 of it if you eat it, so that's the difference. And that was the first thing I learned when I went to Venice Beach 20 years ago and saw the hemp signs up and everything, went overlooked at their literature from Jack Herer and everything. And they were saying, "People that smoke cigarettes and smoke marijuana live a lot longer than if they just smoked cigarettes." And it turns out the ones that smoke marijuana, live longer than the ones that don't. [Chuckling]

Rick: [Laughing] Yeah…

Ian: All that BS they used to tell us about, "It kills brain cells and makes you stupid, the stupid stoner." That was false propaganda. It actually builds brain cells. Now I wouldn't… I didn't… won't tell kids to do it… I waited… I never… I waited until I was in my late twenties to start. So, I wouldn't mess with it when I was a child unless you have cancer or something. But as far as adults go, I mean, forget Prozac. Forget all that… ahh… Paxil and filth they give ya.

Rick: Yeah.

Ian: Just get a little cannabis oil, smoke a little herb and chill out at the end of the day, you know.

Rick: Well I would agree, Ian. But today, I mean, they're always going on, you know, "We have to keep it away from the children." But that's… that's just nonsense too. I mean, that study that Melanie Dreger did back in the 1980s, The Healthiest Babies Born on this Planet are born to mothers in Jamaica who use cannabis a great deal. So, if it doesn't harm a baby in the womb, you know, I mean, during the developmental stages. I mean, it's good for children of all ages. But look what the medical system does to our children today. You know, all these vaccines and then, "Oh God, they got attention deficit disorder." So, let's fill 'em full of amphetamine-like Ritalin. You know, I mean, it's just insanity that we're allowing them to do this to our own children.

And… if… you know, if our own children were, actually taking small doses of this oil every day the way they should be, it would prevent diseases like cancer, multiple sclerosis, diabetes from ever occurring. You know, we have a preventive medicine here that's good for all age groups.

Ian: Yeah, you're right. I… I'll have to look into that, I just… cause a friend of mine just had a … I couldn't believe it, like a 14-year-old going to rehab for marijuana.

Rick: [Laughing] Forced there, you mean.
Ian: Yeah. [Chuckles]
Rick: Well that's what they do. I mean, you can go to jail or you can go to 'rehab', you know. But… I mean, I've known two or three people that actually went into the hospital, cause they took too much of that oil and the doctors… when they went in and they told the doctors what they did… the doctor just told 'em, "To go lay down and read a book." There's no treatment for this because there's no harm.

Ian: [Laughing] Yeah, I know. I know, it's also… just weird how the… the way people look at it. The way it's always been, because… I mean, that's… when I grew up…yeah, the pot… the potheads, you know, they were always the long-haired guys and the tough guys that listened to the metal. Well, you know what, you don't have to be… actually… the best way of saying it is, "You can't fix stupid!" So, if you're stupid and you smoke weed, you're still going to be stupid. [Laughing] You know.

Rick: Well I mean, 2,000 years ago there was a long-haired guy that used this oil too…and his name was Jesus Christ. And I mean, it's a proven fact that the holy anointing oil was full of cannabinoids.

Ian: Yeah.

Rick: It wasn't the power of God he was using to heal people… it was the power of cannabis.

End of interview.

For some reason as those words left Rick's mouth the recording mysteriously ended. There were 20 more minutes of an interview, but it was only for the live show. The "Zen Live Show" in NYC archive, cuts after that statement. Lmao. God's like uh what? Okay. Click. End of interview. Lol!

CHAPTER 13:

DR. VICKERS ON THE IMPROVED GERSON THERAPY!

Ian: Alright, we are live. This is IcureCancer.com. Sorry about the delay. I don't know if you guys are, actually able to see this live on YouTube or not. It'd be totally cool if you could. But, if not, you'll see the archive and that's what you'll be watching now. Anyway, so it just took us a little while to get going, but we are rocking and rolling today. I've got Organic Guru Lynette here from the speaking engagement I'll be going to. And, we also have Dr. Vickers, who my friend, Tony Dudley, who is one of my favorite researchers, just loves him and was telling me forever to get this guy on my show and luckily Lynette already got him on for me. So, Lynette, let's start with you. Who is this guy, what's going on with him?

Organic Guru Lynette: Yeah, absolutely. Thanks for having us on Ian. This is my amazing friend, Dr. Patrick Vickers. He is one of our keynote speakers, well actually he is the keynote speaker at the Live Happy Be Cured Dinner Gala that we spoke about before, coming up in April, which nobody wants to miss!

In fact, you cannot afford to miss this event. It's the Natural Health Event of the Year supporting all kinds of amazing speakers such as Dr. Patrick Vickers and the one and only Ian Jacklin, our kick box champion of the past.

So anyway, we have Chris Wark, we have a whole array of amazing expert speakers to fuel your brain with amazing information on how to help your family take control of their health. So|I am introducing to you my awesome friend, who runs a Gerson Treatment Clinic in Baja, Mexico. Dr. Patrick Vickers... Yay... (clapping) thank you, Dr. Patrick! Love you!

Dr. Vickers: Hello Lynnette. Nice to see you. Thank you for inviting me to the show.

Ian: Right on!

Organic Guru Lynette: You're so welcome.

Ian: Yeah, and it's great to have you on. As I said, I've been wanting to get you on for a while and you are with the Gerson Therapy. And Gerson therapy, I'll let you explain it because I'm sure you're quite good at doing that after all these years. But we'll go into exactly what you use specifically. What is... who is Gerson? What is Gerson? Just in a nutshell, real, quick!

Dr. Vickers: Well Nobel Peace Prize winner Albert Schweitzer, he won the Nobel Prize back in 1952. He called Dr. Max Gerson the greatest genius in medical history. Dr. Gerson between 1920 and 1959 when he died, he was reversing a vast majority of degenerative diseases, including terminal cancer. But in 1959 he passed away. And from that point on, for about 18 years the therapy had remained dormant. And then in 1977 it was picked up again by his daughter, Charlotte, and she continued to do the therapy essentially to this date, but many of us have branched off and we've added to the Gerson Therapy by adding advanced protocols.

But in a nutshell, Dr. Gerson was a German doctor. He was suffering from severe migraine headaches and back in university when he was studying to be a medical doctor he cured himself of his migraine headaches using a no fat, no salt, no refined food diet. And then when he graduated, he ended up opening a practice in Freiburg, Germany or Bielefeld, Germany, excuse me. And he started giving this migraine diet to his patients. When one of his patients returned to him completely cured of skin tuberculosis. And Gerson then began to treat tuberculosis. And in a major study of 460 tuberculosis patients, terminal tuberculosis patients... now, this is at a time when tuberculosis was killing a million people a year in Europe. Dr. Gerson completely reversed 451 out of 460 of those tuberculosis patients.

Ian: Right.

Dr. Vickers: It was at that time that a cure for tuberculosis had been announced throughout all of Europe. So, he moves to the United States when Hitler comes to power because he was a German Jew. And when Hitler came to power he fled to Manhattan, where he set up a practice in Manhattan. And a woman came to him from New Jersey that was dying of terminal stomach, gallbladder and liver cancer and she begged him to give her the tuberculosis treatment, but he refused because he understood the political consequences of treating cancer naturally, even back in 1930-1932 whenever that occurred. And she was persistent. He denied her time and time again and then finally he agreed to treat her in secret. And he cured her. And he said at that time he could no longer turn his face away from this deadly scourge of cancer regardless of the political consequences and he continued to treat people with cancer and to this day, the Gerson Therapy remains essentially the pinnacle of treatment of advanced disease and terminal cancer.

So, what does it consist of? Well for starters, our patients are consuming 20 pounds of organic fruits and vegetables, on a daily basis. They get that mostly in the form of juices, but they do get three meals per day. And then we couldn't give the juices without the coffee enemas. Anybody who is juicing, they've gotta do coffee enemas, because when you juice, you create massive amounts of toxins from the release of toxins from inside the cells from the breakdown of diseased tissue and the rebuilding of new tissue. Those are all toxic processes. And if you don't eliminate those toxins you're going to actually cause more harm to the body than good; if you're just juicing and not eliminating using coffee enemas.

So anyway, our patients are getting five coffee enemas per day. And then the last thing, they are getting a myriad of supplements. And those supplements are specific for one thing and one thing only. And that is to increase the production of energy on a cellular level by the mitochondria. The mitochondria produce something called ATP and that's the energy molecule that the body uses to eat, sleep, drink, walk, talk, you need it to maintain a healthy immune system. And you most certainly need it to secure a sick and dying one. So that's the crux of the Gerson Therapy. Now we do other things as adjuncts to the therapy when you're at our clinic. We do ozone, we do laetrile. We do shark cartilage. We do something called Coley's, we do autologous treatment, dendritic cell treatment. We have added things to the basic Gerson Protocol that have taken the Gerson Therapy to a new level.

Ian: I was just going to say, so wait a minute... are you at the regular... is this a different clinic than the other Gerson Clinic. Is this more than Gerson... or...

Dr. Vickers: Absolutely, we... I lived with Charlotte Gerson. And I worked with Charlotte Gerson for 10 to 12 years. If you read in Dr. Gerson's book before he died in 1959, he published it in 1958, a year before his death. He theorized the direction he wanted to take the therapy in and he started mentioning very specific therapies. One of those therapies was the Coley Therapy. And to this day for whatever reason, Charlotte Gerson has refused to build on her father's treatment as he himself wanted to.

So, we are a different clinic. We had to alienate... separate ourselves from the Gerson Institute just for the simple fact that we had to continue to build on Dr. Gerson's work, which as I said, for whatever reason I can only surmise, Charlotte has refused to do it to this day. And much to the dismay of people who are suffering and dying. Because these advanced protocols are enhancing our clinical outcomes. And, so at some point, it's our hope that Charlotte will begin to take on those changes that even her own father mentions in his book on page 128, in his book of cancer therapy results of 50 cases. And hopefully someday if she does that, we can rejoin our forces and start to work together again as a unit.

Ian: Well I can't tell you how pleased I am to hear that because I wasn't sure how I was going to get through this interview if you weren't doing exactly what you just said because I know there are a couple of different kinds of Gerson's out there, and I love Charlotte, I interviewed her for ICureCancer.com, she's right there on the poster. But you're right, gotta keep moving man, gotta keep up with the Jones's and one thing I have learned about Gerson it has like maybe a 50 percent success rate, which is okay, it's the same as leukemia and chemo basically and so it wouldn't be as horrible for you. But, you know, like what I've learned over the years, you need more than just juicing and things like that. So, let's get into that. And if I may, really quick, do you believe in any meat at all? Or are you almost vegan or just totally vegan?

Dr. Vickers: Well personally when I'm at the clinic or if I'm cooking for myself, I hardly ever cook meat, maybe once, twice, three times a year maximum. But if you're accustomed to traveling you know that when you're traveling sometimes it's hard to get good food, in a quick period of time. So sometimes I succumb, not to fast-foodness necessarily, but not eating the best food.
But in regard to our patients, plain and simple, if our advanced cancer patients have meat in their diet with any kind of regularity they won't survive. They simply will not survive. There are varying reasons for that. The saturated fats in the meat, particularly red meat as you know, but even in chicken, there are saturated fats in the skin and I'm sure even in the meat itself.
But those fats, those cause tumors to grow. Plain and simple, fats will cause tumors to grow. That's why we can't even have avocado on the therapy. If we give our patients avocado and they leave out avocado on a regular basis they can run into issues with their tumors not regressing or going away. So, you have to be very careful about that.

Then the other issue, obviously, as you well know, is when you eat meat you generate acidity. And the true definition of acidity, you know, we're talking about PH and stuff, but the true definition of acidity is improper utilization of oxygen, because when the body is built up with hydrogen protons which are the definition of acidity, oxygen cannot enter the cells and mitochondria cannot produce ATP as efficiently as if the diet were alkaline. So, between the increased fats that are causing tumors to grow and the buildup of acidity in the body, you simply can't eat meat if you have advanced cancer.

Ian: Yes.

Dr. Vickers: I'm sorry, just one quick thing, if you're an early stage cancer and you really make a radical diet change to fruits and vegetables 80 to 90 percent of your diet then you can probably get away with a little meat. I know Chris Wark did, but Chris Wark, you gotta be careful with his cancer. The kid was 26 years old, he had all his cancer cut out and then he made the radical lifestyle changes he did and he'll tell you that, you know, what he did and what an advanced cancer patient, inoperable or severely advanced, when they have that then they're not going to get away with what Chris was able to get away with.

Ian: Right, okay. Man, I was freaking out because I put up a video and I'm like, "Should I put avocado in that blending video?" (chuckling)

Dr. Vickers: Hey, avocado, avocado is a great food. It's one of the healthiest foods you can eat. But when you are dealing with advanced cancer, it's a completely different monster.

Ian: Okay. That's very interesting because I remember Dr. Bernardo, actually had a concoction where they would squish the avocado in with something else. But that's okay. Cause I was totally against being vegan for many years, call me a macho meat eater or whatever you want. Thanks to lots of research I found out that going vegan as Chris did for two months, I did for two months. I definitely would do it if I was a cancer patient. I think I was recently, my PH went down to 5 for over 6 months and you know I wasn't healthy so I snapped out of it and got on the Blend-fast and alkaline diet. I cut out the meat for a couple of months and boom, PH back up to 7.4, healthy as a horse!

I'm just wondering, now... here's the thing... and I have to say it. I've got a very good friend, his name is Dr. Raber, and he is from Tumorx.com he's there at their site. They sell the bloodroot, good bloodroot, internal right, external for skin cancers, gets it right out. I was talking to him one time and I will have him on my show again, but he was saying something about this ATP, the reason why vegan diets work for cancer patients for two months or so, it's good, cause you're cleansing, you're detoxing. But there is something about the ATP energy isn't the same without the meat and vitamin B's and all that and I think if people are to go vegan don't you have to do things slightly differently add in your B's. I mean, aren't you missing something if you don't eat meat, I guess is what I'm saying?

Dr. Vickers: Adding your what?

Ian: And remember I'm talking organic meat folks, organic, not grocery store crap! And I'm sorry what was your question?

Dr. Vickers: Do we have to add in what to make up for the lack of meat? B, did you say B vitamins and stuff?

Ian: Yeah, like shouldn't non-meat eaters be doing something to give them what they're missing because they don't eat meat anymore?

Dr. Vickers: Yes. Yes, we do! Six weeks into the therapy we start allowing non-fat organic yogurt. And that takes the place essentially of having to eat meat. And it doesn't generate the same acidity as eating a big beefy steak or a big, you know, half of a chicken. It's a completely different form of a protein and it doesn't generate the acidity as eating meat does. And it does give the body that added extra protein that is needed. And, also on the therapy, especially since we are doing the advanced protocols, we add in lentils. We add in quinoa. We add, we have oatmeal on the therapy. And believe it or not carrots, potatoes, they're loaded with protein. Okay. You know a common question that I get, "But if I'm on this diet, how am I going to get my protein?" And the simple answer is, "Well where does a cow or a horse get their protein from?" I mean, they're not meat eaters. And, look at how they are able to maintain the definition and tone of their bodies without hardly even having to exercise. Why? Well because nature is loaded with protein, greens are loaded with protein.

So, you know, look in the Bible, you read the Book of Ezekiel, Chapter 4, Verse 9. It tells you how to make your bread. Well if you make your bread that way, it becomes a complete protein, you're not dependent on meat to get a complete protein. So, there are other ways to get protein than having eggs, meat, chicken, you know, milk. So, we supplement with a natural non-fat organic yogurt after six weeks and, that comes from actually a study by Robert Good at the University of Minnesota. He showed that if you deprive a body of any animal protein for the first six to eight weeks, the immune response goes through the roof. But at 6 to 8 weeks if you don't start adding a little bit of protein into the therapy or into a therapy, that immune system, will actually start to decline a bit.

So, it was based on that work that Dr. Gerson was... and Dr. Budwig because actually, Gerson got that protocol from Budwig. I'm sure you've heard of Johanna Budwig.

Ian: Yeah, yeah, of course, the Budwig Protocol.
Dr. Vickers: Yeah.

Ian: Yeah. Well now you just helped me out big time, man. That will be more to talk about too with Dr. Raber down the line. Because I was wondering, because he said the same thing as I said, "Like after about two months," you know.

Dr. Vickers: Yeah.
Ian: just didn't work anymore. But that was Gerson, that wasn't what you're doing. You're saying... and all you need to do is add in a little bit of the protein that's yogurt, you don't even have to go to the extent of meat.

Dr. Vickers: Right. Our patients are getting about 4 ounces a day, at the 6 – 8-week mark. So, that's ample. You know, I mean, that's a good solid quality protein that the body can use to maintain its general needs. But you don't need a lot more than that. I think there's a big protein neurosis. We also have a calcium neurosis. You know, I need my protein and I need my calcium. Well you know, the body does not need that much protein, believe it or not, to sustain itself. So, you know, you just gotta find that equilibrium that meets the bodies general daily needs.

Ian: Yeah, that's what I'm learning myself now that I'm working out again and trying to... you know, like lifting weights. And I'm used to just, you know... protein... like shakes and egg whites and steaks and you know. But this time, as I say, I'm almost vegan. I only have meat a couple... few times a week now comparably speaking to like three times a day before. And so far, so good, I'm feeling pretty good, pretty strong. I don't seem like or feel like I'm missing anything. So, there must be some method to your madness there, brother.

Dr. Vickers: Well I mean, look... I don't know when it was, like maybe back in the late 90s, the top three triathletes in the world at one point were all strict, I don't know if they were non-lacto, non-ova vegetarians, but they were strict vegetarians. And they are the ones who abuse their body the most, so you would think that they would have to replenish their bodies with protein more than anybody. But these guys were strict vegetarians and they were the top triathletes in the world.

Ian: Yeah.

Dr. Vickers: The knowledge is out there.

Ian: Right. Right. Okay. Why don't you tell me a little bit about yourself? Whatever got you interested in this? Did you have cancer, a loved one? How did you get into helping people this way?

Dr. Vickers: Well I'll tell you I wanted to be a chiropractor ever since I was 11 years old. A friend of our families was a chiropractor and they were staying at our home for the weekend when their five-year-old child who was sleeping in my room with me woke up at like 3 in the morning with a cough that wouldn't stop. And his father came up after about 15 - 20 minutes of this kid constantly coughing, laid him onto the end of the bed, adjusted his neck and he stopped coughing immediately. And I said, "That's what I'm going to do for a living." And so, I went on to chiropractic school at New York Chiropractic College and when I had a year left, Charlotte Gerson came and spoke at our school for the weekend, and the moment she opened her mouth I knew that's what I would spend the rest of my life doing. And so here I am now 16 years later, 17, that's pretty scary, seventeen years later, doing what I do. And I mean it just has come naturally. It's a passion and it doesn't seem like work, except, you know, when things get a little stressful at the clinic, you know. Like today.

Ian: [Laughing] Yeah, I heard you had a rough day. We had a little bit of a rough time of getting this happening. I don't know if anybody's watching live or not, cause, I've never got on google roots, but if not, they can catch the repeat. Now I wanted to ask you. A friend of mine that cured herself of cancer, Cynthia Brooks, the beautiful blond girl, right there, from I Cure Cancer.com had started this whole thing, for me. She swore on having a chiropractor in her cancer team. What would you think? I would never think chiropractic would be for cancer. Why would you think that would help?

Dr. Vickers: Well I mean, look, your brain is your central nervous system. Right now, as we speak our brain is trying to communicate with every single muscle and organ in the body and how does that work? Well, the brain, off the brain comes the spinal cord and then off the spinal cord come nerve roots. So, if that spinal cords not aligned properly the information coming from the brain to the body can't be transmitted properly. So, it's very important that from childhood your children are getting adjusted and certainly someone who is sick. Because you need, you need the maximum amount of support from the brain, in order to heal the body. And so if, those vertebras are out-of-place, and they are twisted and torque, they're cutting off the individual nerve flow going to individual organs and tissue.

So, whoever that woman is, I mean, that's a wise choice because chiropractic is very, very powerful as it relates to healing. I mean, look Hippocrates... Hippocrates who we know to this day is the greatest physician who ever lived, he said, two of his most famous quotes are, one, as everybody knows, "Let medicine be your... or let your food by your medicine and let thy medicine by your food." Well, his other famous quote is, "Look to the spine as the cause of disease." And so those two aspects are what are the primary causes of disease today.

Ian: Wow, I was not aware of that. Excellent.
Dr. Vickers: Yeah.
Ian: And cause, I'll tell you what my mentality was and maybe some can relate to it. I thought, okay, I'm going to go to this chiropractor check it out, because I used to be an athlete, get some kinks out. And it worked, it was beautiful.

But, the next day or a couple of days later, gotta go back to him. So right away... and even now, I'm a little more evolved and I'll say, "Did it work?" "Yeah." "Well then, shut up! Keep going." But it just seemed like a scam to me cause you had to keep going but, duh, to keep good health you have to eat well every day, you can't just eat well one day out of the week and then... you know what I mean, so anyway I've evolved, thank God. And then thank you, thank you for explaining that to me, cause, I would never... I thought that was just structural, I didn't even think that that would connect to your organs and the cannabinoids probably all flow through that, right?

Dr. Vickers: Yeah. It's, you know... a look into the human body and it just makes logistical sense on what a chiropractic adjustment can do for the human body. It's one of the most powerful things you can do. And yeah, you do have to keep going back on a regular basis, just like you have to take your car in to get the oil changed on a regular basis. I mean, look it's not a scam or fraud, just because you have to keep going back in and out, you know, maybe once every two to four weeks. It's just normal.

Ian: Yeah. And lately, I've been getting rehab on my hip because I was scheduled for surgery because I used to be a kickboxing champion and so that was going to be taken out, a replacement put in. But luckily I met a friend of mine, Raul Rodriquez, who rehabs the Lakers and guys like that. So, he's doing that for me as a favor because I do this for people for cancer and he's fixing my hip which is beautiful. And he was basically saying that motion is lotion if you don't use it you lose it. And that would make sense with the chiropractic as well.

Dr. Vickers: That's exactly right.

Ian: Yeah, and I just joined a yoga club and now I'm going to get chiropractic! [chuckling]

Dr. Vickers: There ya' go.

Ian: Cool. Now, where else do you want to go with this conversation? I've got a number of people, watching, that have cancer. So, let's speak to them for a bit. What do you recommend to them the ones that are freaking out right now? "Oh my God, I got cancer. They want me to do chemo, radiation, and surgery! Some people say chemo, radiation, and surgery is not good." Ehh ehh... you know, anything that you could maybe help them out, relax a bit.

Dr. Vickers: Well anything with the foundations of mustard gas can't be good for you. Chemotherapy... the foundations of chemotherapy are mustard gas. That's what they use in biological warfare. And the whole paradigm and premise of chemotherapy are, "Let's see if we can kill all of the cancer with the hopes that there is still some of the body's ability to function left." And usually that is not the case and that's why most people end up dying of the chemotherapy before they end up dying of the cancer. That's well known. That's why they've never double-blinded studied chemotherapy because the evidence is very clear that those who don't get chemotherapy live four times longer than those that do. So why would you bite off the hand that feeds you, shoot yourself in the foot, if you publish some kind of a study, that will clearly reveal that anyway? So, no, chemotherapy clearly is the most barbaric, ridiculous option when treating cancer and you have-to-do something based in the foundations of what Dr. Gerson discovered.

Now, in regard to what we do; at the beginning of this interview I mention the advance protocols that we're doing. For example, the greatest thing that we do, I think, is Coleys. Coleys is very powerful. Coleys is the bacterial toxins of staph and strep bacteria. Now the toxins, not the actual bacteria. They've been cultured and then they're injected into the body. And the body sets up a huge fever reaction, an inflammatory process which all healing requires an inflammatory process. You can't heal without it. So, when we give Coley's to our patients an amazing reaction occurs for about... anywhere from two to seven hours, they get really large fevers and you can hear them telling you that they're getting pain right where the tumors are. Why? Because when you put the immune system on high alert with the Coley's it's going to be awakened to the fact that there's a tumor in it, and it's going to actually seek-out that tumor because it's the most imminent threat to the body. And so, it'll go straight to the tumors whether it's an ovarian tumor, a colon tumor, a pancreatic tumor. The patients will almost invariably tell you, they can feel pain, right where their tumors are.

It's absolutely remarkable to watch and it happens religiously. And, if we can get into a tumor directly, like let's say a breast tumor, the results are absolutely phenomenal! I've got two breast cancer patients here right now, we're putting Coley's directly into their breast and within a week already, in two weeks, their breast tumors are significantly softer, more mobile and reduced in size and this is only two weeks.

So, the advanced protocols that we're doing they just take cancer therapy to a new level and I can go into more like we do dendritic cells, dendritic cells are like generals in your body, Dendritic cells around your body seeking out threats to the system. And then they present that threat to the immune system, to the white blood cells, to the natural killer cells. And then it's those cells that rally the attack against the disease. So, in dendritic cell therapy, we draw out the blood, we separate the dendritic cells of the patient and we culture and multiply exponentially, the amount of dendritic cells, and then we reintroduce them into the patient four to five days later.

So, if we extracted one million dendritic cells out of the extraction process, we probably inject 10 million, if not more. And the immune system response, especially when done with Coley's, there's nothing like it in the world, plain and simple.

Ian: Wow. Now. Coleys. I haven't heard that one, so it's throwing me. It's like, what do you mean, like, now is this like... it's not a vaccine.

Dr. Vickers: Well you could technically call it a vaccine. It's a dead vaccine. Where the staph and strep bacteria have produced their normal by-products of metabolism which are toxins. And then when you give those subcutaneously, the body responds as if it has a staph or strep infection, even though it's not the actual bacteria. It still responds to the toxins. And that's what... Coley... Coley just did that? And he was able to achieve some permanent cures. But not nearly on the percentage basis that Gerson could with the diet and the detox alone. So, Gerson theorized that if he could do Coley's with the Gerson therapy the results would be phenomenal. And it was the diet and detox that Coley overlooked. Had he included something like the Gerson therapy with his discovery, his results would have been phenomenal.

Ian: Right. I've always said, in a perfect world, if I had cancer I'd... and money wasn't an issue, I would definitely... well, I now would go to your Gerson Clinic. Because that's... I mean the juicing folks are the most serious thing to do... there's a difference between blending and juicing too.

Dr. Vickers: That's right.

Ian: Blending is like definitely for, stage 1... I don't know, well I'm not the guy to say, but when you get... I'll let you say this. I'm assuming the later stages your organs can't handle the digestion... blended...

Dr. Vickers: You can't. That's exactly right.

Ian: Yeah.

Dr. Vickers: You cannot handle the amount of fiber, for the amount of nutrition that you must get, in an advanced stage cancer. The body requires energy to break down, utilize and draw out the nutrients that are in the fiber. So, as you said, if you're a stage, one cancer patient, you might be able to get away with it. But I'd still be hesitant to do that.

The juices have-to be pressed. They have to go through a two-step process of being grated and then pressed and so that there's no fiber in that juice and then that juice it enters the bloodstream almost as quickly as alcohol does to have energy produced. Whereas as if you had eaten the fiber, it would take you hours. And the amount of ATP you would have to use just to create ATP, it just wouldn't make cost-effective sense. So those juices have-to be pressed.

Ian: Very interesting. Now, but please help save a few people right now because they're going to be freaking out cause the kind of juicer you're talking about the presser is I believe a two-thousand dollar machine, whereas I just recently went and bought one for a hundred bucks and it spins and I know it's maybe not the best but it's all I could afford. Is that okay? Is it better than nothing?

Dr. Vickers: Well no. You're wrong, it's not two thousand, it's actually $2,700! [Laughing]

Ian: Okay [laughing]

Dr. Vickers: [Chuckling] But look, there's something called the Champion Juicer which I'm sure you're aware of, and a separate press. So, a Champion is $220.00, and a separate press is around $350.00. So, for $600 bucks you can get the same exact thing.

Now with that said, that juice... or that juicer, the Norwalk or the Champion and Press that's going to pay itself off within a year. The Champion is going to pay itself off within three months on a therapy like this because the amount of juice that does not get extracted out of the pulp when you use these other juicers is a waste of money and when you're dealing with all the organic produce that you're dealing with, you simply have to be able to extract as much of the juice out of that produce or you're going to lose money. And, so we tell people and it's probably true, that the amount of juice that's pressed out of these fruits and vegetables is exponentially greater than these other juicers that people are buying.

Ian: Okay, but what I don't understand 'cause I've done it. I mean, I prefer the... I don't have cancer now that I know of so I'm back on just shakes 'cause I want the fiber. I want to feel full. But for the people that have the cancer, when I may... even though they're cheap old blender I mean it took tons of stuff and extracted it, obviously, and just left the juice. I mean is that not good?

Dr. Vickers: Okay. Good point. Good point. Gerson discovered that he couldn't get the same results using centrifugal juicers. So, he sent a centrifugal juicer to a physicist. And a physicist analyzed why that would be the possibility, the reason. And what he discovered was that the juice is negatively charged, and the centrifugal force is positively charged. And the centrifugal force was deactivating the enzymes in that juice so that the juice was not as powerful as a fresh pressed juice using a grating and press mechanism. So, the enzyme content of that juice is not the same. And those enzymes are what are needed to literally break down tumor tissue and rebuild new tissue and break down disease tissue. So, it's pretty much well known now that centrifugal juicers cannot produce the quality of juice that the grading and pressing juice can.

Ian: Okay. Yeah, I mean, we've always known that. It's just, you know, people that are on a budget. Well, would it be okay for them to do that? I mean, you're not saying don't do that if that's all you can do and then maybe take some enzymes as well, some proteolytic enzymes.

Dr. Vickers: Well the enzymes in juices aren't necessarily the same enzymes that you and I would take as a supplement. Okay. There's different... there are varying enzymes. And I couldn't honestly tell you the names and their significance. But no. I mean we do give proteolytic enzymes on the therapy in massive amounts. But it's not the same... it's not the same as a fresh pressed juice.

Ian: I gotcha. Oh, so that's good, you're doing both? You're doing those high enzymes.

Dr. Vickers: Oh, yeah absolutely. Our patients are getting loads of pancreatic enzymes in this therapy.

Ian: Wow, man. Are you able to say what kind of percentage you guys are getting? Cause, I mean... I know Charlotte was at 50 percent, but it sounds like what you guys are doing, you guys should be out there, like 75 - 80...

Dr. Vickers: Well... No. And anybody who does give you percentages, it's usually pretty false information because it's never been peer reviewed studied and they're giving you the quote statistics that they've accumulated in their clinic. That's why if you go on, I don't know an MD Anderson site they tell you, yes, we have 45 percent or 50 percent cure rate... or no, they have outrages numbers like 75... 80 percent, yet everybody's dying. Okay.by... what I mean by that is peer-reviewed study. Meaning that a non-biased jury of your peers went over the data and said, "Yup, this is legitimate, it was done correctly. It is true and trustworthy!" To answer that question, we're the only ones in medical history to have a peer-reviewed study proving the ability to reverse advanced terminal cancer. It's called the Gerson Melanoma Study. It's the only study done in medical history proving the ability to reverse advanced terminal cancer. And, well in that study we were able to prove in malignant melanoma, terminal malignant melanoma the deadliest cancer you can have. We proved a 40 percent cure rate. Now, this was back 20 years ago almost. Okay. Things have changed. That was on the basic Gerson Therapy and it was 20 years ago. Those numbers have probably gone done five to ten percent because the environment is more toxic, the tumors, are more deadly... they're more aggressive and you know... so... anyway...

Ian: Yeah, well I mean with all the Chemtrails in the sky, the GMOs in the food I mean [chuckling]

Dr. Vickers: Yeah. And chemo... chemoradiation. You know, and it's just one thing on top of the other. So just with the basic Gerson Therapy, being able to reverse cancer it's getting harder and harder. But with the advanced protocols with melanoma, ovarian cancer, cervical cancer, lymphoma, we're probably taking those percentages up to about 50 percent again.

Notice, you said at the beginning of this interview that Gerson was getting 50 percent results or probably a little bit better when he was alive 55 years ago.

Ian: Right.

Dr. Vickers: You notice our peer-reviewed study with melanoma was only 40 percent.

Ian: Right.

Dr. Vickers: So in that two generation span, or generation and a half, the human body had degenerated universally so much that it had dropped the percentages probably by 10 percent.

Ian: Right. Now, what are your thoughts on the power of the mind and body-soul like positive mental attitude, meditation? You know, people that could possibly cure themselves with this, do you believe in that at all?

Dr. Vickers: I don't think they can cure themselves with their minds. I think it plays a huge role. I see it in my clinic. The patients that come in that are grumpy complain, you know complain about the food, complain about the service, you know this and that, chronic complainers... they're not going to get better. And, typically they're not. The ones that come in grateful that they've found what they found, grateful they have a second chance, grateful they have the opportunity, to change their lives, those are the ones we know they're going to survive. So, the power of the mind and the attitude that speaks volumes for who we're going to cure and who we're not going to cure.

Ian: Yeah, exactly. I would still use my power of mind before I would do chemo, but [chuckling]... I would definitely.

Dr. Vickers: Well, if you did a study between the two, I'm sure the power of the mind would win that study in a heartbeat. I mean, Good Lord, chemo... chemo can't do a damn thing to anything... whoops, can I say that on here?

Ian: Yeah. Oh, fuck it, say whatever you want! [Chuckling] It's my show. Part of me, sorry I shouldn't have said that. Keep going.

But okay, I was... what did I want to say... is there anything you want to say Organic Guru Lynette before we take off? Let me un-mute you. Right on! Sorry I had you muted, couldn't figure it out. Let's... I think we're almost going to wrap up so let's get the information because Dr. Vickers and I will both be speaking at your show, your gala. Give us one more time, what that is again.

Organic Guru Lynette: Absolutely. And it is everybody's gala. It's everybody's show. It is for everyone. We have the privilege of having you Ian Jacklin, having you Dr. Patrick Vickers at our amazing gala. We also have Mary Tocco, the National Vaccine expert, we have Chris Wark coming in. We have a lot of speakers coming in with a wealth of information. You will have two-fold the information from Dr. Patrick Vickers, so this is an event that you will not want to miss. You cannot afford to miss the Live Happy Be Pure Gala, black-tie dinner gala, Thursday, April 3rd. It is a fundraiser for the Gerson Treatment Center, as well as to keep the tours going.

So, we'll have a black-tie dinner gala, farm to table, organic. A silent auction. The two days following will be the two-day organic festival with many more speakers, lots of entertainment and lots of vendors. So, come. Shop. Get Empowered. Get Inspired. And get healthy, so you can live happily, be pure at the event of the year. April 3rd, 4th, and 5th.

Ian: Absolutely. Thank you very much. You know it just popped in my head, I have to ask you cause' I got a couple of people I know that got pancreatic cancer. You guys, what are your rates like that... do you find...

Dr. Vickers: Oh, that's one of the harder cancers to cure.
Ian: I know.
Dr. Vickers: But if you're going to try to cure it, it's gotta' be the Gerson Therapy. Because it's such a deadly cancer. There's nothing out there. I mean, Nick Gonzales... Nick Gonzales' mentor William Kelly who we cured of pancreatic cancer, did a little bit of a twist on the Gerson Therapy and developed his own therapy for pancreatic cancer. So, Nick Gonzales might have a little bit of success with it, but nothing remotely similar to what we can get on the Gerson Therapy especially the advanced protocols.

But that's a harder one to cure and on the basic Gerson Therapy an advanced stage pancreatic cancer I'd probably give it a 25 to 30 percent. If you lined up a 100 in terminal states, like let's say, 6 months or less to live. I could see the advanced protocols could probably get it up a little, 40. Yeah, that's the hard one to cure.

Ian: Okay. That's very interesting. Just so you know, I don't know if you've looked into the cannabis hemp oil yet. That is really working well. It does kill the THC, the THC kills... does kill cancer cells from what I've seen. It doesn't work for everybody. But I've seen a pretty good success rate with that. So... and my friend, actually swears by it. He is one of the two percent still alive from pancreatic cancer because most of them don't live more than a year or two and after a couple of years he still there. And he says the cannabis hemp oil is doing it. And he can't afford Gerson unfortunately if he could, I'm sure he would be down there with you guys and doing much better. What are we looking at astronomical amounts of money for somebody to come to something like this? Do you have any kind of programs?

Dr. Vickers: Okay. To come to our clinic and the price includes the following. We require a two-week minimum stay and in advanced cancer, we really prefer three weeks. We just have seen that a three week stay the patients seem to respond a little bit better for some reason. Anyway, to come to our clinic and the price includes airport transport to and from San Diego Airport to our clinic. It includes a companion. Companion gets to stay for the whole entire stay. They get three meals, three juices per day and they get to stay in the room with the patient. It includes three months of all the supplements you need to go home with. We send you home with three month's worth of Coleys. We send you home with three-months-worth of the autologous treatment. You get IV vitamin C, IV chelation, IV L-carnitine, you get shark cartilage, ozone, laetrile, and hyperthermia. You, get all of those things.

One week is $5,600. And so, two weeks would come to roughly $11,200 something dollars. Okay. Believe it or not, that sounds expensive. It's unbelievably cheap when you see everything that you're getting for that. There's a guy here right now, he comes down every morning and he says, "I can't believe this cost's me this much. You're giving this away."

If you saw our facilities. Our facilities are the best in all of Tijuana. Right on the ocean. Your own private beach, a luxury home, luxury condos. Absolutely impeccable facilities. So, most people see it more as a resort than as a cancer clinic. So, you're looking at a two week stay about $11,200, a three-week stay approaching $16,500 - $17,000 somewhere in there. But again, you get all, of those things included, and you go home with three months of all those therapies.

Ian: Wow. That is a really, good deal folk! You're looking at least $25,000 - $30,000 grand for most treatments down in Mexico. So, that's actually not too bad! And that's... I'm really impressed actually! I'm so glad we had this interview because I said before I love Gerson but I myself, I know that I would need more, much more, you know. Especially for something like pancreatic.
So excellent getting to meet you.

Dr. Vickers: Thank you.
Ian: Oh, what's your website sorry. Your website before we go.

Dr. Vickers: Yeah, my website is http://www.GersonTreatment.com./ If you want to send us an email, just send it to info@GersonTreatment.com or you can call us at 715-299-5070. And usually, I get back to you. I try to answer all calls personally and I usually get back to you within 24 hours. Very rarely that I don't.

Ian: Excellent. Excellent. Okay. Well thank you Organic Guru Lynette and thank you to you, Dr. Vickers, it's a true honor, pleasure, thank you. I'm definitely... we'll put all this information up on the event page that we have this on. And I'll forward people to you if they can afford it and need that kind of help. And I'd highly recommend it. But I would always... always add in some cannabis hemp oil if you have cancer. I've seen it with my eyes too many times that that stuff does work for a lot a lot a people so. Okay Dr. Vickers, anything before we go; really quick?

Dr. Vickers: Yeah, you know, regarding the price. Look we don't want to turn somebody away cause' they can't afford it. I mean we can't give the therapy away obviously it's not how business works [so curing people is a business... that sucks...

Unfortunately, you know, we don't have a fund set up yet where we're able to, you know, divvy into a fund for somebody who doesn't have enough money to come [where a non-profit comes in]. But I'm willing to work with people on pricing. I don't want to send people away cause' they can't afford it. So, anybody who can't afford it, you know, maybe we can work something out where you know it's good enough for both parties. So, with that said, I've had patients raise up to $35,000 in a three to four-week period on a website called GiveForward. It's a website that tries to raise money for medical purposes and it's linked somehow to Facebook, and my patients were getting donations from people they had no clue based on how connected to friends on Facebook and this and that and I don't know how that works. But GiveForward.com. It's an excellent resource for raising money for treatment.

Ian: Wow, excellent. Well again, true pleasure. Thank you very much, Guru Lynette, I'll talk to you soon. And ladies and gentlemen this may be our format from now on or we may be back on ZenLive next week, we'll see how it goes. But thank you and God Bless. Peace.

Dr. Vickers: Thank you.

Director and Founder of NORTHERN BAJA GERSON CENTER
715-299-5070 www.gersontreatment.com Patrick@gersontreatment.com

[See Pic 13.1]

CHAPTER 14:

A TESTIMONIAL WITH J CYNTHIA BROOKS

Ian Jacklin back at the keyboard. Cynthia Brooks is the reason I made iCureCancer.com. FYI. A short clip from iCureCancer.com: the feature documentary. Terminal Cervical Cancer Stage 4 diagnosis.

My name is J. Cynthia Brooks and I was diagnosed with cancer ten years ago now. What turned out, is I had, ten years ago, what they called the fastest moving cancer that they knew of and by the time we got to biopsies the cancer was everywhere and had already made it into a lymph node. So, started talking about the options, you know, what I want to say also is that I had "the BEST" supposedly in the country, oncologist gynecologist. First, the cancer was discovered in my uterus or in my cervix. So, these are the top-notch guys, some of them are Rhode Scholars, Harvard grad, top of the class, right there in the heart of Beverly Hills.

So, the options were surgery and chemo and radiation et cetera, et cetera, et cetera... When I asked, "Well, you know if I do all that is that going to be the end of it?" And they said, "No." And I said, "There's absolutely no guaranty that this cancer isn't going to pop up somewhere else, as it has, with so many people." And, of course, they agreed.

Now, I was just barely starting to study alternative medicine. I had stumbled upon some tricks in my life, something to relieve my migraine headaches. I never get headaches. So, I knew there was something to this business of, you know, this combination of food, herbs, et cetera, et cetera over the course of the years I had heard about a rife machine. I was already at a meditation center; I was studying with the Essenes. The Essenes who wrote The Dead Sea Scrolls and Jesus Christ is one of the most famous Essenes that they have. And, it was actually everything that Einstein ever said, it was all about moving energy, everything is energy, this particular kind of meditation, how to move around energy. So, I was six months studying with them pretty, pretty, heavily, three to four times a week. And, of course, they were very into, the Essenes have always been into body cleansing. That's how I was getting more and more interested in alternative medicine.

Once these doctors told me what my option was… It just wasn't… I just couldn't do it. [Shoulders cringe] It wasn't acceptable! I just couldn't do it. And knowing what I knew, the small amount, at that time, what I knew of alternative medicine, hearing miracle story, after miracle story. So, I rejected everything … to the fury of my doctors [smiling] and, actually went out and sought another oncologist gynecologist, who is probably one of the more famous ones. And again, right there in the heart of Beverly Hills, and claimed to have one foot in eastern medicine and one foot in western medicine. When I went to him and told him what I wanted to do, what I was trying to do, he discouraged me. And said, "You can't do it, not with this kind of cancer." And I was sitting there in his office and he was sitting across the desk from me and he says, "I know what you're trying to do, but, all of my patients who have treated your kind of cancer the way you want to, are dead!"

So now I have this, you know [skeptical giggling] I have this [hands balancing back and forth] eastern medicine doctor telling me I'm going to die too. And I just kind of threw my hands up in the air and I said, "Well then we're going to see if it really works or it really doesn't. I was just very set on my mark. I did have support at the meditation center, everyone there was saying, "You can do this. You can do this! You can do this.

In my opinion, dealing with life-threatening ailments, cancer, AIDS et cetera, I think that's actually the secondary disease, the first disease is fear. And I talk about cancer and the subject of cancer that nobody wants to talk about, what I talk about is cancer consciousness. And so, I went out and treated my mind, body, and soul as one, meaning with the meditation, doing the spiritual work, educating myself, as well as putting myself on a program, a body program.

And so, I just asked questions, asked for help, one person after another came up. And what I stumbled upon doing was I sort of assembled a cancer team, as I called it, or a healing team. One was a physicist, one was a microscopist, one was a kinesiologist and they all sort of hitting these different marks and I would cross-reference any time I found out any new information. I did… I, with my cancer, in treating my cancer, I did not adopt any established specific regiment that other people were doing. I sort of, somehow, managed to piece together from all the information that I was finding out, I pieced together something that would work for me.

I did this routine and went back for biopsies about four and a half months later, 80 percent cell recovery doing this. They sent the tests back, of course, three times [smiling] cause' they thought it was a mistake and it wasn't. And then four months after that, I went, and I was completely cancer free. No cancer to be found. And that was ten years ago. [See Pic 14.1]

CHAPTER 15:

DR. NICK GONZALEZ

(I CURE CANCER II EXCERPT)

Dr. Nick Gonzalez: My name is Dr. Nicholas Gonzalez, M.D. I'm a physician here in New York City. I practice an alternative nutritional approach to cancer and other degenerative diseases. I graduated from Brown University with a degree in English literature wishing to be a writer. My first job after college was at Time, Inc. as a journalist. I worked as a journalist for seven years.

As a result, of several stories, I wrote on cancer research got interested in medicine and changed careers. Turned down a book contract, did my postgraduate premed work at Columbia. Subsequently went to Cornell because I wanted to do cancer research.

While I was a second-year medical student I learned about the work of Dr. William Kelly who was a dentist at that time-based in Dallas Texas who was treating cancer patients with an aggressive nutritional program. And even though I was very conventionally oriented I had an open mind and I met with him through a friend of mine who was a journalist who was thinking about doing a book about Kelly.

As a result of that meeting, I began to suspect that he might indeed be reversing advanced cancer. Went down to Texas to start going through his records and within a couple of weeks realized that he had hundreds and hundreds of cases in his files of patients with appropriately diagnosed advanced prognosis. Cancer patients who had done well on his therapy.

I went through over a thousand of Kelly's patient charts, interviewed over a thousand of his patients. Selected a group of 455 patients that had done well with appropriately diagnose of poor prognosis cancer, done well under his care.

Put all of that into a monograph form in 1986, 500 pages long where I wrote of 50 of Kelly's patients with 26 different types of cancer including a series of pancreatic cancer patients that had survival that was unheard of in conventional medicine, would still be unheard of today.

Unfortunately, in those days if you mention nutrition and cancer in the same sentence it was considered just about a felony. We couldn't get it published, even though I was being trained as an academic researcher in Robert Good the most published author in the history of medicine was my mentor couldn't get it published.

There were two responses from editors. One, this couldn't be real, I had to have made it up, it had to be fake. Or second, editors believed it and said, this is extraordinary, but this is 1987, if we publish it, it will be the end of my career it would create so much controversy with the AMA, The American Cancer Society, NIH and all of that. So, we couldn't get it published.

Finally, in 2010, I rewrote it. It had an introduction and finally published it as one man alone which is my investigation of Kelly. So that's how it started as a medical student I had through a serendipitous chain of events had the opportunity to meet Dr. Kelly and changed my career. I was being mentored by the guy who was President of Sloane Kettering at the time.

But after meeting Kelly I realized that he was reversing cancer nutritionally and as a scientist who thought he had some level of ethics I couldn't turn my back on it. So, despite the political harassment that being involved with alternative therapy, it would entail I chose that as a course of my future work. I was offered two jobs at Sloane Kettering, well true, turned both down because it would require that I give up my controversial crazy nutritional work.

But that's how it started. I was being trained to be a very conventional researcher, trained to do bone marrow transplant, but as a result of my own investigation of Kelly's work realized that there was, other ways to approach cancer that are non-toxic nutritional and even cheaper and with results that I had never seen in conventional medicine.

Ian: Comparing your kind of money you're made doing alternative compared to what you would have you ever thought of that?

Dr. Nick Gonzalez: [Deep belly laugh] I think it's a joke when the critics of alternative medicine, "They're in it for the money!" Well, there may be people in alternative medicine that are in it for the money. That may be true. But this is not the way to make a living.

First of all, you're being harassed by your colleagues all the time. You know, during the early 90s it is well known you know the Medical Board began to investigate me. That cost me over about a million dollars in legal fees. It ended up fine. In fact, the person sent by the medical board to investigate my practice Julian Hyman was a very well esteemed oncologist in New York, still alive. His brother was a Columbia Professor in Oncology, his nephew was an orthopedist. He comes from a very eminent family.

He came in here as a skeptic from the medical board with the power to shut my practice down. Became a good friend, a strong supporter. And as a signed affidavit says, he said he saw miracles in my practice. So, he became one of my biggest supporters. You don't make money being an alternative practitioner treating cancer. I guess... I mean, some people might. But this isn't the way to do it. You want to make money you do bone marrow transplants which I was trained to do. A single bone marrow transplant in the days when I was doing it and this goes back 30 years when I was training on 25 years ago, it cost $450,000-$500,000, up to a million dollars depending on how sick the patient was. And a lot of it was profit. Pure profit. So, if you want to make money you set up a bone marrow transplant unit.

During the 1990s there was a big push to set up franchises for bone marrow transplant. They'd be like McDonald's, you know, every town have their own bone marrow transplant franchise and they'd just run patients through it to the tune of you know $500,000. Insurance companies were being forced to pay for it even though it didn't work that well. The lobbying groups, here's where lobbying groups for patient advocacy can be misinformed. It was the patient advocacy groups that thought insurance companies should be required to pay for bone marrow transplant and they through congressional legislation insurance companies were forced to pay for it even though it's not that efficacious for most cancers. But there were groups that went to set up franchises. So, if you want to make money you go into conventional oncology.

Some of these oncology drugs, like Avastin, can cost $10,000 a month and a lot of that is profit to the oncology. What's not generally appreciated by patients because oncologists are not required to inform patients of this. Is that oncologist's actually make money from the use of the chemo in their own office.

Thirty years ago, chemo was usually given in hospitals, that's completely changed. Now oncologists give it to them in their office. Every oncologist has, you know a set of offices where they administer chemo, the nurse does, and you'll have ten-fifteen patients getting chemo at any one time. And that's pure profit to the oncologist. They don't even have to see the patient. The nurse does all the work. And some of these drugs like Avastin are enormous profit makers event though they don't work very well and the oncologist makes the profit. The drug company makes some of it, but the oncologist makes a lot of it. Oncologists do not make their money from office visits. They make the money from the use of chemo in their office. And they're allowed to do that ethically, morally and legally. They're allowed to do that. To make money off the use of chemo in their office.

The Wall Street Journal estimated that the minimal amount of money an oncologist makes on the use of chemo per year, this is a minimal now as a $100,000 but some of these doctors are making millions of dollars a year from the use of drugs in their office. So, there's a financial incentive for oncologists to use chemo in their office. So, to answer, the short answer to your question, if you want to make money, you don't do what I do, you go into something else.

Ian: I have a person right now that's one of the children that are being murdered by the chemo for their leukemia. And of course, it's not working, the chemo's not working. And they won't let 'em do anything other than that. But the next step is going to be bone marrow transplant, right, isn't that what they for it.

Dr. Nick Gonzalez: usually, yeah. If chemo fails, then they do a bone marrow transplant. If initially fails that they don't go into remission you get more aggressive and you do a bone marrow transplant.

Ian: Could you as an M.D. Expert right now pretend, I'm the Judge and tell me what your opinion is on doing the bone marrow transplant for this child?

Dr. Nick Gonzalez: Well I don't know the specifics of the case. And you know, I try and be really scientifically objective. There are people who have been cured of cancer with bone marrow transplant and they're few and far between. For example, for breast cancer turned out to be a big fiasco and even conventional doctors don't use it anymore because it was proven not to work and it's expensive and deadly.

The problem with bone marrow transplants is several. First, they're very toxic. Now when I was doing them minimally ten to thirty percent of the patients getting bone marrow transplants would die from the procedure itself. It's a very toxic procedure. With a bone marrow transplant, a lot of people don't know what that is. What you're trying to do is use very high doses of chemo and radiation, far higher than you would normally administer at such doses that it would normally kill a patient because it would wipe out the bone marrow. So you use these high doses trying to kill every cancer cell in the body, then you salvage the patient by transplanting bone marrow so their bone marrow regenerates. The limitation with most chemo and radiation is the fact you go into bone marrow failure and die. So what the bone marrow transplant it was the hypothetical and practical thought that you could use these really high doses and then salvage the patient.

Well for most cancers it's proven not to work. But there are some cancers, to be honest, to be fair and to be completely scientifically objective, like acute leukemia of childhood where sometimes it actually works. Now often it doesn't work. I remember taking care when I was under Dr. Good, it was about a 20-year-old kid, a young adult with acute lymphocytic leukemia which is supposed to be one of the cancers that responds to chemo. Well, he didn't respond. And then he had a bone marrow transplant and then he died. And I remember it was a horrible, horrible death. I mean he was swollen like a balloon. He went into liver, kidney failure and I swore when I was doing it, I said, "I don't ever wanna be involved with this!" It was such, to see that young man die. And yes, well maybe if you had the bone marrow transplant, he would have died anyway and maybe this was a last-ditch resort. But it was a very tragic death. So, it doesn't work frequently, but it does work occasionally. So, there is scientific justification to argue with acute leukemia of childhood, it does work sometimes for those patients. But sometimes it doesn't and ten to thirty percent of people still can die from the procedure. With new technology and more knowledge, the salvage rate is higher, but still, a lot of patients die directly from the transplant. So, it's really risky business.

Ian: What would you do if it was you, ya had no AMA to tell you what to do if your child had leukemia?

Dr. Nick Gonzalez: Well, first I admit out front, I'm biased because I believe in what I do. I wouldn't be doing this for the last 25 years if I didn't believe in it. I don't have children so it's easy for me to think hypothetically and give advice. But, you know, if I had cancer I never would do standard therapy. If I had a kid I would never do a bone marrow transplant. I was trained to do them by the guy who did the first bone marrow transplant in history and the guy who was President of Sloane Kettering. So, I know about bone marrow transplants. I would not do it. It would... first, it's too risky. It's toxic.

The other problem, even when it succeeds the doses of chemo and radiation that are administered are so high and chemotherapy and radiation are mutagenic, a lot of these patients that are cured years later develop secondary cancers caused by the chemo.

For example, there's a group at Stanford under Rosenberg, who have been studying cured patients with Hodgkin's disease. Hodgkin's is one of the few, there are over a hundred different types of cancer, maybe six responding to chemo. It's one of the few cancers that respond well to chemo. Trouble is the doses that you use and the drugs that you use are very carcinogenic and mutagenic themselves and it's estimated now up to 25 percent of the patients cured of their Hodgkins diseases by standard therapies are developing secondary cancers years later, sometimes six months later, sometimes 20 years later. And when you develop a secondary cancer brought on by the previous chemo and radiation they're very aggressive treatment resist and usually patients die very, very quickly.

So, the downside of even the cured patients is they live under a sword, you know, dramatically it's hanging over their head that at some point there's a likelihood, a strong likelihood and the percentage keeps going up as more and more patients are out longer and longer developing a secondary treatment-resistant aggressive type cancer, often a secondary leukemia or a sarcoma, they're very aggressive, don't respond to chemo and radiation, patients die quickly.

You might argue, well you got some light. You know, they had a period of time when they were cancer free. That's true. But the point of that story is not to condemn chemo or be like, you know, the conventional guys condemning me, I'm going to condemn all of them, well, yeah.

The fact is, it's not a good way to treat people, there have to be better ways. Even when it works, there's a downside. Even when it does cure people and it does and I'd be lying if I said, "It never works." It does work at times for some cancers in some situations. But even when it works there's a downside, it's very toxic. And you're at risk always for developing secondary treatment-resistant cancers.

So, it's not a wonderful magical treatment. Back in the 1960s when multi-agent chemotherapy first was developed, the first disease they were really using it with was Hodgkins and it had some of these miraculous results and they thought this would be the end of cancer. Well, it didn't turn out that way. Most cancers don't respond to chemo and even when it does there all the downsides that we were just talking about the secondary cancers enormous toxicity, they're never the same. The chemo regimens used for Hodgkin s make men and women sterile, so they can't have kids.

Even if you don't get a secondary cancer, your immune system would be affected forever. So there all these other things. It's not a perfect way to live and the purpose of medicine is not just to get you over the disease but to get you well and doctors forget that. And chemo may get you over the disease sometimes in some circumstances with some patients but it's not going to get you well in the sense of optimal health. We need better ways.

Ian: And what would your way be?

Dr. Nick Gonzalez: Well the way I approach cancer is nutritional. And we have our own approach it's an individualized diet. Every patient we see gets a diet designed for their metabolism. Now in the alternative world, a lot of practitioners have one diet for everybody. My mentor, Dr. Kelly realized different people need different diets.

We have ten basic diets, they range from plant-based, fruits, vegetables to red meat like an Atkins diet three times a day. Every patient gets a diet designed for their needs. Ten basic diets, dozens of variations that we choose from. Large doses of supplements. Every patient we see gets a very aggressive supplement program, vitamins, minerals, trace elements, glandular products like liver or thymus from organically raised beef cattle. We don't believe the vitamins and minerals, trace elements will cure cancer, but they help to regenerate the normal tissues so the body can fight the cancer better.

The main anti-cancer element of our program is large doses of pancreatic enzymes derived from a pig source. Dr. Beard a hundred and ten years ago in 1902 first proposed that pancreatic enzymes have an anti-cancer effect. In orthodox physiology it was known then, it's known now that pancreatic enzymes are digestive enzymes. They break down food. That's how we digest, protein, fats, carbohydrates.

In addition, above and beyond that, Beard said a hundred and ten years ago that pancreatic enzymes represent the body's main defense against cancer would be useful as a cancer treatment. He proved that both in laboratory studies and with human patients a hundred years ago, but he was never taken seriously even though he was a full professor at the University of Edinburgh, very eminent scientist who was nominated for the Nobel Prize in 1906.

But at the same time, Madam Curie with two Nobel Prizes under her belt suggested that radiation was a simple easy way to cure cancer and that's how cancer research really went in the wrong direction. Madame Curie was a media star. She was one of the first great media stars of the last hundred years. She knew how to use the media even in those days. And she had this wonderful story of this Polish immigrant, one of the first women to get a Ph.D. D. In theoretical physics in a Western University and her husband was a physicist. And in 1895, X rays were discovered, and she immediately saw that this presented enormous medical possibilities both diagnostically you could see into the body with an x-ray they never thought you could do that before.

And, also practically in terms of treatment. So, by 1905 when Beard was talking about enzymes, Madame Curie was saying, radiation is going to cure cancer, which she doesn't realize it doesn't cure most cancers even when the tumors regress they often come back more aggressively. And it's extremely toxic and she herself would die from radiation-induced aplastic anemia where her bone marrow failed, as a result of radiation exposure.

So, Beard suggested a hundred years ago enzymes thought would be the main anti-cancer element, the body, we use pancreatic enzymes to treat cancer today. That's out main anti-cancer component.

The third component, first, diet, second, supplements with enzymes, third is detoxification which raises the hackles of my conventional colleagues probably more than any other aspect of our program. As the body repairs and rebuilds and as tumors break down a lot of toxic debris is realized, and that stuff can really overload the liver and the kidney and make people sick.

In conventional medicine they realize this can happen too with chemo if you break a tumor down too fast you can poison the liver, poison the kidney, they call it tumor lysis syndrome the patient can die. Well, it happens in our therapy too that tumors break down, people get sick.

So, we have a series of procedures like the infamous coffee enemas and liver flushes and juice flushes and juice fast that are very simple techniques that are very effective that help a body mobilize, neutralize and excrete the debris that are realized during the reparative process and when tumor breaks down.

So, we have individualized diet, individualized supplements with enzymes and detoxification routines and that's the therapy we use which we find extremely effective and that's why I've devoted 25 years of my life to this instead of bone marrow transplantation. [Chuckles]

Ian: Right!
[See Pic 15.1]

CHAPTER 16:

REV. LYNNE HEROD-DeVERGES (Essene Master)

Phat Boy Slim reigns out!!! Right here right now, right here, right now, right here, right now, right here, right now, right here, right now!

Host: Ladies and Gentlemen… we have Mr. Ian Jacklin. Mr. Ian Jacklin, how are you tonight, sir?

Ian: I am doing great, doing great! How are you guys in New York?

Host: Everything is great. It's actually getting cold here finally.

Ian: Yeah, here too. I can't lay out by the pool anymore.

Host: No, no, we've covered those up.

Ian: Right on, well thanks a lot of guys. I got my good old friend and one of my spiritual gurus, Rev. Lynne with us today. How are you doing Rev. Lynne?

Lynne: Good. How are you?

Ian: I'm doing very good, very good. It's so good to reconnect after all these years. A lot of my friends I brought to you… just so people know what Rev. Lynne does. She's an Essene which Jesus Christ was an Essene. The Essenes wrote the Dead Sea Scrolls. They were the higher sort of more evolved of the people back in the day and always have been sort of from what I understand, and she teaches meditations and course of miracle things like that. So, we have a lot to talk about. This stuff all blew my mind, cause' I was raised in conventional style. My grandfather was a minister of the church, my father was the organist for the church. We were Episco...palian. I can never say it.

Lynne: Episcopalian.

Ian: Episcopalian is America. We call Anglican in Canada. So, and I know, I've got nothing bad to say an about Church. My family were very open and let me believe whatever I wanted. They presented me with what they knew, and they were always open for me to find my own way. And I've studied most of the religions.

And the one that I gravitate most to as far as spiritual connection goes is this one. The Essenes. And Christs. I mean Jesus Christ was the man. I don't care if you're a Christian or not. You gotta' admit Jesus Christ was probably the coolest cat ever to hit earth, other than maybe Santa Claus.

Lynne: [Laughing]

Ian: But it's the same thing, kind of. But anyways...

Lynne: It is the same thing [chuckling].

Ian: Yeah let's try and not offend anyone that's you know old school, Jesus bible thumper style. And at the same time kind of give people something else to look for. The thing I liked about this meditation is that it is proactive. I never liked going to a church and just sitting there listening to hymns and praying and sermons. It wasn't proactive enough. Whereas when I came to your school, I learned that we can, actually physically, mentally, emotionally do things proactive that will stop us from self-sabotaging from whatever it is.

So, we got a lot of good stuff to talk about. Why don't we just start with you introducing yourself and how you got to where you are. Where I come to see you now for spiritual guidance. Give us your history. Thanks.

Lynne: Alright. Well actually as you said, I'm an Essene Minister. Also, and I'm going to talk a little bit about the Essenes in just a moment. But as an Essene Minister there are various things that I do which include spiritual mentoring, clairvoyant and intuitive readings as well as energy healing, and also I am known as the Miracle Maker and I assist people in being able to create Miracles in their lives from a very conscious way. So as an Essene and for those of you who may not be familiar with the Essenes. The Essenes are a very ancient, very old community that was part of the Coumarone? The area along the Dead Sea. And, The Dead Sea Scrolls were actually written by the Essenes. So, the Essenes were mystical, if you will, spiritual community that was made up primarily of Jews but there were also Muslims, there were Islamics, there were Buddhists. There were all different types of spiritual faiths and beliefs that whoever chose to learn more to rise above, whatever their particular teaching for great enlightenment, they were able to join this community.

So, within the community, there were many things that were taught. There were many of the sciences, physics, geology, biology, chemistry which is where you get alchemy from. There were just many, many, many different sciences, astronomy, and astrology. As well as learning how to do other various things such as they knew how to commune with the earth. So, they were very big when it came to gardening, when it came to preparing the right foods, and eating the right foods in order for the body to stay, not only pure, but they recognized and understood that the physical body is living organism and so if you want to have healthy cell tissue you eat living healthy food.

They studied many different things including crystals and the power and the vibration of crystals and they also spoke to the spirit world, angels and spirit guides, ancestors, very much like you and I communicate and talk to each other. So, the Essenes were very advanced from a spiritual standpoint, again, very enlightened. And most people did see them as the mystical sect. You know, they weren't quite sure what to make of them. Well, the Essenes that were the most popular of course besides Mary, Joseph, John the Baptist, his parents, Elizabeth and Isaiah, and also Jesus, of course, was the most famous Essene.

The Essenes are today still practicing some of those same types of teachings. Teachings that involve what we call now metaphysics which is also known as quantum physics were really moving into the realm and that understanding as well as teaching about nutrition, the health of the body. How to basically continue to live and to live from a consciousness that is completely and totally engulfed in the state of being love and connecting with that love with all people and all things.

So as an Essene today there is what's called discernment. Most people would either call that either psychic or intuitive and by the way everyone is. As an Essene, there is energy healing. Everything is energy. Everything! And because all things are energy then that means that we can shift and move and change energy, in many different ways. So, what you think is energy, what you feel is energy, your emotions are energy, what you see, what you touch, your body, the things around you, it's all forms of energy. Of course, we know that science has already proven this. Science has also proven that there is more space than there is matter and in between matter, matter is those cells, they're atomic particles, subatomic particles, the smallest measurement of matter so far are photons which is actually matter at the speed of light and so or that is light.

And so in between matter is energy. And that energy is part of what we know as the divine consciousness of God consciousness, universal consciousness, whatever name you'd like to use, that is indeed what is present. And the statement in the Bible that says, "We can do all things that Jesus did." Jesus, basically he was talking to his people at the time and he said, "All things I do, you can do as well!" And what that means is, that, we all have the ability to use our intuition. I don't know a single person on this planet who before caller ID would know who was calling before the phone... you know when the phone rang.

It's like before we heard or saw who it was, it's like, "Oh that must be Shirley, let me pick it up!" We just intuitively were able to tune into so many things around us. And for many people, just the way that they made decisions, the things that they did, the way that their life is able to flow is based on their intuition whether they're conscious of it or not. So, we all have those dynamic abilities. We all have the ability to utilize our mind as a way to shift energy and so what that means is when we are able to think what it is that we desire and we take that desire and we feel good about it we start to feel excited and elated and joyful and just all of these fantastic feelings then our heart is able to open up and the emotion of love begins to be expressed and it is through this love that then the desire is actually manifested because you at that moment have a connection between mind, between feelings, between heart and because there is no such thing as time, past or future, whatever you desire as soon as you have the alignment and your heart is open to love you can manifest instantaneously because it's always in the present. Yes.

Ian: I'm experiencing this myself in unreal proportions for the first time in my life I've cleansed my body physically. I've been on a blending. And this is what the Essenes did they drank water, not wine. They were very into what they grew and meditation, cleaning everything out and apparently and I also was using Cannabis Hemp oil which cleanses the pineal gland. Then I told you this in our private conversation, I actually, believe it or not, folks, this happened, spoke telepathically to a friend of mine recently. And I just couldn't believe it. He wasn't into talking about it when it was over, but it happened in the moment. I was like, I could have sworn we were talking already, and like I did a million other times, "That's bullshit. It's not true. It can't be real!" But this time I was very, I'm opening up to it now, and I just literally yelled from my third eye at him, "Can you hear me?"

Lynne: [Chuckling]

Ian: He's like, "Yes, I can hear you!"

I'm like, "What?" It's like a little kid the first time you get on a walkie talkie with somebody, you know, I freaked out. I thought, "No, way is this happening." But he wasn't into like figuring out where that went. So, but anyway and just to let you people know from what I hear because now we're in the Age of Aquarius, we left the Dark Ages December 21, 2012, that this kind of thing is supposed to be happening. Our planet is now in a part of the solar system where we're in the light ages, the light is here and many more things like this may be happening. So, don't freak out if it happens to you, we're supposed to be evolving at this time.

Am I right about that, Reverend Lynne?

Lynne: You're absolutely correct! This is a time, we're on a mass consciousness-level, human beings are evolving. We are moving into what we call the upper chakras, okay. And for those of you that may not be familiar, there are seven primary chakras along the spine. The first chakra being at the base of the spine and then you work your way up to the seventh chakra which is at the crown or on top of your head. And so, we are evolving as a human race into those upper chakras of the fifth chakra which is communication and expression of spirit into the sixth chakra which is clear seeing or the third eye. And the seventh chakra which is the ability to know and it's our direct connection to the divine source and to all information, all universal information.

So, we are really moving and raising into those chakras, into those areas, and it's love, that's able to actually magnify it. Did you know by the way, that the heart is five times more powerful than the mind, and that what lies in your heart, is actually what emanates in terms of your power and your energy field!

Ian: Right, for when people are doing the course of miracles or the Abraham thing or the Secret thing which I learned from you long before the Secret... even before I think, oh what was the first one that I liked, the very first... oh, no it's not going to come to me... [finger snapping], the very first... the book that everybody first read when in the early 90s... What the Bleep Do We Know?

Lynne: Okay.

Ian: But... I want to get back to the smallest size I think they found now is quantum, it's even smaller than quantum, it's the quanta but that's just to make your point, there's way more space than there is matter.

Lynne: Yes.

Ian: In that unknown, it's somehow we're able to connect and the third eye sixth sense sort of way and our thoughts are energy just like the wind. You see the wind blow those leaves in the tree. We know what's happening. Well some of us... or I'm learning, and Reverend Lynne knows, and Cynthia knew, and a lot of our friends that are in the know, that there is that out there that third eye, that sixth sense is out there, and they know how to tap into it. And I've experienced a little bit of it myself and I think you're right, I think we all are that way we just so have so many disbeliefs about it, it's too hard to move forward.

Lynne: Yes, well there's a lot of what I call programming and conditioning that has convinced so many of us that at very young ages that what we're seeing or what we're feeling is not true. Even something as simple as a parent that may be feeling, maybe a little sad about something. And the child that four or five-year-old child goes up to their mom or their dad and they say, you know, "Are you sad? Or are you unhappy?" And the parent's like, "Oh, no, I'm feeling great. Everything's wonderful!" Well, the child in that moment has been invalidated as far as his feeling. He knows that there is something that's not quite right, that there is something that is wrong but as soon as you say, "Oh, no, everything's great! It's wonderful! Don't worry about it!" You know, "Let's go play with your blocks", or whatever. That immediately begins to program that child in believing that what they are feeling or what they are intuiting is incorrect, it's invalid. And that's just a very easy and simple example, as you know, it happens, in so many different ways; particularly with the imaginary friend and other such things that may take place that kids tap into because we're so open as small children and then we are slowly told, taught and through repetitious pattern shown that we can't trust our intuition, we can't trust that information. So, we start to shut it down.

Ian: I know. Cynthia brought up something brilliant recent on the show. A lady was asking about her brother who has schizophrenia and it's something that I'd always kind of thought and may be known on a deeper level, but she said... I can't remember how she presented it. But basically said, "He's not schizophrenic, he's just really physics!" And that's the thing...

Lynne: Yes.

Ian: people that are schizophrenic that are hearing voices. They're hearing voices but they're listening, the ones that have problems are listening to the wrong ones and I thought that was so well eloquently put by Cynthia. So those people out there hearing voices, they're connected folks but they're probably listening to the dark voices. Do you want to speak about that?

Lynne: Well they are definitely connected. There are many different types of dis-incarnate spirits that are around us. And although they're not always able to be seen, some people do see them, but many people also hear them. And so, by being open to it you hear everything. The analogy is like Whoopee Goldberg in Ghost. I don't know, for those of you that saw it as soon as she actually allowed herself, to open up.

First, she was pretending it was a con. And then, she actually heard Patrick Swayze's voice and went, "Oh, whoa, wait a minute." And then, of course, all the other spirits are like, "She can actually hear us!" So, what happened, she was bombarded. And so, for someone that does not know how to maintain a level of balance for someone who has a lot of maybe fears of phobias, for someone who is really bombarded that can be an extremely overwhelming situation and some of the dis-incarnate spirits, just like those of us who have physical bodies, you know, not everyone is necessarily working to be closer to the light.

Some people have a passion for murder or robbery or whatever they do. Well, there are dis-incarnate spirits that also have a passion for all different forms of expression. And so, there are times when voices that are heard or dis-incarnate spirits that people hear they may be very, very, very relentless in telling someone what to do or how to do it or whatever the case may be because that's part of what they want, as-a-way to feed them. They don't have physical bodies. So, they get fed by being able to sometimes, shall we say, direct or confuse someone who does have a body.

Ian: Absolutely, and this is something for all your guys out there that have maybe fallen on tough times and you fell into a whiskey bottle. These spirits, these negative spirits love alcoholics and drug addicts and people that are just lost because they can get into your body and stay there, and they are more than happy with the fact that you like to sit there at the bar and drown your miseries and stuff too and they'll keep you there forever.

So, there's another thing if you have any addiction problems you could have a negative entity affecting that. Because I got a reiki healing done by a lady like yourself who's not just reiki like you're obviously is not Reiki, you're connected to the light and so is she. When she was done the healing, she asked me, "If you felt anything?" And I said, "No." And then all of a sudden, I felt like this, like somebody was doing this. But there's a wall behind me. And I kept looking around, I'm like, "What the hell!" And I had a tight New York Yankees bat ball cap on, so I'll never forget it. And I felt something flip, blip, blip, blip and when came out here a flat chip about that big, kind of like what you pop out of a VHS tape fell out of my head, I swear to God, she saw this, so I don't think I'm crazy and it fell on the floor and it disappeared. We both looked at each other like, "What was that?" I'm like, "You're the psychic, you tell me!" So, she had to ask her teacher and she said it was probably psychic plasma or some kind of negative energy, cause I had just gotten out of one of those dark places where I was going to dark seedy locations and just nursing myself to death basically and I had snapped out of it and I was getting myself healthy. I was listening to the Abraham tapes and I was sweating, working out and I got this reiki thing and a literal physical thing fell out of my head and disappeared. What do you say about something like that?

Lynne: You know again I would say that it is obviously a form of energy. When a person is intoxicated regardless of what form it takes. You know, whether it is drinking or pills or drugs or whatever. There is... you do leave yourself more vulnerable for various types of energy to get into your space. Now it doesn't always necessarily mean that there is a spirit that has come into your space literally. Sometimes there are influences that these spirits can have stand being several feet away but because you are so open they can still have an influence in terms of what you might do or what you might say or how you may behave. But one of the things that I think, is really important for people to understand, is that there is no energy regardless of how... I don't use the words negative and positive because all energy is just a form of expression. Some of it is... are forms of expression that you desire, and other energies are forms of expression you never really want to have to have expressed. But the energy that is not for your best and highest good. Okay. That energy can never ever, ever, get into your space or have an influence over you if you are at a vibration if you are at a frequency and a vibration that is of the light. When I talk about frequency vibration it's exactly what it sounds like tuning into a frequency channel on your radio or your television or even your computer and every form of energy vibrates. Some vibrate a little slower, some a little faster. You know, they vibrate in different ways.

So if you are vibrating in a pattern that is really, really high energy and close to and very close to the light or to what I like to call the Godhead. Then an energy that would have you cuss somebody out, beat somebody up, stay in a pattern of always, you know, getting drunk or not showing up on time to work or whatever the case may be those kinds of energies would never be able to take over your space or even get close enough to do anything because you would be at a whole different vibration. Understand what I'm saying. Which is why meditation is so important. That's why meditation is really, really, important.

Ian: Yeah, and I've noticed lately since I've been meditating more and cleansing physically and stuff that I experience almost constantly not quite, but quite a bit love. Constant love. And, it's weird cause it's almost like I'm all giddy and in love and I want to tell somebody about my new girl, but I don't have a new girl. I'm in love with my...

Lynne: With yourself.
Ian: My being here.
Lynne: Yes.
Ian: Yeah, it's hard for me to say, "I'm in love with myself." But I'm in love with being allowed to be in this body and be on this earth at this time. I mean I really learned to appreciate things and have some gratitude and I think I lost it there for a while. I think I got a little high and mighty in my kickboxing days and my karate man days with the movies and stuff and then when that didn't happen, and I had to go back to, being a regular person, working at a bar or digging ditches the really hitting ya on top of some other things. So, in my wisdom, as it gracefully came to me it's like I'm just non-stop so happy I kind of just want to start screaming out and yelling at people you know and singing and stuff [chuckling].

Lynne: And it's okay. [chuckling] you can do that. You can sing in the rain or sunshine. [chuckling]
Ian: I'll tell ya I haven't sung in the rain and the last time I sang in the rain was because of a girl. This time I'm singing in the rain, cause of you know life, god!

Lynne: Yes.

Ian: And that's where ya all want to get to. All you young guys out there, you want to get to that spot where no woman, no anything, no job, nothing can ever affect you. You want to be... get that vibration Reverend Lynne's talking about and once you get it, they can't... the outside forces can't really get you if you stay on that level.

Lynne: That's true. That's very true. And so again, which is why meditation is so important. Even from, you know, everything that I talk about spiritually I also reference in terms of science because science is moving into a wonderful, wonderful space of validating so many things that spiritualists and particularly the eastern philosophies, the Essenes and others have known for years. People didn't necessarily believe it, or they didn't think it was true, well now, science is literally able to validate it through experiments, through sensitive instrumentation that they use. Because when we meditate the brain waves and brain patterns are completely altered and they're altered in such a way that one of the things that have been proven most recently is that when you have a thought about anything and then you have the feeling that goes with it, it is already done and experienced. When you experience it in here when you experience it in here, it will, it must show up externally. And that's because, again, the heart is a giant magnet. So, what it is that you love right here, right now, is what shows up in your experience. And no matter what if you have a thought that may lean toward lack or fear, if you are then experiencing feelings of depression or apathy of jealousy or you know, and again of the lower vibrational type of feeling then what is going to emit from your heart as far as an emotion is going to be fear. And what happens you magnetize or call to you that which you fear. So as soon as you begin a process of keeping your mind focused on what you truly desire. Thinking about what your choice to experience at this moment and then feel the exhilaration of that and as you were just saying Ian experience the Love of that, then you are able to actually call that into your realm or into your own personal reality.

Ian: Yeah. Yeah. Exactly. And I can't wait until... being in this situation now, I can't wait until I do meet the right girl and I'm able to give her this pure kind of love. There's no neediness, there's no like I need you to make me whole. It's like, "What do you think? You like it!"

Lynne: [Chuckles] Yeah. [Laughing]
Ian: Effort, on this and this. So, I hope you like it. Let's rock n roll. Let's make some kids.
Lynne: Yes.

Ian: I'm a little on that schedule yeah.

Lynne: Yes, no. No.

Ian: Did I just say that?

Lynne: No, no... it's...

Ian: [chuckling] Sorry.

Lynne: That's exactly, no that's exactly it. Because you are so in love with yourself and in love with life right now because you are thinking life mate, joyousness, excitement, companionship and you are in love with that. You will be... you are attracting her as we speak.

Ian: Right.

Lynne: In fact, she might be listening to this show right now. [Laughing]

Ian: Hey, baby.

Lynne: You never know.

Ian: Where ya been? [Chuckling]

Lynne:[Laughing]

Ian: I got some dishes back there, just kidding, just kidding.

Lynne: [Chuckling]

Ian: Hope you didn't hear that. Anyway... well yeah, that's... I mean, it's going great. And I want everybody else to experience it too. And what we want to do with this show too, is do this 30-day miracle thing, you guys. This is free folks. I'm going to do it. And if anybody else wants to do it, you know, get on my Facebook... or sign in to wherever this is written down in the Facebook events and for 30 days we can practice this together I'm going to do it too... meditation kind of thing. And I know it works cause I've done it before and right now I'm looking at something that says, "What are you manifesting?" I actually... it was I think a tattoo you rub on somebody's arm, but I put it on my computer because I realize so many times in a day I'll catch myself... like I used to be really negative, I used to be hard on myself. That's how... you know, I became a champion kickboxer for a reason, I had to learn to believe in myself. And so, but even to this day I'll have negative thoughts happening, but I catch them because of what you said, if you think of it too long it may happen. So, I catch 'em I see a light just sort of... we used to be a video game we played was you could hit the button, it just swooooshhhhh bombed the whole screen and cleared everything out, so I just feel that in my head and my heart any time negative things in my head I just [snaps fingers] zap it out white light and I think that's for another movie, not mine. [Chuckles] Right?

Lynne: Yeah. So that's very true. Now, the 30-day creating miracle plan is one that is a series of exercises that are only about 10 to 15 minutes a day. But as you work the exercises, you will begin to notice a shift in the way that you think. In the way that you feel.

You'll be able to notice even some of those energies, such as thoughts or belief systems, habit patterns, things that you've heard and experienced in your life even those will start to come to your awareness that may be against what your desire is. And there's something that you can do about that too. Because on an unconscious level we do have various experiences that may have happened when we were five years old or 15 or you know at whatever age, at whatever time, whatever the experience and if those experiences are going or moving against what we desire as you do these exercises, as you get clearer about what you do chose to create and as you begin the process of creating them you're going to notice some other, what I call, really lower vibrational energies start to surface. When that happens the first thing you want to do is give thanks for it. You have to be in gratitude. Do not resist ANYthing, cause' everything is an absolute lesson for you to learn from for you to correct form and then move forward. So, if you have a thought, something like, "Oh God, I don't have any money. I'm broke. You know, I really wish I had some more money!" That is a belief system and a thought around lack and if what you are choosing or your desire to manifest is to get a big raise at your job or to manifest a lot more money that belief system goes against that desire. Do you see what I'm saying? But instead of going, "Ah, I shouldn't think that. I can't think about it. I have to like, you know, do something different!" That's resistance to that energy, to that lack energy. And when you resist it, you immediately open into an emotion of fear and when you go into fear, you're going to attract more of that lack. So, the best thing to do is give thanks. "Thank you for showing up! Thank you for showing me where I still have this belief system where I am not moving in a consciousness of my true desire. I appreciate you for that and now you may exit!" You know.

Ian: Really? I deal with so many cancer patients, you know and the one thing I can tell where their heads are at? The ones that are grateful, even if they don't believe a word you're saying and are never going to use you again, they're grateful you took time to talk to them. And the other ones, who need it the most, are usually not so grateful and cut up everything you have to say even though you're giving them proof after proof. So, I've learned to deal with that, that's an interesting thing. And somebody that is grateful, they are... talk about high vibration, you know, the level of vibration of a human being. Somebody that gets that is high vibration.

Lynne: Absolutely. Absolutely. Well, the 30-day miracle plan will help you to raise that vibration and move into that consciousness. Now I do want to share with your audience as well that for everyone who is part of your audience and ZenLive TV if you sign up for the 30-day creating miracle plan, then once a week we can all get together on a conference call for an hour and you can all ask me personally different questions that you have, you can share your experiences and I'll also be sharing some additional information and feedback based on where you are.

So, for everybody listening, if you sign up, then we will have a conference call once a week for four weeks and we'll have a … you'll get a chance to really hone in on what your heart's desire is and being able to consciously create that for yourself very quickly.

Ian: Wow, what an offer that is folks for you. You don't have any idea. I mean, she's like a $150 an hour counselor that movie starts come after. So, for her to give us free time like that, that's awesome. And just so you know, she has a ton of services. She does Angel Readings, she can be just a friend to shoot the breeze with cause' they got that whole psychic thing too, so they can help with problems. My one good friend, Julianna she still thanks you to this day. She didn't come to see you, we used your energy healings once a week, Tuesday nights you'd go in. And Reverend Lynne does hits, she closes her eyes, she looks at you, she sees your aura and your chakras, and she'll sit there and clean things out, cut cords off that people have attached to you and stuff so you can free up and then you can ask questions. And anyway, Reverend Lynne saw that my friend had a baby growing in her tube, had she not gone to the doctor and verified that she probably could have died from something like that. That's just one of the many stories.

So this is a really good opportunity, thanks for offering it to me and my friends. So hopefully a few people will join up and you'll see how this works. Now the key point that I learned, you can't use this to manifest things. You have-to-use this as Reverend Lynne says, it has to be the heart. This is the energy. So, you can think it hear and if you send it out to the universe here, you tried that Secret stuff and it never worked for you, you'll get the opposite sometimes cause the way our brains are wired, negatively, positively, you'll get the opposite of what you want if you're all up here.

You have to really think it and feel it from here and I think that's why I've been manifesting things, you know, left, right and center since I learned that. Course, I come from a pure place.

Lynne: Yes.

Ian: A pure place of light, you know, you can't be manifesting, you know, hookers and lottery winnings, I don't think [chucking].

Lynne: Well no, you can. You know what, energy does not know positive or negative. If that's a person's true desire, yes, they can manifest those things too. And that's also part of it, is that in the manifestation process you cannot have any judgment about your own desires.

You know, and so sometimes a judgment can be, "I'd really like to have that Ferrari." And a judgment that may come up is, "Oh, you know, you can't afford that!" Or, "You know, that you're not the kind of person that's sporty like that." Or, "You know, only this kind of person drives that kind of car!"

That's a judgment that you may have against yourself or a judgment that you may feel someone else would have against you. So those are also some of the things through the 30-day miracle plan that are important for you to shift and turn around and clear so that you can just be in a place of, "You know what, I desire a Ferrari because I desire a Ferrari. It is totally okay for me to have that. I choose to have it. I love having it. I love being in it. It's phenomenal." And you feel yourself experiencing it then you're able to really bring it to you.

Ian: Right. I see what you're saying. Whereas some people may think you're selfish for wanting something like that, you're as valid in asking for that like anything else, what your heart desires. And you deserve good things like Ferrari's and stuff, you know, personally I would start a little smaller and draw less attention to you cause' you'll probably get carjacked but you know...

Lynne: [Chuckling]

Ian: [Chuckling]

Lynne: Well...

Ian: [Laughing]...

Lynne: We'll make sure that Ferrari is in a nice safe garage. [laughing] With lots of security.

Ian: Yeah lots of security. Well, that's great so we'll hit on this. We'll do this, people sign up. You know, go to my I Cure Cancer even my email, Facebook or whatever and everybody that was a part of this tonight we'll start a little group and we'll see what we can manifest for ourselves over the next month.

I know what I need to do as far as my production company and I got people out there with cancer. This would be perfect, if you got cancer you're manifesting it. Let's talk about that, how can they use it for healing with their sickness?

Lynne: Well again, everything is about first of being able to have a clear intention. So, it's having the thought and it's having the awareness of being and extremely healthy, no cancer. Then it's feeling, it's really allowing yourself and through meditation, I just can't stress that enough.

It's absolutely changing your brain wave pattern so that your body feels the experience of being healthy and being without cancer and being whole. And so, as you feel that and as you think that and as you envision that and as you intend your health you love it it just... you don't even have to try to love it, your heart will automatically move into a vibration of love and the more you resonant with that every single day the cancer can absolutely change it will absolutely leave.

Now some people are accustomed to practicing these techniques and they've practiced them and practiced them to the extent where, again, they manifest, right here, right now. Because, when you're in the present with the thought, and the feeling energy doesn't know about the past and it doesn't know about the future. If you find it seems to take a long time or it doesn't work it's only because there are some decisions, some belief system, different types of programming and conditioning that you have experienced that tell you it's not possible.

So, what I propose are certain tools and certain things you can do to eliminate and to transmute those belief systems and those patterns that say, "Well that's impossible." Or, "That's too hard!" Or, "The doctor says," or "This isn't supposed to be this way." Or whatever the reason is, those are, again, energies that aren't necessarily negative energies, but they aren't in alignment with what your desiring.

So, there is a way to clear those energies and it's really a form of integration in such a way that you become neutral and that doesn't mean you don't feel, it just means that you don't have any kind of charge on the cancer and you can just simply love being in the experience of being healthy and living your life fully and when you are in that experience that's when it happens.

It's no different than, Ian, you are a spirit in a male body. I'm a spirit in a female body. I don't walk around all day thinking, "Oh, I'm a woman, I'm a woman." You don't walk around all day going, "Well I'm a man. I'm a man." You just are a man. You go about doing what you do. Right? You're not giving any emphasis to yourself being a man or you know one way or another.

Just like you don't think about, "I'm breathing air. I'm breathing air. Oops! I better not stop breathing. I have to breathe the air. I need more air." You don't think that. You're just breathing air. Well, when you are that neutral and when you can be in that consciousness with cancer or whatever it is that you chose to and desire to experience that will be your experience. And so, it's really quite a simple process. It is a five-step process if you will over the 30 days that will start you on your way. Now I am not going to promise at the end of 30 days you'll have a miracle. Some people have absolutely gotten their desire at the end of 30 days. Some people have gotten other desires that they had that they didn't even start off with before the 30 days was over and then they got what they desired at the end of 30 days. Some people may take a little bit longer. We are all in different places along our path of enlightenment so what this will do though is, it will really start to shift your thinking, shift your feeling and shift the emotion from fear into love so that you can begin to really embrace life and love a life that you would like to have. I want to let people know as well if they can also go to the Center of Light Miracles.org. So, you can go to Ian's site at I Cure Cancer and you can to CenterofLightMiracles.org and at the very top of the home page is a banner that says, try the Free 30-day Miracle Plan.

Ian: Right. Yeah and I'll make sure I post that on my Facebook Event as well. And so, this is a perfect opportunity to check it out for free to see what Cynthia and I have always been talking about for years and have had Reverend Lynne on a couple of my different shows.
There is a method to this madness folks, is all I can say. And the way Cynthia got me in to learn it, if nothing else, the thought process of the meditation is stimulating your electrical circuit in your brain and it's good, you're building brain cells if nothing else.

Lynne: Exactly.

Ian: if it's all a bunch of hogwash, who cares. But... I'll tell you what, every single person that's been cured of cancer by chemo, radiation or surgery, to me, that's a placebo effect, cause there's a 3 percent success rate for chemo on tumor type cancers. So, if you cured yourself of cancer using chemo it was probably your brain that did it. And these are proactive ways, again, instead of sitting in Sunday School and singing Jesus loves me, which to me you already know that you actually, can use these meditations you learn on how to bring good things to you, how to protect you from bad things. And again, if nothing else, it's stimulating your mind. The thing I wanted to bring up about the dead sea scrolls, the whole quantum physics thing and the reason why... see the dead sea scrolls, the most important thing in that book, as far as I'm concerned, is the fact that they left... that it had reincarnation in it. It talks about reincarnation.

Lynne: Yes.

Ian: Dead Sea Scrolls are books that were conveniently left out of the Bible that speak about things like reincarnation because the Church didn't want you to know that you have eternal life already. You don't need the Church, you don't need the Pope, you don't need any... you have eternal life already and that was in the Dead Sea Scrolls. And those kinds of people, the Essenes were just like that. I mean, they just knew, again, water instead of wine and meditated and understood.

And so, these are from THEN, these meditations are from back then, before Christ. I mean, it's amazing this stuff. So, this is an opportunity to try it out folks for free and if you like it cool. It'll definitely help you out; I know it helped me out. And so, good, thank you so much for that.

Lynne: Absolutely. Absolutely. I will say that Jesus, again, was the most popular Essene and really did make spirituality popular. But you know, part of the reason why the Church did not want so many of those writings and scriptures included in the Bible... first-of-all the Bible would be, you know, like huge [chuckles]...

Ian: Right.

Lynne: even bigger than that. But with at least, you know, 150 volumes, but beyond that, back in the day, the Church was also the state and so it was always about the state or the government being able to have control over people and what they saw is that people were beginning to believe in the one source, the one God and so if this is what people are believing, rather than punish them for believing that and going that way, let's just jump on that bandwagon and use that as a way to keep people within the confines of the government and under this power and Constance Standpole was the one who really started part of that movement.

So that's the reason why the Church left many things out of the writings that they felt if people knew about it they would... the Church would not have control. Really it was about the government would not have control. So that's why it was formed in that way. But you know, I would love as my experience to be able to read many of the Dead Sea Scrolls, of course, we know that they are spread out throughout the world various different religious and spiritual sects have the Dead Sea Scrolls, they're not in one place anymore. And so... and of course, they're very old, they're very fragile. I don't know what's been interpreted. And I don't even know if the interpretations would be true, to what was actually said. Because it was written in a language that's now a dead language. Nevertheless, it would be wonderful to have an idea of many of the scrolls what was really told and what was taught. Now the Essenes, again, they were a people who were scientists, who were open people of love. And I always have seen Jesus as a master teacher.

When the Jews, you know, from the time of Adam they wanted to really create what's considered a superhuman. They wanted to create someone who was so High and so divine that this person would be able to lift or uplift their faith in their people. And so that's why the Bible starts from Adam. Now Adam actually is a name for the Adamic race. And the Adamic race was a period like Neanderthal and so forth when man was on this earth. But it did not start... this world did not start with the Adamic race. Man was long before the Adamic race. But that's where the Jewish story began. Where it goes from Adam to Abraham. From Abraham to David. From David to Mary and then Mary had Jesus. And this superhuman was to be a man who would be able to embody the full essence and spirit of one who was truly enlightened and like God. That was their intention. And they knew because of their wonderful study of science and so forth. They knew very clearly that based on the alignment of the stars and based on the time period that he would soon be born.

Now, do you know that when Mary was born, Mary was one of three girls that they believed could have been the superhuman as Jesus. And then they quickly realized that it wasn't one of those girls, but that one of those three girls would have that child. And they pinpointed it to Mary being the one who would have that child. And so, it was very nicely orchestrated in such a way for her to become impregnated so that she was able to have Jesus. And there were certain men who were selected to impregnate her and then they narrowed it down to one, because that particular person with Mary they knew... again, they were very advanced smart people. They knew that they would create this wonderful, if you will, superhuman. In the translation where it says, "The Virgin Mary." Virgins during the Essene time was not someone who did not have sex. A virgin was someone who had remained pure in her body and in her spirit. She did not eat certain foods. She did not do certain things. There was a level of education and a level of training she received to keep her heart, her intuition, her everything, very, very open. And so, she wasn't a virgin as in, no sex, she was a virgin in that women in the Essenes prepared their wombs and prepared their bodies in a very specific way to have their children, so they could have high vibrational children. In the translation it came down to virgin, a virgin was translated and turned into a woman who had no sex. But that wasn't actually true.

Ian: Right. Yeah. I've heard that story before. Yeah, there's a lot deeper... there's way more to the story than what the basic church will tell ya' that's for sure, once you do some reading.

Lynne: Yes.

Ian: Interesting. Here's some proof for people that we were talking about as far as quantum physics goes and all that. There's a guy named Gregg Braden, amazing, amazing speaker, guru kind of guy. He's got on tape in one of his lectures... now, of course, I have to just believe that this is true. I suppose somebody could have gone through a lot of work doing trick photography. But, basically, these three Chinese doctors chanted cancer out of a person's body with video cameras on the cancer in their body live. As they were chanting you could see the tumor disappear. I'm just going to believe that this was a scientist's experiment and true and there's no hogwash going on in there.

Lynne: Well it would make sense. Go ahead. It makes sense to me.

Ian: Yeah, well they did it. I mean, as far as I'm concerned, they did it. So... and the quantum physics I don't know the science behind but at somehow it does show how you can dissipate tumors by chanting with your mind.

Lynne: Well, yes. Well even... okay, going back to the fact that matter has more space than it does matter. So a tumor is nothing more than a collection of cells that are forms of matter. In between that matter are more space and more energy. Every energy has a vibration. When you sing, when you speak, when you play an instrument, any form of sound has a vibration. And if you know the right vibration that has the frequency to be able to break up the matter then it will dissipate and it can be reabsorbed into the body.

Ian: Right. Dr. Rife.

Lynne: So... you know, it makes sense. Um hmm.

Ian: Dr. Royal Raymond Rife invented the machine that sends out specific frequencies that he found for cancer cells. And it works, he was curing it from everybody and of course, they buried him, buried the information, as they always do with anything that works. But hey, once you learn this folks, what are they going to do? They can't take it away from you. It's all up here.

Lynne: Yes, that's true. It is. It is. And in all honesty even where medicine is today with what doctors are doing, with what pharmaceutical companies are doing and so forth we do also want to just give honor to them because they have assisted in a process of helping some people through that medium and form of expression to become healed. They have also brought some other people who chose a different form of expression, to become more aware as a way to become also, more enlightened. So, either way we want to just honor the fact that they have played an important role and an important part in the process of healing cancer, whether it's to raise your consciousness into enlightenment so that you heal it in other ways, or whether you utilize their methods, either way, you can benefit and get a healing from it.

Ian: Yeah, it's gratitude. We have-to-have gratitude even for big pharma.

Lynne: Absolutely.

Ian: And I'm glad you just flipped a switch for me because I'm always anti-big pharma and I'm a bit of a fighter, a bit of a scrapper and I get a little angry sometimes but you're right, we have to be... I gotta thank Big Pharma for teaching me this because if it wasn't for them doing it wrong for so long, I would have not figured out what was right. So... thank-you... big pharma. [Chuckle]

Lynne: [Chuckles]

Ian: [Laughing]

Lynne: That is the scrapper in you... [laughing].

Ian: That was a low vibrational, sorry about that. [Chuckles]

Lynne: No, no, no… No Judgment. It is what it is. It was just a form of expression. [Laughing]

Ian: Yeah. Yeah. But I love that. I'm glad you turned that around. We have to be in gratitude for them.

Lynne: Yes.

Ian: That is such a release. It's for health in general when you start... when I lost my attitude that, you know, God or the universe is against me when I finally just started realizing that I'm against me. And then I let that go and it was okay.

Lynne: Absolutely.

Well I want to let people know again they can get in touch with me through your Facebook, through your site, I Cure Cancer and also through my site www.CenterofLightMiracles.org

Ian: Yeah. And definitely. If you guys want to jump on this bandwagon with me, I'll do it. We'll do it for a month and we get to talk once a week for four weeks. And we'll see what happens with that. So again, thanks for that offer that was very kind of you.

Lynne: You're welcome. And it will be announced for everyone who signs up you will receive an email and it will be announced the evening and time. It will be the same day and the same time every week and if you can't be on the call you may email your questions, they'll be answered on the call and you can listen to the replay. You'll have a week to listen to the replay as well. So, don't feel like you'll miss out if it's on a day or a time that you can't listen to.

Ian: Yeah. And this will be just a good way for you to get your feet wet and see what I'm talking about. And you'll see it works. I mean, as I said, I never took one person to Reverend Lynne that didn't just get their mind blown with the things that they learned there. So, we'll all get together and do that. I'm trying to think if there's anything else I'm missing... I have one minute. I think we're good.

Lynne: I feel complete unless there's something else that you...

Ian: No, I think Cynthia helped me realize one day recently that helped, we need contrast. Because I'm wondering why can't there just be light. Why does it have to be yin and yang, dark and light? Why can't it just be light? And she says, "Well I guess we need contrast!" Would you be able to end this on a note like that?

Lynne: Well, yes. I would say that it is important for us to have contrast and because that's how we're able to move into those higher levels of enlightenment and start to become aware. Everything is a teaching tool, everything is an opportunity for us to grow and to learn and to always remember that we can be in a place of love.

Ian: Right on. Yeah. Yeah. Okay. Beautiful. I don't know. I think that's closure. Right on. Thank you so much, Reverend Lynne, I appreciate it.

Lynne: Alright. Thank you. It was great being on.
Ian: Yeah. Right on. Okay. Everybody, thanks for tuning in and come join us and we'll make some miracles. Peace.

Lynne: Bye.

Jesus Christ was an Essene. The Essene's wrote the "Dead Sea Scrolls" hence me studying with Rev. Lynne Herod-Deverges in 96. This meditation aided J Cynthia Brooks in her spiritual side of curing her terminal cancer back then as well. This was one on one with Rev. Lynne on the history of the Essene's and how their meditations still help some today.
http://centeroflightmiracles.org/

[See Pic 16.1]

CHAPTER 17:

SKIN CANCER CURED NATURALLY

(GERSON THERAPY)

My name is Howie Don and I'm 52 years old and I am a downsized environmental engineer. In 2008 after having a problem with a growth on my back, I learned after having a biopsy that I had a pretty serious case of malignant melanoma.

The biopsy report came back Clark's Level Four lesion, which means that the depth was pretty deep! When I went into the dermatologist's office I basically told her that I needed to have this area removed just because it was causing so much discomfort and at the time she looked at me and she said, "Yes, you really need to have that growth removed."

After that time, I have some time to go home and with all the emotional trauma that I was experiencing, I thought, "Wow, you know, what's next. I have experience with cancer in my family. I lost my dad as a teenager to cancer and my mom is also a cancer survivor also." So, it's something that I'm familiar with, but I didn't think that it would ever happen to me. I thought I was on a pretty good course with my diet and my lifestyle.

But really looking back, they say hindsight is 20/20 and I had a poor history of jobs. And between taking jobs that were working with oil and gasoline and mechanizing, I worked for several years as a commercial pool and spa specialist, a water quality specialist. I did a lot of work with chlorine in tablet, powder, liquid form.

I also did a lot of time as a swim instructor. So not only was I inhaling a lot of the chlorine toxins I was also immersed in the water quite a bit of time. I left my job voluntarily in 2008, this was just after I had a biopsy done. I really wanted to have my insurance take care of that particular situation. I had procrastinated about having my insurance in force and when I finally did get the insurance working I had already had my biopsy done and when I went to a consultation at a small dermatologist office he gave me pretty much the conventional protocol on what they do.

I went to a conventional doctor, he was a thirty-year veteran, surgeon, oncologist and he was right near the dermatologist office and he came highly recommended and I think he felt sorry for me because I went into his office and I didn't have insurance at the time.

When I went to his office I was charged fifty dollars and he told me, "Well the next step with malignant melanoma is a wide incision and a lymph node biopsy." He explained to me in detail what that was even though it was a very short consultation. And I understood it completely. I actually have a pretty good background in anatomy and physiology, so I understand how the body works and some of the medical procedures that they use.

So, leaving his office I really didn't feel a whole lot better because of I really... even after having just a small biopsy and incision done, I really didn't want to do any more cutting and when they do a wide excision they take quite a large bit of tissue. So, and then if they can't close it properly they take some time skin grafts from other parts of the body and then in addition to doing a wide excision they do what's called a lymph node biopsy and they take a needle type device and they biopsy the lymph nodes. They actually go to a lymph node which is called the sentinel lymph node and if that comes up positive then the surgical procedure is to start removing lymph nodes.

It's really important to keep your lymph nodes and to keep as much body tissue as possible because whatever we're born with is really needed for a natural healing process. And I really wasn't thinking about natural healing until I started to do my research on the internet after my first consultation.
I had about two weeks between my initial consultation and then a more expensive one at the City of Hope in Duarte California. I was receiving a lot of peer pressure from family and friends to go the conventional route even though I had started seeing information on the internet that was saying that a lot of people are able to heal naturally not only for cancer but a lot of other life-threatening illnesses.

So, I had two weeks to do a lot of research and more and more I was finding out that people were having success with natural healing and alternative methods. I did follow through with my consultation at the City of Hope. So, at my consult at the City of Hope with a younger surgeon oncologist, I finally got the same information that I got in the shorter consult. Again, wide excision and lymph node biopsy.

And I got a little bit more for my money this time, it was an $800 consult rather than a $50 one. And I got some drawings, and, I actually squeezed in a little bit of questioning for him also. I had already started doing some research regarding alternative methods and I said, "Well what happens if I combine conventional methods with natural methods?" And, he actually paused it seemed like it was kind of a scene out of a movie.

And he said to me, "I know people who have tried that before but don't miss the boat. And I think it's a way of the doctor's kind of instilling fear into you, so that you make a decision, to kind of follow through with the therapy. Both surgeon oncologist never asked me what I wanted to do. It was always the next step is and the next step is when you go along with conventional therapy.
So, as I walked out of the hospital through the revolving doors when the valet brought the car back to me, I looked at my wife and I said, "I'm not going back."

I had already done substantial research on the internet and for one reason or another I ended up finding therapy called The Gerson Therapy. And it was really phenomenal that the information there actually made a lot of sense to me. Again, I understand how the body works and then I realized that this seemed like the most natural chose for me to heal my body again.

So fast forward, I'm actually just about two years into the therapy, and early on actually just months into the therapy I stuck with it really religiously by the book and started seeing results very early on. The reason being is that most people who do conventional treatments have already hurt the body by doing chemicals and radiation and surgery. And I had not done any of those things. One of the things that really helped me is that the body's natural immune system was able to really kick in rather quickly. And I saw the results and without becoming overconfident I just stuck to it and over a period of months, I became stronger and stronger and stronger.

Now I'm just under two years into the therapy and I feel in great health and now I'm ready to go and tell others and help others to find more information about alternative therapies. So, I kind of urge people, if you're thinking about doing alternative therapy do it early on because the results are just magnificent for the body to heal and to do it naturally. The alternative is to do conventional therapy and at what price you know, there's substantial scarring and trauma to the body not only physically but emotionally.

So, go ahead and do your homework, do your research and make a good decision, because the alternative therapies now are becoming more and more popular and all you have-to-do is to get on the internet and find out how to heal.

Ian: Alright, I'm the camera guy Ian Jacklin from ICureCancer.com and I wanted to put this up because if you've heard me rant and rave before skin cancer is the one that is one hundred percent curable. One hundred percent. The doctors, the alternative doctors aren't legally able to tell you that, but I'm a camera guy, filmmaker, I can say whatever I want.

I know for a fact, I've got two people I've interviewed that say, fast-growing melanoma, one hundred percent curable. Do not go to your western medical doctor they will just cut it out of you. But they do not cut the roots out. The roots go way deeper. If you get it done alternatively it heals you from the inside out, and it'll go away and it'll never come back and my man, I call him Texas Walker, cause he's like, he looks like Chuck Norris. Walker here did it the right way and I hope you chose the right way too.

CHAPTER 18:

AMERICAN BIO-DENTAL CENTER (TIJUANA)

The following is a short film I made on this place.

Francis Crawford - Mercury is one of the most toxic elements known to man. And the dental profession for a long time and even today there are many, many dentists in the United States that think there is nothing wrong with putting mercury amalgam fillings in the body. But the problem with mercury is it's a toxic heavy metal. Every time you have a cup of hot coffee or a hot drink and you've got a mercury amalgam surface of that tooth in the mouth it is creating out-gassing mercury.

Dr. Garcia: There's a lot of evidence and there's a lot of information that relates certain parts of the mouth with different organs of the body and that's what we can call meridians. So, if I have a certain decay or an amalgam filling in a specific tooth I might have an inflammatory response. It could be liver, intestine or any other main organ and probably I will not have any problems at this point but eventually, I can develop a disease.

Alessandro Procella, General Director: My name is Alessandro Procella and I run a clinic in Tijuana for the last ten years. The clinic is a dental clinic and it's a biological dental clinic. We are into the alternative part of the dentistry which consists of use and materials that are nontoxic. In the industry of dentistry are thousands of materials that do a lot of harm and they're used in like amalgam for the last 150 years and we all know that amalgams are 50 percent mercury, the rest is nickel, copper, silver and different materials. They use the mercury to amalgam to put together the other material.

At the beginning was against the law but for some reason they allow it and now they're still doing it up to today is very, very bad for the health of the general public.

Ian: Hi, my name is Ian Jacklin. I produced and directed a film called iCureCancer.com. And while I was doing that I learned that the mercury in our teeth is very, very toxic for our system, it is not good for you at all. And when I was interviewing a gentleman by the name of Burton Goldberg, who is known as the voice of alternative medicine, he mentioned that I could probably do a documentary just on bio-dentistry itself and how the cancer is involved with it what with the mercury in the fillings, the toxicity levels are just out of this world. Well, I decided to do that for my film and while I was doing it I met Alessandro, who was kind enough to invite me down to his clinic in Tijuana.

Francis Crawford: It can affect the brain. It can affect the lungs. And there's a whole dissertation about the adverse effects of mercury and how badly they affect these elements affect the health of a person because they're grinding on the immune system all the time.

Dr. Garcia: You can see in a lot of patients how they're healing process is faster, when you actually extract fillings, amalgam fillings and if they're having any acute problem like arthritis or any digestive tract problems you can also see faster improvement of the symptoms when you help them.

Francis Crawford: There is a dentist who is praised by holistic dentists and condemned by conventional dentists by the name of Hal Huggins. He's the person that first exposed the dangers of mercury amalgam fillings to the general health of people. And you know, they would put mercury amalgam fillings in kids that are 3 and 4 and 5 years of age that have got cavities because of all the sugar and the sweets that they eat and when you carry a mercury load for that number of years it is bound to be deleterious to the body.

Ian: I learned that in Tijuana they're able to work much, much cheaper and you're looking at one third the cost. I also wanted to get... I had a lot of silver in my mouth. I ate a lot of candy when I was a kid. And I decided to get mine out and an American estimate was $15,000 to get all the silver removed from my teeth and the bio dentistry done to refill it and it was $5,000 in Tijuana so just mental note you're looking at one third the price in Mexico, and it's actually the quality is just out of this world. They buy the best materials; the work is phenomenal.

Alessandro Procella: We work in a very, very safe way, under the sponsorship of Dr. Hal Huggins which he is the one that gives us the, how you call it, the guidelines how to extract the amalgams without hurting people. Because if you don't follow certain protocol, it's better not to take it out. It's better to leave it there.

Ian: What they'll do for you, is they'll actually pick you up right at the border; so you don't have to bother driving, at San Diego, take you into Tijuana and if you're doing a lot of work and you need to spend the night they put you up in a five-star hotel, it's very beautiful. And, they'll go ahead, and they test your... they do blood tests, urine tests, hair tests and one thing that is very special to this clinic is they do biofeedback tests, which is they hook you up with electrodes and they find out your energy, your electric impulses, and everything. And find out what materials would be least toxic for your system.

So, I thought that was very interesting. And when they're taking the silver out they put in a dam, so nothing can fall down your throat or you can't, you know, ingest anything. And they have a special ionizer, they got you on oxygen. They've got vitamin C inter-venous line going in you so it's pumping up your immune system. It's carte blanche.

Francis Crawford: Quantum Bio-Feedback – One of the things I do for the dental clinic is I test materials for compatibility with a patient. The materials that go into a mouth that replace mercury amalgam fillings or other materials that have been removed. We have to be sure that those materials don't at some time in the future have an adverse reaction to that patient in terms of a resonance or in terms of compatibility of materials. So, I test those materials, to make sure that the ones that are used, are compatible, with that particular patient.

Mary Jo Geideck, Health Advocate: The reason I came to Mexico is I'm very close to the border. I live in Bonita, California. The reason I came down here is the dentists are excellent, the facilities are excellent, they are state of the art equipment.

And what is so great is they're very... they're reasonable. They are a fraction of the cost they are in the United States and, yet you get a better quality of dentistry. I've been in the field of nutrition for 38 years. So, I keep up with a lot of the foremost things and they're finding about the heavy metals and all different things and how they affect your body.

Quite honestly, lead and mercury are very toxic, and they are very toxic to your children and they start working within the body. It can affect your heart and your liver and various other things. Such as when I came down here I had a very bad one tooth that had had an amalgam filling and a crown on it that was fractured. And I ending up having to have it removed and as a result, it had already affected my bone and I had to have a bone graft which is unfortunate but that was just because it was so decayed. However, because I practice such good health I didn't even know that it was that infected and as a result, I had a form of diarrhea for two years that the doctors couldn't figure out and the minute I had the tooth removed it stopped.

So that's how the effects, of what is going on in your teeth can affect your body. If a simple tooth that you don't even know is affecting you, you know, it's not aching or something, can affect you physically and other forms in your body. So, meridians of your teeth connect to certain parts, and this tooth actually was the outer meridian, of my intestines and my stomach. So, it more-or-less, makes sense, that that was causing the problem.

American Bio-Dental Center, Tijuana Mexico offers very affordable bio-dentistry of the highest quality. Specializes in amalgam replacement with materials specifically designed for your own biological chemistry. 877-231-5701
http://www.americanbiodental.com

[See Pic 18:1]

CHAPTER 19:

VANDANA SHIVA

(VINICE BEACH)

[See Pic 19.1]

Ian: It's funny I woke up this morning and I got on the internet where I get my news and I saw where they passed a law from now on our government can't even stop Monsanto, our government cannot even stop Monsanto. Okay. So, I was very angry, didn't know what to do. I get a call from my buddy Matt Mullen on Facebook and he's like, "This Shiva lady, she's speaking in Venice Beach." I'm like, "Really, get out of here, what are they going to shut down the streets?" I mean that's how much this lady means to me. She's a Christ-like figure and very intelligent, especially on the war against GMOs. So it was a quaint little gathering in a restaurant in Venice and I got front row seats, sitting right there with my camera and got to even ask her a question too.

Ian's Question: Okay. I made a film called I Cure Cancer so I know a lot about how important nutrition is for people to regain their health if they lost it so obviously, I'm interested in this subject GMO's. I was wondering if you could speak on the law that was just passed a few days ago here in America stating that basically, even if a government wanted to say no to Monsanto now, they couldn't. Has anybody else heard that?

Lady (Marisa Tomei) – Yeah.

Shiva – It's more the court's ruling is what I gather is it.

Lady (Marisa Tomei) – It's a rider.

Shiva – It's a rider but that no court can rule against Monsanto. But that was where I think some things going very wrong because normally, I know my friends who take these issues to court sue the government. Now the government is being sued in a court and the government that's being sued turns around and say, "We won't listen." The courts are supposed to regulate excesses of government. Yeah. So, it's a constitutional crisis of a very deep kind. And I really think good constitutional lawyers... you know this is it, this is the problem. The GMO issues were seen as a particular concern of a very tiny group of people.

As a very specialized concern. But it cuts through everybody's life, whether you are worried about health or you're an environmentalist, it doesn't matter which part of the environment you care about, could be the pollinators, it could be the soil organisms, last showed 22 percent disappearance in four years of beneficial soil organisms. Animals are dying from eating this stuff. So, it doesn't matter which place you enter it affects you. And the GMO question now needs to be put in its broader political context. And I think some good constitutional lawyer should be found to challenge that Rider and I'm sure... I mean, in my basic sense of how a democracy works, if courts rule against governments, governments can't turn around and say, "Sorry, you don't matter."

Ian: Here! Here!

AFTER PARTY INTERVIEWS WITH RANDOM FOLKS

Matt Mullen: So here we are after we just saw Dr. Vandanna Shiva speak at Ax Restaurant, is it Axa? I don't know. And we had a great talk and just talking, exchanging ideas that work with a lot of people and you know, one of the main attacks that we should have not only the genetically engineered foods, you know Monsanto, more Round Up as well. The roundup residue is in the food and that's cancer-causing as it is and anything that's cancer-causing, has to be labeled, right? If it causes cancer?

Second Guy: Absolutely. And what about the bees? Okay. We've seen this colony collapse, not everyone's willing to recognize that Round-Up is affecting the bees and other insects and in our, you know, crops, our pollinators. So, it's time that we go after the dangers of Round-Up itself.

Ian: Okay. (looking at a t-shirt he's wearing...)
Guy: All the different languages.
Ian: Monsanto, Murder.
Lady: Assassinate. That's Hindi? I don't know what they ??/ is.
Ian: All different languages.
Lady: It's all different languages. I got Hindi on there, Korean. I'm trying to use my mushroom it's mandarin.
Matt Mullen: The back says.
Ian: Those are awesome shirts!

Matt Mullen: 85 to 90 percent of soy, corn, canola, and sugar beets are genetically modified. Genetically modified foods cause Cancer. GMO foods are self-replicating genetic pollution that threatens the food security of our planet. FDA, Monsanto are Murderers. Thank you very much.

Ian: Murderers.

Matt Mullen: Hey we gotta' get you a shirt.

Ian: And the coolest thing with Marisa Tomei was there. And when I asked my question in front of the group, she seconded my motion. Hahaha. Came up to me afterward and even thanked me for asking that question. And I said, "Well thank for getting my back there, lady!" haha
Wow, she's even more beautiful in real life! I love my life… ;) My Cousin Vinny was a favorite!

CHAPTER 20:

ROBERT SCOTT BELL OF NATURAL NEWS

Ian: And so that's good and for a change, you're actually going to be the one interviewed, which has got to be different for you?

Robert: Yeah very frightening.

Ian: [Chuckling] Well I got you once already for my film, but I figured... I'm really excited about this new platform, this radio thing on the internet and the web TV thing because the information I have been gathering for my film as you know is life-saving/life altering to teach people how to cure themselves of cancer holistically and then also to wake them up to the fact that you're not allowed to do that for your children, they're forced chemo, radiation and surgery, as you know, cause that's what I was interviewing you on my film about earlier. So, it's good that I'm able to get this information out quicker now with this new youtube platform and then the movie will sum it all up too when that's all said and done. So, how're things going with you? What's new since I interviewed you at the Long Beach Health Festival, right?

Robert: Well, I mean, you know life rocks and rolls. I tell you what broadcasting six days a week it's hard to keep from getting dizzy, once-in-awhile. What's clear is that the feds and the medical monopoly don't know even what cancer is. There's a story, I think we just covered on today's broadcast about the redefinition of cancer. They acknowledge, well, maybe they were all wrong about these cancers and maybe they're not as deadly.

And another story about living next to or near this fossil fuel burning plants, whether it be oil or coal and the benzene released and there's a link to cancer clusters there. I mean these are things that patently obvious what I would call your moment of duh regularly on The Robert Scott Bell Show and yet we're seeing more and more of this kind of news coming out vindicating all that we have said in the natural realm as a homeopath as a natural healer and all the medical doctors who have been persecuted and prosecuted simply for acknowledging that cancer is not a deficiency of chemotherapy, radiation or even surgery.

So, it's just strengthening what we've been doing for many years and I'd have to say the consciousness is shifting, it shifts slowly. They fight it as long as they can until they have to admit it and then they'll say, "Well it was self-evident all along, we knew it! What were you doing all of those years?" Well, they were drinking some pharmaceutical Kool-Aid.

Ian: [Chuckling] Right. [Laughing] Yeah, well let's... for some of those people out there that may not know, I mean you're like The Guy over at Natural News, Mike Adams the Health Ranger's Network and how did you get into being the health guy, I mean, what was it that brought you to doing what you do today on the radio?

Robert: Well I was a boxer and I threatened... no, I'm just kidding. Haha.
Ian: [Chuckles]
Robert: I've done this for so many years. I started in broadcast media in 1999 and got national syndicating in 2002. So, I've been in the broadcast media for a long time. And Mike Adams, I admired him for many years with what he had started with Natural News and to have him on as a guest every-once-in-awhile and his presence on the internet kept growing and he was a fan of the show as well as I was a fan of his. And we struck up a friendship just over the years and mutual respect. And we talked about wanting to get this message out more frequently than just once a week, yet not many in the broadcast, what we call, the traditional, even mainstream talk stream radio if you can call it that, I had a place to accept or understand the message that I was delivering. Once a week they could tolerate. Five or six, no.

Mike and I talked about it, is there a way we could make this, you know the spoken medium of radio available more frequently and discussed the launching of Natural News Radio and we did that about two and a half years ago on the Natural News platform which has grown to be the number one, as far as largest, alternative health media type site on the planet and it's been growing strong ever since and I'll just tell you and your audience now we've been hinting at it now for a while but we're working behind the scenes to bring the Robert Scott Bell Show out five additional days of the week branding with Natural News and a syndicator to radio and that may be happening within the next two weeks. So, we're very much on the verge of an exciting leap out even bigger and of course, the reach is global already through Natural News, but also domestic U.S. Syndicated radio is going to be accessing this information soon as well.

Ian: Yeah, wow, so you help build that with Mike? You've been along with the whole time?

Robert: Yeah, well we were the launched program for it, and then a number of good programs have been added along the way and trying to round out some messages and some voices that would normally get heard in traditional media, so it's been a great endeavor and you know, it's still growing. But at the same time, media is shifting, recognize, just look what's happened with Alex Jones and his success within the traditional broadcast syndication barter type media and it's quite astonishing. So, it tells you that it is possible to bring a message like this out. It is accepted now and there is an economic support mechanism to make it work, cause let's face it, if they can make money off of it they would find a way to get it one there and that's always been the issue. The economics have been too easy from Big Pharma, the other aspects of global corporations with no allegiance to any nation or state, that's what drives pretty much the messaging in the mainstream media, the advertising there is all about drugs and occasionally cars, but mostly drugs.

Ian: Yeah. It's amazing that Alex Jones is busting out the way that he is. And Mike is coming out too, yourself, myself, Ty Bollinger, you know, everybody that's in the health world, you can't really not get involved which some people may call conspiracy theories, but after a while, you kind of gotta' call certain things Facts. And you kind of wonder why would, in the alternative health world... people say it to me all the time... like don't bring up 911 because it takes away from what you're talking about. And I'm like, "But I found out about 911 because I was researching Rockefeller owning the pharmaceutical companies in the early 1900s which he, you know, bought out the medical schools and next thing you know that's what they teach. I mean, you can't have one without the other. Have you found that sometimes people say, "Why don't you guys just stick to the health instead of the political stuff?"

Robert: Well that's been from the very beginning I could never stick to just the health issues because my journey, Ian, and you know from talking to me before has been one of a discovery through the motivation to be well because I wasn't well.

To begin with, the first 24 years of my life I suffered from chronic diseases, vaccine damage, anti-biotin damage and food that was not adequate, not organic and my discovery or my prayers for health lead me to discover some of the things you just mentioned here about the history, not only of America but planet-wide about the collusion and cover-up of natural ways to heal and of course nutritional aspects of that, meaning that most of the diseases that we call infectious disease are actually the result of poor nutrition or toxicological exposures.

So it really is a paradigm, distinct paradigm shift from the way we all grew up in the west thinking that germs were bad and that, you know, it was just a random act of bad luck if you happen to get ill or if you happen to get cancer, which is not something you catch as a communicable disease but they've been working hard, for instance with the issue of HPV claiming that that sexually transmitted virus as claimed will cause cervical cancer later in life. I've disputed that from the beginning as well.

But again, we're dealing with a fundamental paradigm distinction. And that's difficult because a lot of times you're speaking apples and oranges to folks out there. They really have no bridge in. So my talent, if there is one, is an ability to make that bridge possible from the medical side of things understanding or their misunderstandings bringing it into a holistic framework and interacting with that community. At least those that were open-minded. If they weren't, I didn't have a lot of time for time because they pretty much own the rest of the airwaves. So, had to work very hard to balance out any little bit we could from what they were delivering.

Ian: Okay, yeah, the key is how do we get sick and you've got something there about the germ theory and the law of terrain. Do you want to speak a bit about this?

Robert: Yeah, well if you remember growing up those of your audience are westerners, even Western Europe although more so in North America we've been really razzle-dazzled by what's known as the germ theory or to point to Louie Pasteur who was a contemporary of Antoine Beauchamp. Pasteur had the favor of the Emperor, it's all who you know, that's throughout history that's been true.

And because of that what he stole from Beauchamp and others he basically claimed that it was basically the germ that was the cause of disease. They would find some kind of micro something, some kind of life form that they had never seen before, would create disease by its very presence. So, the boiling down the germ theory states that it is the mere presence of or contact with a pathogen that will result in disease.

So, if I were to sneeze on somebody or in an audience and sneezed on the audience and the virus would fly about the room, everybody would contract it, everybody would get sick. That's obviously, seemingly an overly simplistic way to understand it but that's basically it.

Whereas Antoine Beauchamp, Claude Bernard, and others recognized the real way disease was created was not because you were exposed necessarily to a germ, but that you had upset the terrain or milieu or environment from within and that corruption gave rise to new life forms. So, if you change the terrain, you change what grows there.

So, it wasn't so much what you caught, it's what you created via... what? Nutritional deficiency or toxicological proficiency. You know, just talk to an organic farmer about his soil or her soil. Ask them about healthy soil versus soil that is unhealthy that's polluted and toxic and ask them what grows there? They will say visually it's a distinct marked difference. You can look into a lake that is pristine and healthy and clean and you can test the water and see what is there and you can test a polluted lake and you'll find that pathogenic life forms, bacteria, fungal species, viral species will be prevalent in the polluted lake much less so, or almost none there in regards to a disease-causing, as they call it, organisms in that clean lake.

Again, the law of the terrain is something that we have not been taught in the western. They still really don't teach it within allopathic western medical schools which are all designed as you know to look at all life as having a drug deficiency of some kind.

Ian: You're a homeopath yourself, right?

Robert: Yeah, so don't be frightened.

Ian: [Chuckles] Was that how you got started? Were you doing that before radio?

Robert: Yeah, in fact, I was learning about homeopathy, wow, back in the early 90s and partway through my training had appeared on a radio station in Atlanta, WSB750 a.m. That's a 50,000-watt station, with my mentor at the time. We appeared on for an hour. We were scheduled to be interviewed about alternative medicine and homeopathy and four hours later the host said he'd never... except one other show I think he had the switchboard lit up for four straight hours. We talked about a lot of very controversial things, including cancer. The fact that it was not, you know, the result of necessarily genetic issues, primarily, and the fact that it could be cured.

We also talked about AIDS and the fact that it wasn't caused by HIV. You want to talk about outrage on the airwaves, oh my gosh.

But at that moment for me, in 1994 I realized that I had a knack or ability to communicate these principles that were seemingly lost to America or the West in a way that could be understood even if it was outrageous to those who had heard it within, in the medical profession in particular. And I kind of planted that seed in my head I guess, "Maybe I could do this!" It wasn't until five years later, that we actually launched a show in Atlanta, and then, eventually went into national syndication.

So, there were a lot of pathways along the way and then a parallel track in the media, but that media track spoke to me very, very intensely because I felt like my culture, if you will, my country, America, had lost it, completely lost it in terms of its understanding of health and healing.

And in fact, you know learning about homeopathy, I never heard the word until I was 24 years of age, so I didn't realize that the university that I went to, Emory University in Atlanta taught homeopathy in its medical school up until about 1949, one of the last areas to do so. So, if I went back and back into my memory growing up in the south even though I was a New Yorker by birth, I went back into the Civil War Museums after learning of homeopathy and recognized that the civil war troops, in fact, had first aide fuel kits, medical kits and they all contained homeopathic medicines.

So, I realized then that we had been completely lied to. Somebody had erased history from our eyes so that indeed we could be controlled and manipulated to believe that modern medicine had been around forever, even though we knew it hadn't, but anything that preceded it or had a parallel existence was wiped from memory very efficiently and effectually and you mentioned, Rockefeller or Carnegie, The Flexner Report of 1910 set the stage a 100 years later for Obama Care.

But even prior to that the medical monopoly was on. So, it wasn't good under Republican Administrations either. This is nonpartisan or trans-partisan destruction of health and healing in America which still seemingly they can't get their head out of the pharmaceutical pill bottle with the advent of Obama Care or the Republicans attempts to repeal it, they would just go back to the preexisting medical monopoly which wasn't a lot better.

Ian: Now do you think there's any hope for us in our medical system as far as ever coming around? I mean, it's down to the bottom lines, it's the elite that runs the world, we understand, the one percent, the Illuminati, whatever you want to call them, Bilderberg. I mean, the rich are running the show. We can't get good medical care in our own country. They're dumping chemtrails on us, there are GMOs in our food. I mean it's pretty obvious; that they actually just are trying to reduce the population. Is there anything that we can do anymore? Do you think?

Robert: Well if there is hope, it's hopes for bankruptcy, funny enough. I mean the inability to pay for it is something that will eventually cause it to collapse and that's frightening for most but for me I really see, that's where the revival or renaissance happens in healing. Because at this point from the standpoint of a blast into the mainstream, it's not going to happen, there's too much of a police state in force right now, whether it be FDA or even state or medicine and the whole concept of licensure is pretty much guaranteed the limitation on or the elimination of anybody that would try to pop their head up and say, "Hi, you know, I'm a doctor or a non-doctor and I can help you overcome cancer without chemotherapy, radiation or surgery!"

So, the medical monopoly has to collapse in order for this to rebuild. And again, this is a very scary thing, many of my friends who happen to be considered progressives or liberals who still believe in this federal intervention and that healthcare is the only hope that we have don't acknowledge or if they do they kind of turn a blind eye to the recognition that nothing in that progressive, so-called, healthcare, Obamacare system actually has anything to do with healing, it had everything to do with managing diseases and profiting from them and of course bankrupting the average persona along the way.

And this is something that the pharmaceutical industry had to have in Obamacare because too many people were starting to leave the medical monopoly, and in order to strengthen their ability to have a future they needed a way to mandate participation which is what Obama Care is, there is no homeopathy in Obama Care, there are no herbs, there are no supplements, there is no detoxification. There are only vaccinations and mammograms, for instance, and drugs, of course, plenty of drugs.

So the idea that this is a health care system that we have is a false premise at its very beginning but we don't get there because the scattershot arguments from Republicans and Democrats are arguing about privatization of system that is not private, that is not involved in any shape or form liberty or freedom or health freedom and so we're in a mess and that's why I say the collapse has to occur in order for the revitalization to happen, when people realize that healing was nothing that the government had invested in or mandated or enforced by licensure. So, it's sort of a long answer to your question, but yes, there is hope, but inevitably it has to come crashing down for the rebuild to occur and then we'll have a healing revival in this country.

Ian: Yeah, once people see what you and I have seen, you know, it'd be over tomorrow. That's what I always laugh about. It is only one percent of them. You know, all we got to do is what Iceland did, you know, get rid of the politicians and the bankers and bail out the people, not the bankers.
Do you think this is going to happen though, cause you and I know what has to happen, but do you think it's going to happen?

Robert: Well there's no way that it won't happen. It's an impossibility. I mean, as sure as gravity exists ultimately. But again, our power... I should say this for the first time tonight, our power of belief is so very powerful that it seems to be overcoming the force of gravity in that we have such an incredible debt-based system, it's not just the monetary system that is failing but the medical system in large parts are falling as well.

Now I don't discount the fact that you can put Humpty Dumpty together again in an allopathic emergency trauma center, that's brilliance and that will never go away, the need for that. But the idea that they could be utilizing their techniques of poisoning the body in other areas for revitalizing or bringing health back into the body is absurd again on its face.

So that part of the allopathic system will have to crumble and then the freedom of all the healers that genuinely know how to heal, whether they be a doctor or not, whether they are licensed or not. In fact, I foresee the end of licensure as well because once people realize that licensure was never about protecting the public and only about protecting the economic self-interest of a particular industry you'll recognize that what you're looking for are people that are qualified to heal, not based on the fact that they have a license by some state, private, semi-private government organization but by their capacity to have people that have come through their system and they are alive and well and they can speak and they can say, "Yes, this is what I did. This is what I had. This is where I am today." And in this way, you as a human being can actually make an informed decision about the method or the direction you want to go.

You know, as much as I'd like to say, "Let's ban vaccines and I wouldn't argue that that might not be a healthy thing to do, I'm so much a proponent for freedom that as long as there was a free market and not a pseudo-free market, but I mean, where the ideas could flow, where you could speak freely about natural medicine, cures for disease and I don't mean you can out and hang your shingle and lie overtly. But if you say, "I believe that the dirt in my backyard can cure cancer, and as long as you say... "I have no studies to show it's true, it's just a belief I have!" If someone were to say, "Well that's good enough for me!" That's how much I believe in freedom. Freedom to screw up is inherently something given to us by our Creator, that is free will. And the government tends to want to... as they claim, protect us from ourselves, but in reality; what they're doing is protecting the economic self-interest of those who profit off-of disease.

So, the idea is truthful and not misleading and not lying about what you do. If you are a medical doctor, say so, you got a graduate degree, say so, if you don't then say that. Let people know your true background and if you are engaged in fraud and deceit there are laws that predate any medical laws or licensure laws that could be utilized in a, you know, minimal governmental situation that could protect the public or would allow you to be made whole again, barring that you're not killed, but large numbers of people that are killed are not being killed by homeopathy or herbs or reiki masters or acupuncturists or chiropractors, though chiropractors are licensed are being killed by the licensed modern medical doctors, even some of the DO s who have adopted this drug everything that moves methodology.

Ian: Right. Right. Let's... cause we kind of skirted over it, pretty quickly, with the HIV thing because there's a lot of people out there that don't know there's... I didn't know it until recently. And I learned it from you and Liam Sheff about HIV. The HIV test folks apparently it turns out to be bogus. It not only doesn't accurately tell you-you're going to get AIDS it doesn't really do anything, so they give you the AIDS medicine and then the AIDS medicine kills you, and so they say you died of AIDS. This is true, right, Robert?

Robert: Well it's pretty, pretty, simple when you look at it, step back and look at it. Now you have to understand I grew up at a time as a generation X'er that this age thing came on the scene and we were all told that now sex would kill you. It wasn't that you could get a sexually transmitted disease like Gonorrhea or Chlamydia or syphilis and you take an antibiotic or around or whatever and then you'd be cured... the theory was anyway. But this one was going to kill you, they didn't know why, it'll happen in six months it'll happen in a year, then they said two years, then five years, then ten years, then twenty-five years, it kept changing over time.

So initially I had the reasonable belief that, yeah, there was this new plaque that was killing everybody primarily gay people, but they extended it to hemophiliacs and then they said Africans. So just so you know my background was such that as I was raised pharmaceutically and medically, I had no reason to dispute it, the knowledge of this initially.

But as I was trained in homeopathic medicine, talked about the difference and distinction between the germ theory the law of the terrain, my mentor in homeopathic medicine when he saw this said, "This doesn't make sense. What they're saying is not accurate. This is not the way disease happens. This is not the way microbes work. And then discovered the works and writings of Professor Peter Duesberg, who was considered a heretic even though he was the golden boy, I think he was the youngest member ever elected to the National Academy of Sciences and he could do no wrong.

There was no grant that he was ever turned down for and in fact he wrote at a certain point in this new, so-called, gay disease or plaque that these people were killing themselves with a lifestyle, a drug based lifestyle that these drugs that they were on the amyl nitrate poppers which were immune suppressant the vast extraordinary use of antibiotics like no time in history because they really did have a lot of sexually transmitted diseases because of the things they were acquiring and it was literally destroying them from the inside out.

In fact, that population they had predicted that there would be something devastating that would happen to it. Now I'm not saying from what we call it a religious dogma or condemned condemnation that's not where I'm speaking from. I'm just speaking purely from biology, physiology, immunology perspective, you cannot destroy your gut with antibiotics for years and years on end and expect to have a healthy long life.

And so, this was pretty much what Duesberg had said. Now he disputed then the cause being HIV that Robert Gallo and Luke Montonay Gallo stole supposedly some debris or material from Montonay and then claimed he had discovered it, that was a whole ruckus behind the scenes there that came out.

Bottom line they had said that it was a retrovirus that they never even isolated. And then Gallo of course had patented a test that he said would detect it, yet every test if you read behind the scenes or into the inserts or even the FDA's own acknowledgment that these tests as you said, the HIV test, could not be utilized to definitively diagnose AIDS much less acknowledge or corroborate or definitively say that somebody, actually had, or did not have this so-called HIV.

Then we step back more, and I encourage people to read Liam Sheff's book Official Stories, the whole chapter on it is astonishing. See the documentary film House of Numbers as well, that there is no test. It's not a test for HIV, it's nonspecific, it's cross reactive, it'll test positive for 120 different things including pregnancy. And in fact, if they don't dilute the blood extraordinarily it will test... you will get a positive test in a hundred percent of the people.

And of course, the test being determined to be positive or maybe it's positive or maybe it does not depend also on what country you're in. Also depends on the color of your skin in some cases. If you're an upper-middle-class white housewife that's married and you test positive, they'll say it's a false positive. If you're from the inner city and you're a black woman, you could be married, it doesn't matter, they'll say, well no that positive is a real positive and you have it and they'll put you on drugs.

Of course, in the early years, the early 90s particularly when they put people on AZT which was a failed and very dangerous chemotherapy drug that was banned because it was too toxic for cancer patients, it ended up, you know, killing thousands of people and they claimed that was AIDS and then they're packaged it in lower doses and said, "Ahh ha, now it works and now look the AIDS patients are living longer because of our drugs." This has all been a scam and a ruse and it was a pharmaceutical windmill tilt that was very profitable for the survival of the Centers for Disease Creation and Promotion, otherwise known as the CDC.

So, there's a lot of scams in the cancer industry. But the cancer industry was waning, and they needed a new cancer and so-called HIV/AIDS scenario was that boondoggle that would be profitable for many decades to come and we're still reeling from that and the community that still believes in HIV or HIV testing is basically setting themselves up for slaughter over time and we've seen far too much of that. I'd like to see an end to that as well. But end the HIV test and you end pretty much what AIDS is, which is immune deficiency which is real but for any number of causes that pre-existed and had more to do with lifestyle, behavior and drug toxicology.

Ian: Yeah, well look at the Baby Rico? Story. I mean a classic example, right? Do you know which one I'm talking about?

Robert: Oh, yeah. Carol and Steve Nagle? And Lindsey Nagle? I've covered their story many years ago on the air and been following that. It just breaks my heart every time I think about it. But you know, this goes back to some other discussions we had for your film that you're working on still about jurisdictional issues and how is it possible that you can make a decision as an adult not to take chemotherapy, I just get emotional I think about the baby Rico story because this baby, born healthy, they gave an HIV test too because they knew the mother, Lindsey Nagle had tested positive in her childhood, years being adopted from Romania coming over, but her parents Steve and Cheryl had recognized and found from Professor Duesberg that the HIV test was not necessarily a test for HIV and they were the only one of many children in Minnesota at the time so called diagnosed that pulled their child, Lindsey, off of all of the drugs and she was the only one of those children, ten, fifteen, twenty or to have survived. She's a healthy young lady and had a baby.

That baby they took and told her that they would have to force feed this medication or they would steal this baby from her. And so, this is a big disaster that there is no freedom for your children. If you're a parent, a mom and a dad and you have a different perspective on medicine your child could be claimed by the state and will be claimed by the state particularly when it comes to cancer or this issue of AIDS and that means that first amendment is long in effect. What does the first amendment to the constitution of the United States that was the Bill of Rights?

First Amendment being the Freedom of Speech, Freedom of Religion, Congress shall make no law respecting the establishment of religion or prohibiting free exercise thereof and that is the violation there with the state-sanctioned religion, don't kid yourself, America has state-sanctioned religion and it's not Christianity, it's not Judaism and it's not Islam, it is modern medicine and if you don't believe me, you explain to me how they can take children based on the parents belief that modern medicine is not appropriate for their child.

Now I'm not telling you that it's appropriate to withhold medical, let's say interventions in life-threatening situations like accidents and trauma, but in terms of these chronic diseases because they hold the monopoly and the state sanctions that religion of the medical monopoly, you try and define it some other way, it's a state religion.

Ian: That's very true. That whole Baby Rico thing just slew me. I mean, they're basically they said to the child services, "Look we've been through this before. I was a child that was told, was HIV. They gave me the drugs. It almost killed me. I got off the drugs. I was fine. So, the same thing is going to happen with my kid, so we don't need your drugs. Thank you very much!"

And they said, "Oh, yeah, too bad." Cause this is twenty years later or whatever and now they have laws; child protective services can come in and just take your child and that's basically what happened to them and they're doing it to people with cancer as well. There's a couple of families I have been following, you know the one, Jay Matthews? The situation, right? Do you remember that one?

Robert: Yeah, I interviewed Jay and his daughter at the Health Freedom Expo as well. My heart goes out. It's a difficult situation because he's very much involved in the system as a licensed pharmacist and had an awakening, but didn't realize the evil that he was up against in the pharmaceutical medical establishment in taking children. I mean, it's like a ritual slaughter and the worst of the death cults... demonic death cults out there when it comes to children with cancer or these chronic diseases that are life-threatening and that is why we spent such time, you know, your interview of me at the Health Freedom Expo out in Long Beach last year, was it last year, I think, already, or earlier this year.

The fact of the matter is the jurisdictional issue is one that has-to-be explored very intensely because the question is, "How is it possible that the state can take ownership of a child in such a situation?" And |I just don't hear that discussed often enough and that's why we talked about it. And again, I don't know... I sometimes mention it on the air, it's almost too much for people to fathom that certain basic things that they assume are normal and natural and are right to do in America are the very things that put their children at risk when they have children in that marriage and you know, I don't mean to oversimplify it, but it does come down to that aspect because in law everything is about jurisdiction. If jurisdiction can't be established there is no way in, but if it is established then you have no way out just about. So, it's devastating, absolutely devastating. And as I said, I don't know if others have covered it with you, Ian, but I think it is so very important to bring out.

Ian: Yeah, I've talked a bit about it with Joni Cox and hopefully we'll be talking to the parentalrights.org... soon to find out what they're doing. Yeah, and I had a good interview with Dr. Leonard Coldwell recently on this show and he's kind of getting on the up and up with all the contract law and the constitutional law. And it appears and that's what you and I were talking about a bit too that we may be going that way cause once people don't know this but as soon as you get a birth certificate for your child, that child is now owned by U.S., Inc., not you. And same when you get married and you get a marriage certificate, the same thing, now you're owned by U.S., Inc. Am I correct in that?

Robert: Yeah. It's, you know, licensure is something that I discuss often and I'm, you know, I'm vehemently opposed to and why? Because it is a process of subjugating yourself. It's a process of asking for permission where none is required, and you do that as an adult you become a child. You become basically someone that is not able to stand on their own. And that's the concept of medical licensure, the doctors of chiropractic that went down that road because they fought for what they call credibility.

I don't want that kind of credibility, in fact, even if they offered licenses to homeopaths, I would refuse them and reject them outright because I don't ask permission where none is required. Healing is a birthright. It is a primary fundamental human right, the ability to heal yourself or heal others based on the freedom to associate in this way. I get the very concept of asking for permission puts you under, subjugates you, puts you under the jurisdiction of that which we would control and own you or the fruits of your marriage for instance in the context of a marriage license. Why should you ask permission of the government, to enter into a holy union or matrimony between yourself and your loved one? That used to be the purview, if you will, of the Church, if you will, you would go and your preacher or whoever would bless it, you would, how would you do it? In your family Bible, you know these rights of passage, you'd just list it there. It's as simple as that. You didn't ask permission of the state.

Now this is an interesting history lesson because after the so-called Civil War or the War of Northern Aggression, the War between the States however you want to qualify it or call it, the Fourteenth Amendment, the citizenship change that occurred, that you were no longer sovereign, but now you had become subject to the jurisdiction of the District of Columbia, ten miles square. And at that point it changed the nature of the American, the human American who was sovereign not because of any governmental decree or sanctioning but because by your very birth you were acknowledged to be self as opposed to in England the Crown was the sovereign, the King or the Queen and everyone else was its subject.

That was the antithesis of what we the design for the government was in America. Now the idea of asking permission to marry is rooted in a slave type mentality, particularly in a form of evil racism because after that war the people wanted rights, but they really weren't granted rights they were granted privileges by government and at that point this idea of marriage license came into being particularly and only when a white person, a Caucasian person wanted to marry a black person, you had to ask permission before that was granted by the state. And somehow that has transpired over the ensuing decades to a century plus that everybody had to ask permission of the government to get married and it's a false assumption. It's incorrect and nobody should ask permission of the government.

And this is what is also astonishing to me for those who want to have gay marriage. I could care less whether you have that, it doesn't impact my marriage. But why would you want the government to sanction your relationship? Unless you were interested in receiving a benefit from government and if that's the case when you accept the benefit you're going to have to accept the strings that are attached, and those strings are pretty-damn ugly when it comes to having children because those strings as you said to attach to those children, the fruits of the labor... I'm sorry, the fruits of your marriage become property or wards of the state at their pleasure, at their whim and their whim right now primarily is when you reject the religion of modern medicine, that's their litmus primarily. People say it's all about, well if you abuse your children, well yeah, sometimes there are cases where you can point to, child protective services doing a good service and pulling a child out of a very dangerous situation, but that's rarer than reality.

The Reality is they're pulling children out of families who refuse to inject toxic poisons that would kill them in the treatment of cancers that were brought on by things sanctioned by the state including vaccinations, including drugs, including processed foods and additives and preservatives and colorings and flavorings and pesticides and herbicides and fungicides and GMOs, genetically modified organisms, all of these sanctioned by the state, when you reject that they give you a label according to the psychiatric? Bible of orthorexia an oppositional defiance disorder. I'm telling you the only people that are going to survive this is orthorexic and are ODD. If you're not ODD you better become ODD or else you're going to go down with that medical ship. Am I making any sense here, Ian?

Ian: Yeah. Oh, absolutely. Absolutely! It's just insane what's going on. One thing I always wondered about... okay, let's just say, cause even though I'm 44, I still haven't had children and I'd love to if I could find the right woman I would love to have a family and if I do I could be in trouble because I think that I'm allowed... even God says in the Bible, right, you can defend yourself, you can defend your loved ones, you can kill if you have to in self-defense. So, if somebody was to try and tell me that my kid was going to get the chemo, radiation, and surgery, they're trying to kill my kid and I think I'm allowed to use whatever it takes to make sure that, you know, my kid doesn't get hurt, which is probably why I don't have one yet. [Chuckles]

Robert: Well yes, if you're willing to defend your children as any parent, should and would normally. Once you perceive the threat that modern medicine is in these cases, you have the ultimate right to use deadly force and defense of your child. Now am I authorizing and advocating... I mean, this is not what I'm saying, I'm just saying speak... you have to be in that situation, you have to be right with yourself and your creator to recognize that and your right, your birthright to defend your children.

You know, I've often referred back to my good friend, Michael Badnarik, who ran for the Presidency from the Libertarian Party in 2004, he was their candidate and shortly after he got the nomination for the Libertarian Party, I was one of the first that got the first interview right outside the hall there and interviewed him about a number of topics and he was...he jokes, he was a deer in the headlights, cause he didn't expect to win the nomination.

But one of the topics at that time in 2004 was you know post 911, a lot of trial balloons about mandating vaccines, bioterror scares and I asked Michael, I said, "You know, the government is talking about mandating vaccines for smallpox and different bioterror issue things, "What's your perspective?" And he, being the true Libertarian, one who loves Liberty says, "Well here's my perspective, doc you bring a needle, I'll bring my 45 and we'll see who makes a bigger hole!"

Ian: [Chuckles]

Robert: And he was just dead serious. Because he recognized the assault with a potentially deadly weapon that a vaccine is. And until the American people recognize this they will shirk or shriek in fear. They'll be in terror of the authorities and the authoritarians and not stand up. When you do standup, it's like the bully you finally punch on the nose, you find out, that they're actually cowardly. Now that's not to say that I would also not recognize that there is a risk in standing up to a bully. But at some point, we simply must because to not do it is more dangerous than the threat of doing it, standing up to the bully.

And then when one does it, that's the living example for another and another and another and then the cascade arrives and then potentially a peaceful non-violent revolution occurs where people recognize that the sanctity of their home and their family is something that cannot be tread upon by any governmental authority when there is no evidence of harm or intent to do harm particular by the parents who are simply defending their children against the assault of a dangerous religion, again, being the Church of Biological mysticism, John Rappaport coined the phrase that is modern medicine.

Ian: Right. Now for contract laws... or for when... let's just say, I have a kid and I don't want them to be in the system, so I don't get a birth certificate, well then what happens down the line when they gotta go to school and they gotta get a passport because their little league hockey team is going to Europe or like... then what happens?

Robert: Well my kids don't have birth certificates. We don't have a marriage license and they have passports.

Ian: How do you do that, with... and do you not get a social security, as well or...
Robert: They don't have that either.
Ian: How do you get documentation then without having all that?
Robert: Well you have birth affidavits, you have witnesses, you have Bible records, whatever you need to do, you provide it to them and if you've read the application for passports there are means by which you can do that.

I'm not saying it's easy, but we actually-used our congressman at the time to help push that through because we were basically abiding by the laws as they were written in regards to that. So, all of those things that you mentioned, are not required in order to obtain a passport, but I'm not saying it's easy, but I am saying that it is possible because I know first-hand.

Ian: Okay. Yeah, I always wondered about that and how you get. Do you pay taxes?
Robert: All taxes that I lawfully owe.
Ian: Okay. [Chuckles] So that means, no. [Chuckles more]
Alright, interesting; Okay, let's see what else did I want to cover?
Robert: Probably covered some of this with Dr. C. didn't you?

Ian: Yeah, I mean I'm amazed that my one guy Eric his child... the child services have sided with him. Cause the percentage of success rate for her was not good and he said, you know, basically... so you're telling me she's going to hit with, I don't know, 70 out of a hundred bullets instead of you know, whatever. And they're like, "Yeah." And he goes, "Well that's not good enough." And they agreed with him. They actually agreed with them; they're letting him do holistic. They're trying the cannabis oil which I don't know what you're hearing on your end, but that cannabis oil is curing cancer, it's curing everything.

Robert: I've done some interviews about it. But I would rather not have to ask for permission. Follow me here... I'm glad, believe me, I'm glad that she sided with them, but the point is why ask for permission where none is required. That is perhaps the most revolutionary thought, but that was the dawning of the American Revolution. Why should we ask permission of the Crown of England to do that which was our birthright, that was the basis for the Declaration of Independence written, you know, under what we know of as the law of nations.

And so, there's a lot more depth and detail to this than just jumping off, you know, a cliff and saying, "Well I'm going to live differently." Yeah, I mean, that's a starting point, but do your homework. I don't encourage people to do it blindly, but recognize that there is an existence that is yours.

You have been given life by that which is created you and that even goes beyond your mother and father and these are the spiritual issues that I encourage you to look-into because ultimately, it's not a governmental legal issue, it's a spiritual issue. It's your recognition of where you are in creation and how you exist and how you wish to move about the creation cabin so to speak.

So, these are very big issues, your very deep issues and there will always be people in government that are willing to take away your freedom because you don't feel you can handle it and I feel like most Americans don't feel like they can handle it that's why they have the government that they deserve. Question is, are you mandated to participate in it? And if so, then you are a slave and if not, then you have some capability or capacity of regaining a freedom that you didn't even know you lost.

Ian: Now doing what you've done are your children safe if I'm sure I don't know their ages, but I'm assuming if they were under 18 and got cancer would they be safe? Have you set-it-up so they wouldn't be taken away from you?

Robert: Well they're not in any system in that regard and again you have to look into issues when you talk about law, jurisdiction is everything. Is there a contract of adhesion that binds them to the government, that government claims ownership over them, there is no marriage license, there is no birth certificate, there is no number, it would be very difficult for them to claim ownership of this... Now, this is an area of somewhat of speculation because you can do everything right and somebody targets you and does what they want to do anyway because they have the guns.

But the reality is there are more of us then there are of them. And the question is, do they want to take something like that on because that could be the spark that ends them. And so, they're very... they're not stupid on that level. Make decisions about where they go and who they take on based on the ease of access, based on your posture, based on the fear that you may have based on your knowledge. All of these things are taken into consideration and account.

But we have a whole history that is lost as I mentioned about the erasing of medical history in America and because of that, we have a very shaky foundation for liberty. I can talk about it, people might have a superficial understanding of what I'm saying, but it's very foreign to most Americans, this concept. Very frightening in fact, and I recognize that. But ultimately, the government will not be able to sustain its position of domination, simply because it cannot be sustained by the economic system that is beyond bankrupt and when everybody is going hungry there won't be enough FEMA camps to put those people in because the very people that are trying to put you in it are also going to be hungry.

So, there's a different kind of apocalyptic future, one that actually is positive, but it may be pretty ugly along the way, I recognize that. And I urge people to look-into growing food right now. Not waiting for the difficulty in getting it or accessing it or acquiring it based on economic and even energy collapse we've been discussing a lot on the show recently with Liam Sheif about the issue of peak oil and what that leads too. What does that look like?

So, there are a lot of factors here. I'm not painting a Utopian future, but I'm also recognizing, this is life and life will go on barring, you know, another nuclear catastrophe on the order of Fukushima. It may go on for a lot less of us. So, there are real issues that are very dangerous and scary, but while we're here, we plan to do the best we can do and do I provide the healing that is necessary for those who are willing to listen because it is the God's honest truth and I say it every hour of my show that the power to heal is yours and I don't change that because it's an immutable and unchangeable fact of life itself.

Ian: Yeah, exactly, and this is a good way to wrap up the last ten, fifteen minutes. Come back to the cancer thing, you've been in this business for a long time, do you have any particular personal stories you would like to share, of people that have gotten cancer and were able to beat it?

Robert: Well very... really too many, because partly for what I've done myself with helping folks but a lot because I've been in broadcast media for so many years interviewing hundreds and hundreds of doctors and non-doctors alike that have worked with it and lay persons as well.

So I'm an accumulator of information much like you are in what you're doing in media and film and documentation but particularly the reality of seeing folks that have had cancer that has either gone through traditional allopathic oncology or not but either way come out there alive and then have moved more toward or totally toward holistic therapies.

It is clear to me that the only way to overcome cancer is to detoxify the body as a primary starting point, it's not the only point, beyond that is to replenish the nutrients that have been diminished over time or that are no longer in the food that people are consuming and in this way we are talking about, you know, a multi-facet approach but focal pointing many different ways to do the same thing, that is clean the body of the toxic poisons and metabolic wastes that have accumulated and replenished the body, re-nourish the body with minerals, all of the essential elements for the body to function properly.

Now that is the physiology, but we also have to acknowledge the emotional, mental, economic and even spiritual components of all disease including cancer, there are a lot of emotional and even spiritual aspects to it. So, to look at things like Bruce Lipton, The Biology of Belief, very powerful way to also set you on a course of healing even if you're in the direst of circumstances that seem to be untenable and indeed you can overcome them. Again, not because you get lucky, but partly you have-to believe that you can and then with that belief in place things will start to become revealed to you should you be open to them if you ask with a sincere open heart it will be given unto you.

Now you can talk in terms of religious texts or just spirituality, but I've seen that to be also the God's Honest Truth! I had to be open. My prayers were answered not by a lightning bolt that healed me from 24 years of chronic disease but by someone being sent to me who could teach me who to heal then I could, in turn, teach others to do the same or even better and that's what we're here to do and that's what I do on the http://www.robertscottbell.com six days a week.

Ian: Yeah. Yeah. Right. Wow. What... now you never had to fight cancer yourself, right? It was pretty much everything but [chuckles] when you were younger?

Robert: Ian, I had many family members die of cancer, aunts and uncles and grandparents, it was very common in my family to look at my elders and see them diminish over time with cancer, scary C word and they all had gone through traditional allopathic oncology because we were a medical-pharmaceutical family. And I knew of their childhood just from talking to them, because I respected my elders, I was fascinated by it, their childhood. I would meet with them and ask them questions about it, what it was like when they were young and all of them were healthy, every one of them. None of them had allergies as I had, none of them had muscular skeletal inflammatory disorders as I had, none of them had chronic digestive disorders as I had, none of them had chronic recurring infections of the ears, the sinuses, the stomach, intestines, none of them had the things I had.

And yet they died of cancer. Mostly in their sixties and seventies, I think one in their fifties. Now I could put the math together. It looked to me very bleak and dire in my circumstance because the first 24 years of my life I had been ill with something, chronically ill and so I could see if they were dying in their fifties, sixties and seventies I don't know if I would make it to my forties, but I was sure that if I did that I would also have cancer-based on not having a healthy childhood as they had. And so that drove me as well to recognize that this just wasn't about the suffering I had temporarily as a young person but that I would not grow old.

And so, I really was motivated and because of that the undoing of all the things that I mentioned and more here I am in my later forties and I've undone those diseases and I find myself healthier than at any time in my life previous and getting stronger. So, this is quite an extraordinary transformation and I joke to people sometimes in my lecture how I got all of my old age diseases out of the way first now I'm going in reverse.

Ian: [Chuckles]

Robert: I'm so cocky as to believe that as I grow older there won't be other issues that I'll have to deal with, but I recognize it's not necessarily because I'm growing older it's because I'm not keeping up with the toxic accumulation and I'm not replenishing that which I have lost, you know, via nutrients bringing into my body.

But there we see people that are very old and in very good shape that have incredible livers, strong livers and they sustain a lot of assault over time and then they die of not a disease but they're simply old and they're done. They've lived a long life and they're ready to move on and they live and move on in a very peaceable way, we rarely see that we rarely ever hear about that. But that is a natural way of moving on after you've lived your mission in this lifetime.

Ian: Right. Right. I just... have you ever heard this talking about homeopathy, have you ever heard of this stuff, it's a buffer, PH buffer.

Robert: Yeah, there are PH buffer, homeopathic remedies that work with PH issues, there are also cell salts that work with a lot of the minerals on a homeopathic level that revitalize, replenish some basic life force as we talk about. When I work with homeopathy I work on the basis of dranous. Which is the French word for drainage or detoxification and I do that in conjunction with of course other mechanisms like increasing selenium levels from food grown sources or food grown supplementation, utilizing other foods that can enhance glutathione production, the One World Way is a wonderful non-de-natured whey protein that can assist in that.

So, there are a lot of mechanisms with which we can cleanse the body and there are a lot of mechanisms with which we can replenish the body. It's not mysterious. It is accessible to most everybody and there are more aggressive and sometimes very expensive means by which to do this with, you know, for instance, intravenous chelation therapies or other things. But it's not to say that's the only way. If you can't afford that, you can't succeed it as well. There are other ways to go. And that's why... I can't be a show just about homeopathy it would be too narrow, and I don't narrow-cast, I broadcast and that's why I cover all of the aspects of healing including sometimes the allopathic things, if they're necessary interventions, I'll acknowledge that as well.

Ian: Right. Okay. I was just curious because I'm personally trying to get my saliva PH has been 5 – 5.5 for the last six months which is bad as you know. But the urine is like off the top, you know, it was good before I started taking this, now it's like way above 7 or 8. So I didn't know if the homeopathy medicine could actually help; is it just masking it and making it look better, or is it really boosting my PH?

Robert: Well it's altering what you call cellular or metabolic metabolism if you will, cellular metabolism. And there is a function of status in the body that tries to find that balance. I will say that if you take a PH remedy or homeopathic medicine and you consume you know a high acid type diet, animal proteins to excess of your needs, you're still not going to overcome that with homeopathy, it's not a powerful sledgehammer in that way. It's not a drug in the same sense of an allopathic drug that can kill you or stop something or force something to start.

But in conjunction with other dietary shifts, cleaning up what goes into your body and altering the foods that you know impact PH in certain directions it can accelerate healing and accelerate a normalization in those areas that you're looking to do.

Ian: Okay. That's good to know. Yeah, and anybody out there you should always be checking your PH level folks to make sure you're not acidic. And I guess that's about it for our hour today, Robert, I really appreciate your being on. I've looked up to you for a long time now and you've got a lot of wisdom and appreciate your sharing it with everybody out there, man. Do you have anything you want to talk about before we go?

Robert: Well, Ian, just gratitude for you and all the work you're doing and ask you to come on my show tomorrow [chuckles].

Ian: Oh, okay.
Robert: Some of these things and I can turn the tables on you for a bit.

Ian: Yeah, alright. Let's do it, man. Well, right on. So, anybody watching if you want to go to I Cure Cancer.com we still are taking donations to help finish this film. And if you need any help from anybody just let me know people. Appreciate you tuning in. Robert Scott Bell from Natural News.com and The Robert Scott Bell Show appreciate you being here with me today, sir and I'll talk to you soon.

Robert: Alright, thanks, Ian.
Ian: Bye everybody. Peace!
[See Pic 20.1]

CHAPTER 21:

INTERVIEW with DR. MATTHEW LOOP

Ian: It's so exciting to have you here man, 'cause if you said once to me recently that I'm an inspiration to you, and I was like, 'what! No, no, no. You man, you!' I got your book. It was one of the first books I read when I was getting into this whole alternative cancer thing. And it really helped lay down the groundwork for what I do now. It was the same things that Dr. Bernardo was teaching me—from my film I Cure Cancer which was from Professor Brian Scot Peskin. And that was the Otto, Warburg. So, I mean I think we're still in the same school of thought as far as health and longevity go, right?

Matthew L: 100%! And I look at you as a fellow health warrior. So, I'm grateful to be on this call today. And like I said, I really admire your work. You know it's a lonely road to walk sometimes, especially when you're getting out there and you're going against the grain of the masses. People are programmed to do and to think in a certain way. So, just to try and empower them to live healthier lives is just … I mean, that's always been my mission, and really, I have a passionate heart and very enthusiastic about that and I can tell we're of the same blood. So, again, I'm grateful to be here today.

Ian: Yeah, right on! Who'd have known! (laughter) . . . the name of the book that I first read that you wrote was…

Matthew L: It's "Cracking the Cancer Code." I wrote it in 2006. A little background about myself: I graduated from chiropractic school in 2004, and – a lot of people don't know this – but chiropractors are actually trained as primary care physicians. I remember when I was young distinctly that my grandpa and grandma were on all this medication. And I was like, you know … I can't say I was totally wise at 16-17 years old, but I think I was wise enough to know that that wasn't the way it should be. And so that's when I really started to question about health and what I was programmed to believe. Then once I had a chiropractor come into our health occupations class when I was a senior (in high school), he started talking about homeostasis, auto-regulation, that is, your body is programmed to heal itself.

He used the cut as an example, you cut yourself and it automatically heals. You don't have to consciously think about it. And a lot of what he said just resonated with me. And I'm like, "you know, to be in a drugless, surgery-less profession to where you could actually help people recover their health and reverse chronic disease is pretty darn cool!" So I just decided to get into that. Of course, I developed and studied extra in nutrition and biochemistry, and really all the ways in how to optimize your immune system; because we all need certain things to thrive and survive. And I just became really inspired around 2004. That's when I started working on "Cracking the Cancer Code". I finished it in 2006 and got it published. It was kind of cool because I ended up getting a pairing with "The Secret" – the book that dropped on Amazon. It really allowed my book to take off and get it into maybe similar people's hands who also knew that the mind was involved in healing. So, I'm really glad it got into your hands because I know that it has helped inspire you, and obviously we're part of the same mission. We have the same goals. We want to empower people who want to save lives.

Ian: Right. Cracking the Cancer Code. I'll never forget that. See now…we haven't actually met though have we? Physically.

Matthew L: (laughter) No. It's kind of funny how the internet works. But, I was going to tell you: I'm going to be in Orange County…is that where you are?

Ian: Los Angeles…close enough.

Matthew L: I'm going to be speaking there in mid-January. So maybe we can connect when I'm out there

Ian: Absolutely! Yeah, I'll throw the big camera on you too, to get a quick little thing for my new film. … and you're asking about it so I might as well tell you, there may be some who don't know it; I made the "I Cure Cancer" film. I think that came out in 2006. And then I've been shooting part 2 ever since. It's up in the air as to what to call it. I want to call it "Baby Killers" 'cause to me, that's what the oncologists have started doing. They're murdering our children with their chemo, radiation, and surgery; 'cause we know it doesn't work. 3% of the time it will work for tumor-type cancers. We know this now.

Oncologists, unfortunately, don't know it! And I'm making part 2 to impress that to people and let them understand that when you take your child in—with the exception of some of the leukemias which have up to a 40% success rate with chemo. That still means that 60 of the 100 bullets are still going to hit your kid. That's why not too many people make it out of that.—But I know so many people, obviously more adults because children are locked into our system and you go to jail if you don't let them give your child chemotherapy. This would probably have happened to me. So, I'm making this film and it's coming along great.

And then out of the blue comes this Cannabis-hemp oil. Or more commonly called Cannabis Oil. OMG! There's no silver bullet as everyone knows, and there still isn't because sometimes it's just your time to go. Or, you like being sick and you like the attention you get and you don't follow instructions, so there are a few ways you can still die of cancer, but the treatments (chemo, radiation, surgery) shouldn't be one of them. As you and I have figured out, and I've seen with my own eyes hundreds of times, people 1) get on an alkaline diet, 2) get their PH level up above 7.2-7.4, or, if you happen to have one of those weird cancers where you have too high PH – more acidic fluids to bring it down – you can talk to my friend Dr. Gonzales about that in New York City; so there are many ways of treating this cancer. So cannabis/hemp oil came along and I've got to throw this in the mix. So that is going to be a big part of the film as well.

It's ridiculous. I talked to Rick Simpson, who is a friend of mine, the guy from "Run from the Cure", and Ronnie Smith who is an old school guy, and I've talked to a number of old school guys; And between my friends with one connection – just one person – I literally know over 10,000 people that have been cured of cancer using cannabis/hemp oil. I'm going with what I see and what works. If I was out there and had cancer and was too busy with my life and family and job, and didn't know this, I would want somebody to get on the internet and say this stuff. I don't have any kids yet, so I have some time on my hands. So that what I've been going, and it has come along great.

I haven't got any major investments as usual – so it's wherever I can drive to from where I live in Los Angeles basically. But I want to thank my fans out there for all your donations and for buying the DVD of "I Cure Cancer" which you can do by going to ICureCancer.Com.

You can get a DVD. This just goes back to what I'm doing. This is my life folks. But to update you, bro.: Part one went great. It's kind-a-like a hit on the internet. And part 2 will be too.

Matthew L: Yeah . . . it's a great empowering movie. That's why I say you're a true health warrior. The message is getting out. People are starting to become more conscious nowadays. I think that … when you start to learn how you're being manipulated throughout…I felt like I was asleep for 20-something years of my life when I started to realize and wake up that, 'WAIT A MINUTE – you mean the FDA is not really protecting my best interests?! You mean we don't really need to be on all these meds?! You mean the AMA functions more like a cartel and the Gestapo than anything else!!??' I mean you start to really question a lot after that, and it drew me into asking like: "How are people being persuaded? How are people being manipulated? What is the science of propaganda? Because when you understand the science of propaganda you can spot it instantly on the news, the radio, the TV.

When somebody says it, you don't have to buy into that. And if you understand the principles there, you can use that to ethically help influence people into actually doing something that will save their life, that will save their children's lives; or, to better humanity. Do you know what I mean? Like, there are certain predictable patterns that people live by, and people are predictable to a certain extent. There's a guy whose name is Edward Bernaise. He wrote a book called Propaganda; Sigmund Freud's cousin. He literally tells that he was using the course to manipulate the masses. But, bottom line is, you have to understand how you're being programmed, so that you can slowly come out of that, or, as I did, just suddenly drop that old paradigm—that I bought into my whole life—cold turkey. I was probably, three weeks straight, devouring information, because I just felt like, "where the hell was I the last 20-something years of my life?" And then as I started to get in practice and see cancer reversed numerous times, numerous times, I mean it just blows your mind that this information is not out to the masses. But, you realize why, and if you understand the history of the business of disease like I talk about in chapter two of my book, it makes a lot of sense. You've got to know the history before you can actually…before it really clicks and you say, "Okay, here are the connections. Here's where the money goes. And here's why these "alternative therapies" are not the mainstream."

Ian: Right. Let's go through that chapter right now. I know, but my people want to know too. Want to give us some basic history of why we are so screwed up today?

Matthew L: (chuckles and Ian smiles) Sure. It's interesting. Without getting too deep into the one percent, the elite, and you know who I'm talking about obviously: there's this controlling hand over society. And they've been in control for a long time. It's so funny when people talk about the richest men in the world, they never mention these certain names, like the Rockefeller's, the Rothschild.'s Yet they were so integrated and integral in shaping how society is right now, they literally stack the chips in their favor. As I talk about what I'm about to go into, the history of medicine and the business of disease.

I'm all for capitalism by the way because I'm an entrepreneur, but I believe in conscious capitalism, helping people, delivering strong value into their lives and you're compensated upon the value that you bring to somebody; not because you're manipulating them into 'this toxic sludge is good for you' crap, which is what's going on with Big Food and Big Pharma. So there's a huge difference there.

But, if you understand a little bit of the history…you go back to 1910. You have a guy whose name was Abraham Flexner. He was commissioned by John D. Rockefeller to go around and evaluate all the medical schools in the country at that time. Rockefeller, a Standard Oil tycoon, was looking for ways to diversify his empire because the only thing that people like that in power want, is more power. So, he partnered with his competitors JP Morgan and Andrew Carnegie. They decided to go into this pharmaceutical interest. Everyone that was not as high as they were, were basically made stockholders.

This snake oil, this new stuff, didn't have any research behind it, because at that time doctors and medical schools were run by alternative practitioners using nutrition, homeopathy, chiropractic, magnetic therapy . . . all these other modalities, these other treatments now considered alternative, were the mainstream before. So all the medical doctors were using them.

However, Flexner went around evaluating all the medical schools in the country – as an employee of Rockefeller – and he came back with this infamous "Flexner report." Basically what he found was that there were a certain number of institutions that were using these alternative therapies (as we call them now), and they (Rockefeller's) wanted to have their pharmaceuticals in all these institutions; because there were petrol-chemicals in all the pharmaceuticals which were a way to get the oil in other places.

So, they wanted to diversify their empire. So what they did after this "full evaluation" (the outcome of which was rigged from the beginning!) is that they closed down roughly 60-70% of all medical schools at that time! 60-70% that did not follow these new guidelines, these pharmaceutical drugs, these wonder pills, were closed. That's how it started.

So they basically blacklisted all those medical doctors and practitioners, put them in jail, created these fear and propaganda campaigns that literally shaped the news how they wanted it; because at that time, of course, they still owned the media, they knew how to manipulate the public, and that's just what they did.

So, that kind of in a nutshell what happened with the history. You had the Flexner report that came out and, of course, swallowed it hook-line-and-sinker because they are lobbied by these industries (who bought them!). And you had that whole machine that took place, the medical cartel – the AMA monopoly – that came into being. So, there's just a lot of history that people need to understand about these organizations. It wasn't all unicorns and altruism.

For lack of a better word, it was a conspiracy. It wasn't a theory. These people wanted to dominate other industries so they took over. Now you have these companies that train the medical doctors and control what information gets pushed to the public. That's how after decades and decades and decades you indoctrinate/shape opinions of the masses (medical profession and public), through these PR campaigns and everything else. Even chiropractic in the 80s there was a case called the Wilk case. It was a federal case where the American Medical Association (AMA) was found guilty of conspiring to contain and eliminate the chiropractic profession! This was a federal court case.

So that just gives you an idea of the history of medicine, and why these groups are 'not your friends'. I think the average medical doctor, and I'm sure you would agree to Ian, they get into medicine because they truly want to help people. Do you know what I mean? So often they really want to help people, but once all the interest and the private money comes into play into their lap from pharmaceutical companies while they're in school, and they're literally trained by them, their perception is a little bit jaded when they come out (understatement!). They only believe what they're taught in school, and also "what the leading researchers" teach them anyway. So they are not taught to reason or ask questions as you would think. It's very disappointing, but as we mentioned before, I think more and more people are not coming to the realization that something's not right. We have one of the sickest nations in the world. How is that when we have the best trained medical specialists? Do you know what I mean?

Ian: I know! Here myself and a number of friends on Facebook and stuff, we speak about studies. Somebody is taking cannabis oil for where they're at, and they're jotting down what's happening so they can help others. We just found out about CBD oil. The THC oil we knew about. That was curing cancer, crone's disease, and many, many things. And again I want to throw out "take it easy on the 'cure' word" because I don't know if it has actually cured crones, but I know people that couldn't leave the house before, and now do work out, do yoga…have wonderful lives. Regarding macular degeneration or definitely some eye issues that cannabis is good for too. And for cancer. . . it works.

Matthew L: Yeah, I've heard a lot about cannabis oil. I personally don't have any experience using that, or even know somebody in my close circle that used that. But the research is there, and actually, with all these cases coming out of the woodwork, it just makes sense from a physiological perspective, once you dissect the biochemistry and how it works and everything. So, it's showing great promise.

I've always been under the impression . . . you know there are environmental toxins, emotional toxins and physical toxins that get into us that we need to get rid of, obviously, through a good diet and detaching from environmental stress and having just a good environment free from emotional stress as well. But there are other, I would say, nutritional power boosters; like vitamin D, probiotics; just some basic things of life that we've forgotten about in our type-A American society that really go a long way. So, cancer, while it is complex, I think sometimes we actually forget about how simple the solution just might actually be. Like, how many of us detach and get outside and really focus on deep belly breathing to oxygenate our bodies to help create that alkaline environment?

How many of us eat living foods from the ground all day? How many of us drink really clean water? I mean sometimes it's just the basic things that can dramatically boost your quality of life. And I know you and I have talked just a little bit about fasting. It's been around for thousands of years. Tumors have to grow too. Cancer needs food and if you don't feed it, it's not going to grow. And there's been a lot of research, two guys in particular: one is Herbert Shelton, the other is Paul Bragg. They wrote great books on the power of fasting. So I strongly recommend that if you haven't incorporated that into your regimen, it's just something that will help knock cancer out. It's just another added tool that the masses should know about, yet it's been suppressed for a long time. Because the media is owned by the sponsors it's very difficult to get air time, but there is hope like you said, and even with the Cannabis oil, I mean that's just fantastic the developments.

Ian: Yeah. Yeah. Just to finish that thought about the CBD for anyone out there listening, there's an amazing documentary on CNN, so just go to YouTube and google the CNN with Sanjay Gupta. Amazing documentary. It'll blow your mind folks. Watch it. Watch these kids go from having seizures, like multiple times a day to zero! ZERO! This is CBD oil. It doesn't have the THC in it that gets you high. There's a newer one coming out now.

My buddy Brad Mossman of https://www.hempremedies.com has been educating me on this. They can make CBD oil out of industrial hemp plants that have zero THC. And it's not illegal in America, though it's illegal to grow the plant thanks to the scumbags that we were talking about earlier that demonize marijuana.

So, I found a loophole folks, a way around. If you live in a non-legal marijuana state and you care—most of my friend don't—I say it's your life, it's your sovereign right to have your two feet planted on this earth, I don't care what country you're from or whatever. You're a human being and got God on your side, and He said you have free rights. So, do whatever you've got to do. But, if you have to stick to the "legal thing" you can order CBD oil that is made in Europe, shipped to America, tested and then it's legal.

So, it's crazy expensive. It's even more expensive than THC oil. But anyway, it's working amazingly well. Also if money is not an issue for you, get both CBD and the high TC oil because they complement each other like no other. And the CBD oil takes the "high" away from the THC – if you don't like getting high.

What started this rambling is: why should we the people have to call each other and say, "yeah I've tried this and that…" I mean it should be DONE. Instead, they're (Big Pharma) spending billions every year on more chemo which we know doesn't work! And we're tired of people having to stand up and … I haven't figured out how, whether it's got to be a revolution or if the light is just going to keep coming to the masses and we're just going to suddenly sneeze and blow them away. I, I haven't figured it out yet, but I'm working on it.

Matthew L: Yeah, … I used to be a lot softer in my approach (laughter). And once I got a purpose I really decided: "You know something? 1) Chemotherapy and radiation and chopping off organs or body parts – it's just barbaric. It's fucking barbaric!" Once I started to really connect back with my purpose and my mission in terms of like: people need great information. Especially children. The topic of this conversation is cancer, but another issue that fires me up is the psychotropic drugging of kids! It's just like, 'what the hell is going on here!' The side effects are obviously in their face, and I think that we as we evolve as a species, this is so antiquated it's ridiculous. The reason why it's still pushed out there is because of very clever marketing and propaganda by these groups in power. That's why it's so important to understand how you're being spoon-fed this stuff.

I literally watch the news. I gotta tell you, I don't watch a lot of TV. I like to go to the movies sometimes, but I know when I watch the television that there are corporate interests being pumped down my subconscious and even as educated about these things as I am, if you're in that environment all day long, whether with friends or family with the radio or TV you start to believe some of this bullshit. It wears on you. Even if you're firmly grounded you've got to stay out of that and you have to do your own homework and research, and you have to look back to certain scientific principles. Auto-regulation homeostasis, that's fundamental to science. Your body is programmed to heal itself-period! All you need to do is get the junk out. Your body will adapt.

I've seen stage four cancer reversed numerous times. It doesn't matter how far along you are, cancer is not a death sentence. That's something people need to understand and know. But if you look at this pinkwashing – everything that goes down the propaganda machine today – they want people to feel like cancer is a death sentence and that you have to go through the system. Then they try to glorify this chopping off of body parts. It's sick and disgusting. And these people need to be stopped.

So, you're right. Maybe there needs to be a revolution because the time for just pussy-footing around and saying, "Oh well, maybe you should do this…" No. You've really got to do this for the sake of your children – to live a better life. I try to be very direct now in my communication with people. I'll give them the background, I'll give them the history so that they know that I'm not just fanatical about this. I'll give them science as well. But you know we're coming to a point where something has to go. We have to take hold and create this momentum. I believe that we are. It's just that it needs to happen a lot faster.

Ian: know somebody that cured their kid with cannabis oil. You want to give my kid chemo?!!" What's even worse is that two or three of the stories I'm following, the children look like they have already been cured of cancer by the cannabis oil, yet they're being forced to have chemo for another two years! Get that: forced to have chemo for another two years even though they're cancer free! The one lady—I don't remember her name—I want to have on my show. CNN is going to do a show on her too.

She basically has her kid cured and she moved to Colorado so she could get the Cannabis legally, and it didn't matter… the hostile medical profession said, "Sorry you're still getting chemo!" They went to court three times. They beat them twice. The third time they brought in a different judge and they got them . . . so they're on the run. They're running from the law (a bad law) right now. I told them, "Come down to Tijuana man. I'll hook you up."

Matthew L: It just blows my mind that this is America. Honestly, it really does. You think about the perceived freedom that we have, but you realize that there are a few puppet masters in control and it's because people have been so . . . . to a certain extent, we have to accept responsibility. All this stuff went on under the table and people have just been so comfortable in their own little lives, getting their knowledge off the tube (TV). It is just one of those things from which we have to wake up. It's time to wake up. Our children's lives are . . .

Ian: it's the suffering, the suffering. OMG! The suffering! This one little girl that I've been following Jay Mathews kid—she could be in my film—just had her arm cut off. This girl was totally healthy. Except she had bone cancer. The parents took her to a place in Arizona, a holistic place; got her going, got her PH level up good and high (7.2) . . . she'd be cancer free now if they'd left her alone! But the cops caught up to them, forced them to do the chemo-radiation-surgery, and then, of course, through the complications due to the chemo – which just destroys everything – she lost her arm because of infection recently. I mean, that's really got me upset. So, they're going to be hearing from me. But that's what's going on man! I can't take it anymore. I want trials. All you oncologists out there right now, expect trials, in my lifetime.

Matthew L: This is a criminal act. It really is. I don't know how else to put it. It's barbaric and it's criminal. You know I can't recall the exact source that I saw this study, but they did a study with oncologists. They asked the oncologists, "If you had cancer, would you take chemo or radiation?" And the overwhelming majority (85%!!!) of them, said, "No way." . . . . I've had a couple of oncologists buy my book and one, in particular, started giving it out in his reception area! I was blown away because usually oncologists and neurosurgeons are very set in their ways many times! I was just blown away that he did that and he was trying to be more holistic in his approach, which was great. But chemotherapy, besides being unproven and being unscientific it is just so barbaric. There's no other word for it. Most people die of the actual treatment than the actual cancer.

Ian: Yeah. And I always tell my people when they come with that, "ask your oncologist, 'Does it get the cancer stem cells?'" Because that's what kills you. Sure with chemo and radiation, you can take off the mass, but they're not the ones that kill you. It's the cancer stem cells. And not only does radiation not kill them, but radiation also makes them stronger! I got one guy contacting me – I hope he's listening – I would NEVER get radiation. You don't need it. And the one radiation that little girl did get actually — and this is why I was so upset — even though they found a real western medicine person that was doing cyber-knife. And that's a legitimate thing. He said, I just saved your daughter's arm because I killed the cancer in the one spot with the cyber-knife. Now, I don't know enough about that to recommend it to anybody. The point is, this MD doctor said, "I just saved your daughter's arm." And now it's gone a year later because the other scumbag oncologist — he's lucky I don't remember his name right now — kept pumping that chemo into her.

Matthew L: Unreal! This just goes to show you where the professionals are so indoctrinated into a certain belief system, that even though they know chemotherapy is toxic to the body, they know it causes cancer, yet if you talk to them they say, "well it's the best we have right now". Or, they'll say that the studies prove that it's "higher." It blows my mind that more doctors don't acknowledge 1) the conflict of interests. The fact that the overwhelming majority of major medical journal studies are funded by drug companies (that get richer on the sickness of people)! This is like the fox running the hen house.

Ian: Yes!

Matthew L: And to believe and to even say that this Pfizer, you know, Merck- funded research is anything but reliable . . . given this massive history of the drug companies of lawsuits of putting profits before people . . . is absolute lunacy. It's ridiculous.

Ian: Yeah, yeah. And any of you out there that had this happen to you or your family, and you want to do something about it and think you can't . . . I'm just learning this stuff about international laws, contract laws. Little things I've been hearing say, "Sue the judge." Not the court because they have their own lawyers. Sue the judge that did it as a human being, as well as the cops, the oncologist(s), pretty much anyone who ruins your life or murdered your child. Sue them personally.

That's the best I can come up with now. I'm going to Dr. Caldwell's seminar in December to learn more about this stuff. I'm just giving people a way to fight back. You're right, I can't believe this is America either. It sounds like Germany back in the days of Hitler, or Russia you know. They're freer than we are now or so it seems, you know!

Matthew L: Yeah. I just am blown away, especially as the years go by and I mean there are a lot of changes happening. It's been expedited so we really need to get on the ball. I think that that's why I love social media in my alter-ego life per se because it allows you to connect and reach the masses very quickly if you know what you're doing. You know what I mean. You can take a message that resonates and get it spread virally to a lot of different people in a short amount of time with a very small shoestring budget. And that's where people need to hear that because unfortunately to rely on major media outlets like television or radio — even if you had the big dollars to spend — there's a good chance you'd not get much time just because it's such a monopoly. So you really have to take matters into your own hands and I think you're doing all the great things, and I really enjoy the fact that you're featuring these leaders; these doctors that are treating and curing cancer. It's amazing. Did you hear about Dr. Burzynski in Texas? Have you interviewed him, or no?

Ian: No, I haven't yet. But I know all about him... I'm limited about where I can shoot and can only do that around Los Angeles until I get some investments or something. But I would love because Burzynski...if anybody hasn't seen that film, please go see Dr. Burzynski. I think it's called "The Movie" or something. Right?

Matthew L: Yeah. I don't recall. Actually, was his "Cut, Poison, Burn"? Was that his?

Ian: No. No. that was actually my friend Louis. Louis Cimino made that. That's another amazing film. If you haven't seen that you have to see that: "Cut, Poison, Burn". It'll just disgust you with what is going on and hopefully make you do either what I do, or, somehow get involved because "Cut, Poison, Burn" and the first twenty minutes of Dr. Burzynski will blow your mind. There's a sheriff that gets on there, and he tells the whole story about twin daughters; beautiful blonde little girls, and there's only one left because the one died of cancer. But she didn't die of the cancer, she died of the treatment. Dr. Burzynski cured her brain cancer with his antineoplastons and she still died because of the original treatments!

Matthew L: Yeah. Again, cancer has been cured several times throughout history. There's another great documentary called The Forbidden Cures. You can go to YouTube and watch the whole documentary. It does go into the history — kind of what I was referring to in chapter two — it goes into very detailed accounts of several practitioners that have cured cancer and that have been really pushed out by the AMA medical monopoly, or medical drug cartel as I like to refer to them as. It'll blow your mind. So, you've got to understand the history and why things are the way they are.

Yes, there is a conspiracy. No, there's no theory. There is a big business that is profiting off of sick people everywhere every single day! Yet, the average cancer patient is worth over $200,000 (two hundred thousand dollars) to a hospital as they walk through the door (and at least that much again to the oncologist). So this is very big business as opposed to someone going let's say getting treatment at Dr. Burzynski's clinic for one-twentieth of that. So, we're talking about much less expensive to get a competent treatment that actually cures cancer and enables you to live an optimal and healthy life. So there's a lot of money on the table and that's why something needs to be done. You just have to get mad as hell and say to yourself 'I'm not going to take it anymore.' When I see little children dying needlessly, it just enrages me so much and that really fuels my passion. It makes me stronger and makes me commit to this mission even more so.

Ian: Aw yeah man! I hear you, bro. I had that little Celina in my arms one day, and I could've just booked (run out of there) and brought her somewhere and took care of her and she'd have her arm and everything. But then I wouldn't be able to help anybody else. It was a hard decision to make at that moment because I had her... in my head. I was like, he wouldn't care, he'd be cool and I'd tell him I'd bring her back in a few months . . . but I just couldn't go there. Anyway, so, I'm getting too angry. Let's talk about something brighter, or I'll start punching the bag behind me.

The cleansing we were talking about, you're saying if I understand you are that the body in its normal state would never have gotten sick, but if you get it back to the normal state then it will cure itself. What are some of the things you like to do? A lot of my friends out there are just thinking 'oh, cannabis/hemp oil, that's it, that's all I need' and I say, I hate to say this but it's kinda true because Rick Simpson told me most people take the oil and that's it and they lose their cancers. But I say, 'don't take any chances. Get on the alkaline diet, get your PH up, detox, do coffee enemas', you know. Let's play with that a little bit. What do you like? What would you suggest to somebody that wanted to start preventing cancer or curing cancer?

Matthew L: There are certain health principles that are universal that have been around that will always be around. I believe there are 10 or so principles that are really true. 1) is having a strong spiritual connection. Whatever that is for you. I think that you have to be connected and grounded in some way shape or fashion. 2) Be grateful and appreciate all of life. I think that that is very important. I think you have to have a positive mental attitude because that's been proven to affect your biochemistry. Experiencing love, gratitude or laughing a lot. Optimism. I get passionate about a lot of these subjects, but I try not to dwell on negative sides so much as opposed to being in the moment, loving my family and friends. Serving people from a position of love. So, again your mental state is extremely important. 3) Obviously, nourishment, nutrition, organic and living foods and correcting any nutritional deficiencies is like the lifeblood of beating cancer. 4) Freedom from emotional toxicity. If you have people in your life that are emotionally bad for you, you need to make a decision. I don't care if they're family or close friends, but you have to do what's best for your health and wellbeing. That just wears and wears especially if you have negative relationships in your life. So, again, you've got to have your positive emotional influencers as well.

5) Obviously, we need water, clean water. You'd be surprised at how hard it is to find good clean water nowadays. I like to opt for spring water more so than anything because it goes through the ground. But, again, know where you get your water from. I don't drink tap water. Now they're finding prescription drug residues in tap water and publicly acknowledging that! I remember an instructor about twelve years ago talking about the fact that he had a friend that worked at the local water treatment facility. And he said, "Hey, we're finding Prozac residues in the public water treatment and we have no way of filtering the stuff!" Freaking antidepressants in your water!

Ian: One of my girl's friends was a nurse and she said that's what they did if they ever spilled the medicine, they'd just put it right in the toilet. So, think about how many hospitals, and how many spills. We're talking about millions of and billions of pills every year being thrown down the drain. Of course, it's going to go in there.

Matthew L: Even when people urinate, I mean, it just doesn't break down accordingly. They have no way to filter it. There are a lot of ways that it gets in there. But it's nuts. Aside from all the crap fluoride and toxic chemicals, you're getting an extra dose of prescription meds if you don't have clean water.

6) Sun rays are important for you. Here again, you have all this media saying that the sun is bad for you. And, hey, everything in excess could be bad for you, but the sun is essential for life! When the sun's light hits your skin it produces vitamin D. Vitamin D is quite possibly the most important vitamin for immune-system function. I mean it's extremely important. It helps to boost your immune system and helps you absorb calcium and a lot of other minerals. A lot of people are running around vitamin-D deficient and they don't even know it. So, don't be afraid of the sun. You need it. It's essential for life.

7) I talked a little be before about oxygen. You need clean air to breathe. If you live in let's say Atlanta, Los Angeles, New York City, Chicago, Dallas, you might be a little hard-pressed to find clean air at times. So you've got to get out, away, and really focus on deep belly breathing and try to get some fresh air because that's an essential factor of maintaining a healthy life.

8) Physical activity: You need exercise. And there's no getting around that. I deal with people all the time. They'll put on these nutritional detox diets, they lose a lot of weight and they're much healthier, but you need physical activity. We are made to be active and it produces and secretes a lot of chemical and hormones in your body that make you healthier.

9) Sleep. Rest is another one. You should be getting eight hours of sleep every single night. That's when your body rests and repairs itself. If you're not getting adequate sleep, you're not going to be 100% healthy. There's no way, it's impossible, it's essential. You don't want to shortcut that if possible. And then 10) I like to talk about fasting because fasting is a key way to detox and get a lot of junk out of your body that doesn't need to be there. You know you find in the wild that animals instinctively fast when they're sick or when they're not feeling too well. If you look back thousands of years in different civilizations, many did have fasting practices. But what I'm referring to is more like a water fast, just water for several days. You can kind of mix that up.

Sometimes I'll actually go on a water perfect food fast with just an alkaline supplement. It's just an all-green food supplement. So if you have an organic whole green food supplement that tastes like grass you can just mix that with water and literally alkalize your body for three or four days just doing that alone. I've done that for a week before. But it's a great way just to clear your body out, give digestion a break, give all your internal organs a break and you find that your senses, your sense of sight, your sense of smell, they're all heightened after you break your fast. It's great. There's a lot of research to support it.

And as I mentioned before, you want to pick up a book by Herbert Shelton called Fasting Can Save Your Life. It's so powerful. An amazing book. In my opinion, those are probably the ten principles of health. There are certain nutritional components or oils like you're talking about earlier. They can accelerate this process. But I firmly believe you have to address all these areas if you truly want to be healthy.

Ian: Absolutely. Yeah, I just finally did a juice-blend fast myself. So, I guess that wouldn't be a total fast because I kept the fiber in there. But basically, I didn't eat anything but organic, or drink organic shakes for two months. I dropped 30 pounds, got shredded.

Matthew L: How do you feel?

Ian: Feel amazing, unbelievable. And the craziest thing happened. I'm going to say it on air because I said it on Facebook: First time in my life last night I spoke telepathically to my friend and he frikin' heard me! Most people probably won't even believe me. And I didn't believe it, 'cause I kinda had done it before, but I just said "Nah!" But I got pissed off because somebody said, "Can you fuckin' hear me?!" and he said "Yeah!" Out loud. I said "Can you fuckin' hear me" in my head and he said "yeah" out loud. 'Cause he was already talkin' to me out loud when I was talking in here (pointing to his head). I couldn't believe it. Pardon me for my French there, ladies. I got a little carried away, but I mean this has never happened to me before. But he didn't want to talk about it. But I've been talkin' to a lot of people like that around here. Down in Mexico the healers, like healers of the light, believe in God, Jesus … all that and they know how to work the light.

And so it's just something I'm getting into and I wonder, 'cause Rick Simpson told me when you take the Cannabis/hemp oil it cleanses your pineal gland. That's your third eye. That's your connection to what's really going on. So, anyway, just to throw that out there folks.

And I hear . . . that's going to keep happening. Our planet is going to get more light, become more awake and that's why I'm not too worried about the one percent. I think they're just going to disappear. I think there are going to be trials for them and all that, but hopefully, in my lifetime, the earth will be the way it's supposed to be. That was fun. (Laughter) I can't believe I just admitted this on air. Everyone is going to think I'm nuts.

Matthew L: The truth is when you really clean your body out, there's so much capability and potential that we possess that I think we only tap into a fraction of it. And, I never ... you know I've always been of the mindset that just because I don't understand it doesn't make it impossible. I mean it's like whoever thought a hundred years ago that they were going to fold up a piece of metal and throw it across the ocean? I mean we have airplanes. It's like the thoughts are already there, the stuff's already there, it's just we have to get to that level of consciousness where we can tap into that. Make sense?

Ian: Yeah, yeah. That may help other people too like artists, musicians, actors. I mean we tap into that all the time. Your subconscious, your super-conscious – whatever. I guess what I learned is that the super-conscious is kind of like god, and subconscious is the stuff around here, and the conscious is our inner. I've interpreted dreams like an unopened letter from God. I always like that one too. Let's see what else do we need to talk about . . . We've talked a little about the nutrition, supplements, doing the fasting is amazing, everybody should try that; the juicing, uh, How long can you do the fast for without doing fats and proteins and stuff? I guess, can people do it for a couple of weeks? What do you say, a week?

Matthew L: The most important part is to realize, 1) you can go months without food. You can. You can only go a few days without water. So, you've got to stay hydrated. That's the big portion. You have to keep enough water in your system. I've done a water fast for seven days. I know people have done a water fast for over a month. I think that's a little extreme for a water fast, but they've done it before. I would say if you're just starting out and you want to try to get into a fast you can do a juice fast to kind of get your body prepped. And I do recommend keeping maybe a third of the pulp in there just to give you that fiber to help give you that digestion. That's totally cool. Do that for maybe a day. See how you feel. You should be perfectly fine.

The hardest part of a fast is just not eating. It's breaking the habit of actually reaching for food because food is such a social occasion in America. I mean, if you think about it, when you're with friends all the time or doing whatever, even when you're not hungry, you're probably snacking on something half the time. So, it's just a habit and I find that while I've never been a smoker, I've never been addicted to any serious drugs, but I would contend that not eating, or actually eating is probably the hardest addiction to break.

Staying away from food. And it really gives you a sense of empowerment as well because if you can fast, the only other thing I can equate that too is my sky-diving experience when I jumped out of a plane. If I can do this I can go ahead and talk to this beautiful woman who is now my wife. You know what I mean, it's like comparing this to many instances in your life which can make it seem a little easier.

So fasting is a challenge at first. But, start off slow. Juice fasting is the way to start off fasting one to two days. You can go easily for five days on a juice fast. It's just breaking open that initial barrier. You're probably going to be hungry for the first day or so. That's fully normal. And depending upon how big you are you have to realize that … I like to equate it to a bear that goes into hibernation. I work with a lot of patients that are just fat, I mean they're big people. And they haven't taken care of themselves. And I say, "Listen, the great news is that your body is going to convert a lot of this fat back into sugar to feed your brain and to keep you going. You might be hungry for the first day, but after that you're fine.

One of my better friends used to be over three hundred pounds. I fasted him a week on just water and he was just fine. He didn't get hungry at all. And then we broke him (i.e., the fast) on raw fruits and vegetables afterward and —— he had eczema and a bunch of all these problem conditions and even one autoimmune condition, and they totally cleared up after this fast because the gut was able to heal itself. The gut, in my personal opinion based on the research and a lot of what I've read, is one of the keys, if not the major key to a healthy body. You've got to be able to digest, and not just digest but absorb things in your body and then be able to assimilate into the cells to get optimal uptake in nutrition.

Ian: Right, right. If anybody wants to see the blend fast diet, you can go to YouTube and search or click: Ian Jacklin blend fast instructions. And I put a new one up too. The audio is a little better on the new one so I'd choose that one. But it's really simple, you just go to your local store, wherever they have organic and get all the cruciferous vegetables, kale, broccoli, the dark lettuces. Put them in there. If you have cancer stay away from the fruits for the time being. I'd stay away from the fruit until your PH is up to about 7. Just mix it with water and add some Stevia and green apple and dark berries are okay because there's not as much sugar, and that will help you (and juice these). If you don't have cancer which I now know I don't . . . I was kind of freakin' out there man and I didn't really tell anybody, but when my PH was low for a while I got it up but still, I just wasn't feeling… I was worried you know. And so I'm down here at Tijuana filming a clinic for my film and luckily for $67 bucks I went and got everything (in my body) checked out. And I'm totally cancer free. My PH is good so I'm happy

Matthew L: That's awesome!

Ian: So, oh I forgot where I was going with that one. I think I got too excited knowing that. I remember that feeling because it's kinda heavy walking around helping everybody else with their cancer and I was a bad boy when I young. I did drink. I did smoke. I did you know everything. After I won championships, trust me we partied hard too. So who knows, but it all came out good.

Matthew L: I think it's important to realize that regardless of where you are or even what you've done in younger periods of life, our body is always capable of regeneration and in healing itself. I don't care how old you are.

Now there is a certain window of opportunity for each and every condition and disease, and if you go past that window you start to develop permanent damage. So, to reverse early on is the ideal scenario. But even in later stages of cancer or diseases where you actually have scar tissue built up in the system, the human body is an amazing, amazing structure. I think that we've been just convinced that we need outside intervention to optimize our health and that's really not the case at all. We don't need to go to the doctor every couple of months. We don't need to take these pills that actually . . . almost . . . what did was it Voltaire that said, something along the lines of "medical doctors amuse the disease with medication, while nature cures it." Something along those lines. I think it was Voltaire. It goes along with the point: Your body is going to heal itself and you've just got to give it those optimal conditions to let it heal. You talked about the clinics in Mexico. There are some really good ones down there. I even reference a couple in my book, and unfortunately, it's hard to get good clinics here just because of the laws as they are. But I know you're affiliated, or, are you affiliated with cancer control society?

Ian: I'm their friend. I mean I've gone to every one of them for the last probably ten years.

Matthew L: So you've gotten a lot of good information and resources through these practitioners. The bottom line is, even for people listening to this, that there are options. Cancer is not a death sentence by any means. It's just that we have to open the blinders a little bit and look beyond that paradigm that we've been conditioned to believe. Like I've said, I've seen cancer reversed way too many times to allow some skeptic or some arrogant doctor (oncologist) to tell me otherwise. If you or your family or loved one or child or whoever has it, it's time that you do your due diligence and make a good decision and realize that there are some foundational principles to health and healing and it's not as complex as we've all been made to believe and you know the newest thing it seems like, over the last, I would say ten years, is the medical profession seems to be putting so much weight on genes nowadays. And while genes are important, if you look at an objective source, it would say five to seven percent could be genetic and the rest of that could be overcome with epigenetics; the ability of your body's DNA to adapt to heal itself. We have time-tested principles that work. So, just make sure that you're well informed. When you go to the doctor or get a second opinion when you start to do the research and do the homework on your own because it's just horrible to watch and hear about stories where lives were lost needlessly to this medical system.

Ian: Yeah. And this just off the top of my head . . . Cancertutor.Com folks, my good friend Webster Kerr runs that site and probably one of the best web sites on the net for information. He addresses the fact that some cancers you've got to do other things to save your life first. You can't just go in and try and kill the cancer. He'll explain that to you if you have a fast-growing cancer there are ways of keeping yourself alive long enough so the other alternative things can actually get to you cancer. Just a quick note here.

Man, this flew . . . I only have a few minutes left. I wanted to see what you are doing now? Tell us a little about how you can help people out there . . . any of my friends that are holistic people. You're helping them with their businesses now. And I believe in this because unfortunately 'ask gas or grass' you've got to pay. Now unfortunately if you're getting western medicine it's probably free if you happen to have medical insurance, but I wouldn't be doing that myself, personally. You do have to pay and the healers should get paid because they're saving your butt. So, how do you help them maybe not be starving all the time and keeping a roof over their head?

Matthew L: Well you know it's really like I was talking about earlier when I realized that marketing influenced communication – works extremely important understanding how I was to see you in terms of what I believed for the first twenty years of my life – there are a lot of doctors and professionals and practitioners that have a very strong message of health. I'm using the medical profession with these principles can be applied to whatever business you're in if you're a film-maker, actor, whatever. You have a message that needs to be heard. And there's a certain way to get people to build an audience, to get them into your pride (lions) so that they know they can trust you, so you're able to deliver value they can connect and you can build a relationships with them, and they can eventually buy your stuff so they can transform their lives.

Example: The I Cure Cancer is a fantastic DVD. But if that can't get out to the masses, it's a great product because it helps people live healthier lives and saves them from this medical system. But if it doesn't get into enough hands . . . what good is it?

My main mission is to really help doctors and people who have a strong message of empowerment to get that message into the hands of their community. So, 1. To build a community, whether it is thousands, hundreds of thousands or millions or what have you and to understand how to effectively communicate to that community so they can get to know and trust you. You become the expert in their eyes and you understand how to bring other people in that deliver value into their lives. Then, making a good income is a by-product of all that stuff. If you have all these pillars lined up, if you're clear on your purpose, on why you want to help people and why you do what you do, if your mission is very strong, if you have that "why" behind you, if you have the tools and resources, if you take action you can achieve that. And so I basically show these doctors and professionals how to do that, how to build their practices and their businesses, and really make a difference in people's lives.

You can learn more about that at my blog. Just go to www.MatthewLoop.com and when you go to the blog, you're probably going to see a lot for entrepreneurs. But realize that all this stuff that you can use, whether it's the Facebook communication, the Facebook marketing, the Twitter, you can use it an apply it to increase your communication to get more people to hear about your message, and you're able to influence them and transform their lives. You know marketing and sales are not dirty words. It's how you approach that. If you really believe in what you have, if you believe that your product or service, or you and your message of health are going to transform someone's life, then it's your obligation to get it in their hands. And there are ways that you can do that to ethically influence people to take the action that is best for them as opposed to what we've seen so many times on television like Big Pharma does as they unethically manipulate the public into buying this toxic sludge crap. So, again it's kind of a similar mission as the Health-and-Wellness to empower people to better lives. I've just taken that into communication and marketing because that's an integral component that many people, doctors, and professionals, they completely forget about. But it's essential to be able to build your message; get it out to the right people and transform their lives.

Ian: Absolutely. Right on Matthew Loop. I really appreciate your being on the show. Before we take off, go to my Facebook page folks, I just posted it. My friend Lilly, she's … fighting cancer in the gogo site, if you can donate a few bucks, she'd appreciate it. I'm actually going to be doing a calendar (Ian show his six-pack abs), and whatever anyone can help her family because her child, her son is taking care of her and her husband and three kids. It's unbelievable what's going on. So if you can donate to that I'd greatly appreciate it. Matthew man, what an honor and respect as always brother.

Matthew L: Ian I'm very proud to call you a friend man. You're a true health warrior and I look forward to connecting in person.

Ian: Right on! Okay. Thanks to everybody. This has been ICureCancer.Com. Peace!

CHAPTER 22:

INTERVIEW WITH TY BOLLINGER

Ian: We're live on IcureCancer.com and on ZenLive.TV. I'm really lucky today to talk with our next guest whose name is Ty Bollinger. He's one of the top guys for knowing what's going on and he wrote the book, Cancer, Step Outside the Box, which everybody has to do, or you will not even come close to the mark.

Ty B: Thanks for having me on today my friend. I appreciate it.

Ian: Right on. It's an honor to have you here. You're one of my heroes, so I appreciate that you are here. You work for NaturalNews.com now right, with Mike Adams over there?

Ty B: Yeah. I know Mike. I do a radio show once a week on the National News network. Outside the Box – Wednesdays, on actually the Robert Scot Bell show. I don't know if you're familiar with Robert Scot Bell. I started about 8 or 10 months ago doing one show a week with him. So, we actually co-host the show, and we have a lot of fun, and we go back and forth on the health issue, political issues, you name it, nothing is off limits with us, and so we'll hit 8 or 10 current events, articles each and every week, man. Just having fun with it. Keeping it light and still hitting the serious topics. I mean you gotta be able to laugh and, so we make it fun, but we address the important topics.

Ian: Yeah. Robert Scot Bell, I interviewed him for my film. I'm pretty sure he's had me on his show. I know Joanie Abbot Cox has had me on, and you had me on your show, I've had you on my show, so we kind of know each other – for those that are watching. There are a group of highly intelligent people that have a passion like I do for getting the truth out. Then you make your own decisions. Now, you yourself, did you ever have cancer, Ty? Or, how did you get into this?

Ty B: That's a great question. I've had some skin cancers that I've taken care of with some black salves, but never had a life-threatening cancer. But I did get into the cancer research arena because of my parents actually. 1996 my father was diagnosed with cancer, and it took the medical establishment about 25 days to kill him. And he was a relatively healthy 52-year-old, went in for surgery on what he thought was gall stones and within 25 days he was dead. Nineteen blood transfusions later they removed his whole stomach, because of stomach cancer and he died. So that was my initiation into the medical mafia; the current cancer industry that kills people better than they treat them. Over the course of the next seven years, after Dad died, I lost both grandfathers, a grandmother, cousin, uncle and finally my mother all to cancer. It was at that point that I said, "Enough's enough! I've been doing research. There are all kinds of treatments out there that are natural non-toxic that could be healing people, but many people don't know about them because the medical mafia is hiding them and suppressing them and running people out of the country for using them. And that's when I published my book.

Ian: Right on! That makes sense. I myself never had cancer, but I have some little brown spots here (pointing to his forehead) that I'm putting cannabis oil on just in case. If you think you have skin cancer the bloodroot that Ty used is amazing, it works, but I'm pretty sure that it hurts right? It's very painful right?

Ty B: Yeah. It is a little bit painful when it kills the cancer cells underneath and they come out, it is a little bit painful. It does burn a little bit. But it's very successful. But cannabis oil is a very good choice as well.

Ian: Yeah. That's why I tell people—before I always told them to use bloodroot because of its 100% success rate. I've never heard anyone not curing their skin cancers using bloodroot, or even the Gerson therapy. You can do it inside out by using Gerson therapy. So, for anybody out there listening, skin cancer is 100% curable. You do not need to die from it. I know some who have. One guy came to me one time, he had a spot somewhere and I said, "whatever you do, don't just get it cut off, because it won't go away, it won't get the roots. And what does he do, he gets it cut off, calls me a year later and says, "Ian, you're right." So, I sent him to an alternative doctor, but it was too late. It had already spread. All he had to do was put some salve on there. But it's like giving birth. Women have told me that when it's drawing that cancer it out, it's really painful; but it works.

Ty B: Yeah it does. And it's funny that you mention that. My grandmother, she died when she was 89, but before she died—she didn't of cancer—she had some cancerous lesions on her forehead. She had a big spot here (pointing between his eyebrows) and a big spot here (on the nose) and I think three big basal cell carcinomas. They were black, and they were clearly basal cells. The doctor said, "yeah this is just "BCC" and we're just going to cut them off." I said, "Why don't you give me a few weeks. Let's wait, I think I can get rid of them." At that point, the doctor laughed at me. But she (the doctor) said, "Okay, fine" and she looked at me like I was an idiot. So, we used the salve on Grand mom; And, within three or four weeks we went back to see the doctor again. The spots were completely gone. She (the doctor) wasn't laughing then. Of course, she didn't ask what we did either. So, you'd think that a doctor if she were competent and really wanted to heal that she would have swallowed her pride and said, "I don't know what you did, but I'd like to learn so that maybe I can help my patients in the future." She never asked.

Ian: I know. Unbelievable. The reason why I made my film and got into it is because my ex-girlfriend Cynthia Brooks, she cured herself of "terminal cervical cancer" 19 years ago. She went back to the doctors – a medical miracle – at UCLA hospital and she says, "Don't you know what I did?" And they go, "No!" Of course, he (the doctor) can't do anything anyway. He's in America. They're legally bound to give chemotherapy, radiation and/or surgery. Sad, but true, state-of-affairs. So, it did hurt, right? You know what "childbirth" is.

Ty B: (laughter) I don't know that it was as painful as childbirth, but it does burn, and it hurts. I've heard from people who had bigger tumors. There was a guy I know named Bill Trucks that had pancreatic cancer and he used the salve on his back. And it literally drew the tumor out through his back, and he has documented it in a book with graphic pictures of these enormous cancerous tumors coming out his back. But it healed and he's well. Yeah, and he says it was painful.

Ian: Yeah, yeah. I've seen that before. Dan Raber is the one that introduced me to bloodroot years ago. It pulls out from one-and-a-half centimeters so it's perfect on skin cancer because it's right there. But like you say, another tumor . . . I've had women with breast tumors when they bend over in the morning to pick something up and it fell out!

At least it's gone even though it hurt. I'd recommend trying cannabis-oil first to you listening folks because it's not as painful. It just depends on what State you're in, whether it's legal or not. But I would never let laws get in the way of your life. Where there's a will, there's a way. Have you been hearing about the mad success cannabis oil is having on your end?

Ty B: Sure! Yeah. A lot of success. As a matter of fact, Robert and I just talked about it on our show a couple of weeks ago. The "Marijuana Moms" out there in California – the big groups of moms that are not only using the hemp oil but they're also taking it and mixing it up and making ice cream, using it in salads, eating it, smoking it, I mean I've got no problem with people eating it, smoking it, using the oil; any of it. I mean it's just a plant. It's a plant that grows naturally and I think it's really good in a multitude of ways, even not just solely for medical uses. It's a great hemp fiber, I mean there are so many good uses for hemp. But you grow it and you could go to jail. I mean it's pathetic the state that we live in.

Ian: Oh, I know. And of course, cannabis oil helps decalcify the pineal gland. That's the "third eye." That's the reason why they got rid of marijuana in the first place, on top of all the money reasons, they knew it would wake people up. I think. Anyway, more people will fight the system when they start thinking and questioning. Which is what we need.

Ty B: Well, we can't have that can we! (tongue firmly in cheek and laughter) Just shut up and do what you're told. (laughter)

Ian: Exactly. Unreal. Well, you still have your show going on right.

Ty B: Yeah. Still got the show. Had a great time this last week, and I traveled up to Huntersville, N.C. I'm good friends with Dr. Rashid Buttar up there. He's a very well-known doctor for treating cancer, detoxification; as a matter of fact, over the last decade it's cost him over $14 million to fight the North Carolina medical board who was trying to take his license, and he beat them. They dropped all charges, but that's a lot of money to have to fight someone when you're not guilty. But he has beaten them. But we were at his advanced-medicine seminar out there in Huntersville. He does these advanced-medicine seminars all over the country. That was the first one I was able to speak at. Robert Scot Bell speaks at them.

I don't know if you know Liam Scheff? Liam speaks at these advanced-medicine seminars as well. So, I had a great time up there. Then I was also a couple of months ago in Chicago at the Health Freedom Expo and that was really cool! It had like 3,000 people there. It was wonderful just to be able o meet people and shake their hand and it was very humbling quite honestly, Ian, with the number of people that came up to me with tears in their eyes and said "Thank you for your book. Thank you for your research. I was diagnosed with terminal cancer five-six years ago; I'm alive. I'm healthy, and it's because of the research that you did." So, it's very rewarding to see the results of the book and you know, that's my passion, to help people. So, I don't take credit for it. I give God the credit for it and the people the credit for being smart enough to learn and use the knowledge that they've been given. It's not me. I'm not a miracle worker. But it is a blessing to be able to help people and see people alive that would have been dead if they'd listened to their traditional oncologist.

Ian: Yeah! I know exactly what you mean. I feel the same way. I'm not at your level yet, but I know exactly what you're talking about. It makes it all worthwhile. I've always done things for free. When I was a kickboxing champion, they didn't have the money like the MMA guys have today. There was nothing like that. I was paid $2,400 for my world championship fight against Javier Mendez. But I always do it for the love of the game. And that's like here too. This is the best. This is even better than that title belt that's sitting back there. Because when you get that phone call saying, "The cancer's gone!" You're like 'YES! – ROCK ON!' (big smile on both). And it's sad when some of them don't make it because there's no silver bullet. But I find there are no accidents or mistakes: you cross paths for a reason. So, maybe I'm helping that person make the shift to the other side. Whatever I can do, I'm just a friend. You do whatever you can to help them out just as if it was you treating your neighbors the way you like yourself treated.

Ty B: Yeah. Yeah. Absolutely true. I think that there are probably far more people that you and I— and the multitude in this industry—are helping. We're not going to know half of them. We're not going to know even a small fraction of the people that you help. But that's why we do it is to help. So, whether-or-not we know it, I think that we're helping a lot of people. And I'm seeing a massive awakening from people that are waking up to the fraud that is modern cancer treatment, and just the whole medical industry is a fraud. People are waking up and becoming aware of the fact that there are options out there, and there are much better ways to be healthy and much better ways to treat a disease than what we've been told.

Ian: Yeah. I do believe that we're at a turning point. Like December 2012 we shifted from the dark ages to the light ages. I'm trying to be positive you know. The chemtrails in the sky, the GMOs in the food, the fluoride in the water, you name it, the mustard gas they give us for cancer instead of cannabis oil you know. We get it, folks. You want us all dead, or at least 6.5 billion of us dead.

Ty B: Yeah. 85-90%.

Ian: Yeah. Yeah. So, I saw a great thing on Facebook the other day. It was a picture of Texas and said, "They say we're overpopulated. If you stack people like you do in New York City, you could fit the population of the world into Texas." So why are they trying to tell us that there's too many of us? It's bullshit. They just want us out of here. They realize that with the masses and the internet we're on to them. We see the little man behind the curtain—Wizard of Oz. I hope and pray that's what's happening.

Ty B: I agree with you. My wife and I have often talked about that literally everyone that is currently alive today could fit into the state of Texas, comfortably. But no, they tell us that the world is overpopulated. It's just a bunch of malarkey. It's a complete fraud.

Ian: Yeah. I'm glad I'm alive at this time to see what happens. I'm just hoping that everybody wakes up as we have, and the tables turn, and we be able to live as we're supposed to, you know. Let the good guys be in charge of the world for a change. Because the bad guys, they've had it long enough.

Ty B: Yeah. You know I think that over the last seven years or so, since my wife and I really woke up to what's going on, not just in the health realm but in all realms of life, the way that we're being lied to and manipulated, we've seen a mass awakening among people. They're on board and are telling us that they see what we see and whereas six or seven years ago we got laughed at. We got mocked. They said, "You're crazy. You're a conspiracy theorist." And now the same people that laughed at us, today are on board and saying "Wow. You are right!"

Ian: Yeah. I had to take a lot of flack too. We're talking 19 years ago was when my girlfriend cured herself of cancer. I didn't even know what an alkaline diet was. She didn't know what it was. She was a pioneer . . . she just ate what God told her or whatever and from people she met. and basically cured it. What was my last point?

Ty B: You were just talking about people are just waking up. It's been 19 years . . . and I've seen a big awakening of people on board that didn't use to be. And you were ameliorating that point.
Ian: Exactly. People who didn't know what an alkaline diet was, know now. I ask, "what do you know?" and they tell me. "I've got to get my PH to 7.2 or 7.4. I'm like, "Wow! Good! Right on!" And I tell them about the apricot seeds, and the bloodroot and the cannabis oil. I'm not the doctor guy, I just send them to doctors with this healing protocol.

Ty B: It's funny that you mention the apricot seeds. That was really my first awakening to natural cancer treatments back in the mid-90s. When Dad got sick, it was Jason Vale. You know Jason the arm-wrestler guy that ate the apricot seeds and cured his cancer; he was the first guy to make me realize that there are options out there. Because I got a hold of a videotape of him. He was on "Extra." You know the TV show "Extra." So, you know I watched that and watched the fact that he had cured his cancer. He had eaten apples and their seeds and apricot seeds, and I actually called him back, then but by the time we got in touch Dad was already gone. It was like three weeks, and they killed him. But I stayed in touch with Jason and I know that you know his story. He was thrown in jail in New York and he did five years in a New York State Penitentiary for selling apricot seeds! So, just a crazy story. You can be a big pharmaceutical drug company and market a drug like Vioxx and kill 60,000 (sixty thousand) people no problem! But you have somebody like Jason Vale who is trying to help people treat their cancer naturally selling apricot seeds, and they're going to make you do hard time in the New York State Pen. It's just absurd.

Ian: Oh! It is! And I don't know if you've heard, but in those five years he was in prison, his cancer came back because he was eating jail food. And even when he got out of jail, he was still pretty messed up and it took him a while and his cancer has been back, but he's taking cannabis-hemp oil now as well as apricot seeds. He's in my film and we're waiting on him for an update to see how that's going. What a nightmare! Could you imagine?! If the judge put me in jail for five years for something I didn't do, trust me, when I get out of jail, I'm going to find that guy! (light-hearted laughter) I won't do anything to get myself in further trouble, but I'm going to let him know how he hurt me. Anyway, with the film I'm making now, I'm going to let the world see what they did to Jason Vale, what they're doing to Jay Matthews. You and I both know Jay Matthews. And there's another guy, Eric here in California whose daughter was being forced to have chemo. So, hopefully at the end of the day, through our radio shows and media, not everyone gets to sit down and watch one of these, so it'll be good to have a DVD of it. I'm still working on that and I'm almost done. I basically just have to get the follow-up stories to the people I've been following. And I'm hoping it'll be out sometime next year. And I'm going to try and get my book out at the same time and we should probably talk sometime afterward, and you can help me out with it because I don't know anything about books.

Ty B: Yeah sure.

Ian: The knowledge I have should be in a book.

Ty B: Yeah, yeah. No doubt. I'll help you out with that for sure Buddy. One of the things you mentioned was Jay Matthews. I was able to meet him for the first time when we were up in Chicago. He was up there at the Health Freedom Expo, so I got a chance to shake his hand. Great guy. And what they've done to his daughter is just criminal.

Ian: Yeah. Do you want to give the facts in a nutshell for the people who are listening, Ty?

Ty B: Sure. Jay's daughter, eight-year-old little Celina was diagnosed – but I don't remember the type of cancer, do you remember Ian?

Ian: It was bone cancer.

Ty B: Bone cancer. Okay. Yeah osteo-carcinoma, you're right. So, they wanted to do some natural treatments. They began to do some natural treatments if I remember correctly. But somehow, you know they're from the Chicago area, the CPS – Child Protective Services – somehow got involved. And I don't remember all the details, but basically, they forced him and his wife to take his daughter to the hospital and to force chemotherapy on her. They said, "I don't care if what you're doing is working or not, you're going to do the protocol that we prescribe." And so, for the last year plus I guess, she's been doing chemo against the parents' wishes. But the State says they should do that, despite the fact that statistics show that the treatments that they're using are not as effective as the natural treatments that the Matthews wanted to use. That didn't matter! So, they're effectively potentially going to kill his daughter!

Ian: Yeah. Oh yeah. It's murder, is what it is.

Ty B: And they had the audacity to tell us that we can't mention her name or put her picture up on the web site. So, you know what? I'll say "Celine" as many times as I want, and I'll leave the picture up on the web site. (Ian laughs) They can't tell us what to do. They're not God.

Ian: That's right.

Ty B: It's ridiculous!

Ian: I don't know if you ever heard my story there. I stayed with them for a couple of days in December or earlier. The first time I was there I heard her screaming so loud in the morning that I thought one of the kids was being murdered by a knife attack or burning them or something horrible, it woke me up. And I remember Jay telling me every morning they do that two or three times during the day because it's a form of medication they have to give her. I was ready to jump and kill somebody because I thought somebody was dying. Every day since I was with them in December, she's had to go through that, and that's just unreal.

Ty B: It's criminal. It's criminal.

Ian: And she did get the "proper care." They got her PH to 7. 2 … 7.4 in that month she was in Arizona she was doing good. I guarantee I would bet my life on it that she would be alive and with no cancer, today had the government not stepped in.

Ty B: Yeah. But hey, you know, "Trust us, we're from the government. We're here to help." Famous last words. It's too common Ian. You're familiar with the "cut, poison, burn" movie? the story of Thomas Navarre with the Burzynski clinic the way that they killed him in about 18 months. For those who are not familiar with that story: Jim and Donna Navarre's son Thomas was diagnosed with brain cancer about a decade ago. They wanted to go to the Burzynski Clinic to treat it down in Houston. Burzynski, it had a very good success rate with that type of brain cancer much better than the chemo, radiation, etc., the big three treatments in the medical profession. The FDA would not allow them to take their four-year-old to Burzynski Clinic until they exhausted all the traditional remedies – which was the chemo and radiation.

Well, the chemotherapy took about eighteen months to kill him. And then on the death certificate, the reason for death was "toxicity due to chemotherapy". I have it posted on my web site. So even the coroner admitted that he died because the treatment killed him. And the treatment was forced on him. Why is that not a criminal offense Ian? Why are the oncologists that forced chemo on him, not in jail? I don't understand that.

Ian: Yeah. I don't know either. Anybody who hasn't seen Louis Cimino film "Cut, Poison, Burn" check it out. As a filmmaker, I'm jealous because I don't know that I'll ever match it. It was such an amazing film. And it explains the whole story about the Navaro's. There was another child that was in the same movie. And they kind of going at the same rate as the chemo and it was horrible. And then the one child had to keep going with the chemo and the Navaro's got him to the Mexico clinic or whatever. And he was doing better, while the other kid that did the chemo died. And the Navaro's kid was still alive, and if they'd have left him alone, he would still be alive. I guarantee he'd be alive today. They murdered him. That's another case of murder.

Ty B: Yeah. I can't remember the boy's name from the film.
Ian: Neither can I now. I've got so many new ones in my head. We have baby Rico with the HIV story. That's an interesting thing many people probably don't know about. The HIV test turns out to be bogus, folks. You get an HIV test that comes back positive, it doesn't mean you're going to have AIDS. The test is screwy.

Ty B: Exactly. You're right. As a matter of fact, Liam Scheff wrote a book called "Official Stories" and he details the fraud that the HIV test is in that book. So, I recommend if you're not familiar with HIV-AIDS link, or the lack thereof, buy "Official Stories" by Liam Scheff and read that chapter because it's a big fraud. I had a good friend that was HIV positive in 1992-1993 back when I was a competitive bodybuilder. I trained with this guy. He was a body-building stud. The guy seemed like he was in perfect health. He went in for an HIV test, he came back, and I remember the day that he came, he told me "I'm HIV positive – they say that I have AIDS." And they started him on treatment and it took him six weeks to kill him on AZT. He was dead as a doornail in six weeks. And he was healthy before he went in for the treatment.

Ian: Yeah. Look what they did to Tommy – the boxer – Gunn – in the Rocky movie. He has a major career in front of him and then to find out now that he didn't have to lose his career. I mean, because I'm a fighter and I know he had a way more illustrious career than I did and to lose that because of some stupid test. I mean I don't know how he's handling that.

Ty B: Yeah. It's a shame, but I'm trying to think of the documentary that Robert and Liam were telling me about … House of Numbers. Check out House of Numbers, a very good documentary on AIDS.

Ian: And again, it just goes to show you that the people in charge, the one percent, the elite, the Illuminati, whatever you want to call them, they're running the show. Everywhere, everywhere, the oil, the food, the skies, I mean it's . . . I don't even know what to do anymore.

Ty B: I know. It's like their hobby is to figure out more ways to try to poison people and make them sicker. I mean it's really disgusting.

Ian: We ought to let more people know I guess. That's the only thing I can think of. Just keep telling people.

Ty B: Yeah. That's what we've got to do. We've got to keep telling people because people don't know. I mean there are still a lot of ignorant people out there that just don't know. And that's by design. The mainstream media lies regularly, and they're good at it. So, the mesmerizing, the propaganda, the brainwashing that we undergo on a regular basis is all by design. So those people that are unaware, they're unaware because the scumbags that are running things want them to be unaware. So, we've got to keep sounding the alarm and waking them up to the truth, otherwise, they'll never know.

Ian: Yeah. Yeah. I had a joke on my Facebook earlier today that, you've probably heard of them, they're called Galactic Federation something-or-other. They've been saying for a long time that they're going to come down and clean up the Illuminati and let our world be run the way it's supposed to. (both smiling) I'm believing in aliens now because I want that to happen. (laughter) When are you coming? (laughter)

Ty B: When is it going to happen? (laughter) Yeah, I'm with you.

Ian: So, all you can be is your own best advocate, basically, in this day and age, let's hear what you would do because that's what people always ask me. You've been studying this forever, if you got cancer what would you do? I give them two answers, 1) if I had money, and 2) if I didn't.

Ty B: Good idea. The main thing that you want to do is to correct the imbalance that caused it. I know that sounds overly simplistic, but hey, the theory of modern conventional cancer treatment is that if you have a diagnosis of cancer you overload them with poison! So, it's like, what was cancer? Was cancer a deficiency of chemotherapy? That's what they treat it like so, that's the problem with the modern treatments is that they don't look at the cause. Because the cause of cancer is not that you were short on chemo! The cause of the cancer is that you have a compromised immune system that resulted from something. Whether it's the toxins in the air, toxins on the food, toxin in the water that we're drinking, whether it is any of those things, whether it's the pollutants from the chemical companies, I mean it could be a whole host of things; the fact that you're eating genetically modified foods that are really not foods that are causing all kinds of issues in your gut; whether it was the vaccines that you took as a child; I mean the list goes on and on.

Something caused those cells to go haywire, the DNA in those cells and for your immune system to fail so that you're diagnosed with a cancer that could kill you. And so, you can pump somebody with as much chemotherapy as possible, but it's not going to correct that underlying condition. So, the number one step that you need to do is to correct the condition. And so, the way that you do that is that you make sure you get your body to an alkaline environment. Get rid of the crap that you're eating, the genetically modified foods, the processed foods, all the things that could have caused the cancer. One of the things I would do is begin to use a rebounder (mini-trampoline) each day, a great exercise for cancer patients. You know jumping up and down on that stimulates your lymph system and helps to detoxify it. I would get in far infrared sauna and sweat to help your skin to detox and to get rid of the toxins from your body. So, there are some really basic things.

Get on a clean organic raw diet. I can't count the number of cancer patients that I have been contacted by over the last six/seven years that have completely controlled their cancer by doing nothing more than just eating a raw organic diet. So, those are really, basic simple things; not-really expensive things that you have to do that could be a good start to correcting the imbalance that caused the cancer. You see, the problem is not the tumor. People think that your problem is your tumor. You know, "I've got a tumor what are you going to do?" "I'm going to cut it out, then I'm going to radiate it. Then I'm going to take chemo just in case...!" Well, you know, none of those corrected the imbalance that caused the cancer in the first place. The tumor is not the issue. The tumor is the symptom of the cancer. So, by cutting out the symptom of the cancer you haven't corrected any of the imbalance that caused it in the first place. So, it's probably going to come back. And it usually does.

Ian: Especially the way they do it in America. You'll find this interesting. The clinic that I'm working with now in Tijuana, it's brand new; they used to be American Bio Dental run by Alessandro Porcella which is still there but also have a clinic attached called American Holistic Care that I actually came up with the name for him myself, lol! That's where I get my teeth worked on and got all the silver (mercury) out. Well, he's expanding it to an alternative cancer clinic, which is perfect timing because we just lost Camelot. Camelot in Oklahoma got shut down.

Ty B: Yeah. The raid on Camelot. Yep.

Ian: So, thank God, I found this place, because now this is the only other place that I know that people that have the money can go and be pampered for six weeks. Which I would if I had the money. Have a pretty senorita nurse come and give you your meds instead of crawling all over the floor to get to it. I know people... my friend and cancer curer   Tamara St John who wrote: Defeat Cancer Now and Healing Through Detox, slept in the kitchen next to the blender; wake up, pull out some veggies, blend it, drink it and go back to sleep. That's how tough this can be sometimes.

Ty B: Sure. Speaking about Camelot (Laetrile, B17) – so you're familiar with what happened with Maureen Long and the people there? Criminal. Just criminal. I was doing an interview on, I think it was Bob Tuscan's show a few weeks ago, and he had talked to a guy that was literally there in the cancer center in Tulsa when the FDA raided it. And they literally pulled the IVs out of people's arms that were undergoing treatment. I mean, it's criminal what they did to those people and what they did to the owners of the clinic. For doing what? For using vitamin B-17 to cure cancer.

Ian: It's unbelievable. They're like family to me because I went and spent a few days there and interviewed them all for my film. It was the best one around! But, it's even better now for the movie. It sucks for them because they held all her bank accounts and she's losing everything because of what they've done to her . . . and for curing cancer! And Michael McDonnough who was the lab guy there, he's a friend of mine, he got roughed up. The FBI lady said, because he came back in to get his laptop, and he was leaving with his laptop, she stood right in front of him and he moved to avoid hitting her, and she screamed to make it look like he was doing something, even though it was she that jumped in front of him. And a big 6' 4" guy jumps him, takes him down cracked his shoulder and ribs and everything. Horrible. The jail wouldn't even take them because they took them to the hospital first. And he had to cop a plea and he's hoping and praying he doesn't go away for a year.

Ty B: Yeah, I heard about that story. I didn't know that was a friend of yours.
Ian: Yeah, yeah. But he found out the other day that he could do a year, for what? Curing people of cancer, and who knows what they're going to try to do to poor Maureen.

Ty B: Yeah, it's sad. It's sad that we don't live in the land of the free and the home of the brave when it comes to health treatments, do we?!

Ian: That's what I tell people now. They don't like it, they go, "You're a conspiracy theorist." I say, "No bro. I first researched Rockefeller, because I had to because he owned the pharmaceutical companies." That's why our doctors today learn what they do because of Rockefeller.

Ty B: Flexner report. Yeah.

Ian: Yeah . . . the early 1900s, and ever since we've been screwed. That's the only way you can get through to people because they think their doctor is a god. And they just can't believe you. It's better now than it was 10-15 years ago. But they usually don't believe you, you know.

Ty B: Yeah, I actually gave about 15-minutes of my lecture this last weekend in North Carolina, about the Flexner Report. Because I want to explain to people, most people don't understand, why their doctor doesn't know anything about natural treatments. And they don't understand why there's such suppression of natural treatments and holistic practitioners. And that really explains it better than anything else. You have to look at the last 100 years and the history of why we are where we are, and it all started by the funding of the Flexner Report by John Rockefeller who wanted to monopolize the chemical industry which later became the pharmaceutical industry.

Ian: Okay now I have the name of it, I couldn't remember the name of it – the Flexner Report. And once people understand that then they chill out a little bit. Because, if 9/11 comes up I'm going to tell them my opinion, it was an inside job. Duh! You don't have to be a rocket scientist to see that building 7 wasn't hit by a plane, but it fell. But I find those guys like you and Mike Adams and Robert Scot Bell . . . y' all are on the same page too. Anyone who is in alternative medicine has-to-be on the same page. All you have-to-do is look at the lineage from Rockefeller to now. And then they understand it. So, I basically found out that 9/11 was an inside job by researching the cancer industry!

Ty B: Yeah, you know it's funny I learned about 9/11, and all of the other what people say are "conspiracies" but it's not, it's a fact not a conspiracy. It's conspiracy fact, it's not a theory. It's a conspiracy fact, it really happened. The conspiracies have been given a bad name, but the fact of the matter is that conspiracies happening all the time. People conspire – all a conspiracy is, is when two people in secret are trying to do something to someone else.

And so, when you have an NFL game that you're watching on TV the quarterback gets in the huddle and they conspire to score against the other team. Conspiracies happen every day. It's not a bad word. But it's a buzz word that it's used when people are bankrupt of an argument and can't debate something they just say, "Oh, you're just a conspiracy theorist."

After I published my book, http://cancerstepoutsidethebox.com/\, the first edition back in 2006, one of the doctors, Dr. David Grey, that I quoted a lot in the book, he emailed me, and he said, "I want to send you a DVD." And I said, "Okay. Send it to me. What's it about?" And he said, "It's about 9/11." I said, "What about 9/11?" And he said, "Well, it was an inside job." So, what had I been conditioned to say at that point from all the mainstream media? I said, "You're crazy." That's what I told him. He said, "Oh really. Well, you're quoting me a lot in your book if you think I'm crazy! Why don't you give it a chance and actually look at it with an open mind before you call me names." And you know, he was right! I said, Okay, I'll look at it." So, I looked at it and my wife watched it with me and at the end of the movie we said, "He was right. It was an inside job without a doubt." And all of our research since then has confirmed that, and much, much, more. So that was really my awakening about what's going on as well as was through my book through to health. I began to learn about everything else.

Ian: Yeah. It's just a major denial that everybody else is in. I can see now because I have friends all over, I have Facebook friends who are pretty much on the same page as me and you. But then go out into the world, and they don't know anything. And they're professors from UCLA . . . I mean they're highly intelligent people! They don't believe there is any kind of economic collapse coming up, they don't believe that cancer is curable, they don't believe anything (that's factually true about these things)! Come on man! Wake up America! I think that's the bottom line. Now I don't spend with people like that, I just think – whatever, you'll figure it out on your own. I have bigger fish to fry.

Ty B: Yeah. What I typically do is I'll just throw a couple of things out now. And I'll say, "what do you think about the chemtrails?" Or, "what do you think about the fluoride in the drinking water?" And I've kind of become a little bit less in-your-face with it. Whereas when I first learned about it I'd say like, "9/11 was an inside job! What about the Gulf of Tonkin? What about JFK? What about Waco? What about Oklahoma City? Ruby Ridge?"

And go on and on with people and you just freakin' blow them away, and they wouldn't even . . . it would just knock them over (figuratively) and the switch would click, and they'd say, "this is crazy, I can't believe any of this" and I would lose them. And so now, I just kind of let it trickle and just see if they're interested. And if they're interested then I'll give them a little more information.

Ian: Yeah… I had to do the same thing. I had a friend tell me that I had his buddy hook line and sinker for the cannabis oil and then since I mentioned 9/11, this guy says, "Oh this guy's a nut." So, . . . being compassionate, I'm learning to skirt around certain issues. It's just like if you're raised racist, you're racist, if you're ignorant about natural cancer cures, you're going to be ignorant. Do you know?

Ty B: Yeah. If you're drinking the municipal water supply, you're getting hit with fluoride and it's making you docile and dumbed down. And that's the purpose of it. They used it in Nazi Germany. That's the purpose of fluoride. I mean, what's Prozac? 90% fluoride? I don't know, but most of what's in Prozac is fluoride.

Ian: Do you have any water filters that you like?

Ty B: Yeah, you know I like the Berkey. We use the Berkey. We actually live on some property here in Texas, so we have a well. So, we're not getting the fluoride and the different chemicals from the municipal water supply. But we still filter the water, so I like the Berkey filter. They have a fluoride element that will take out fluoride. It's pretty affordable. For a couple of hundred bucks, you can get a filter with a fluoride attachment. It's just a gravity filter. So, you pour it in the top and it filters down to the bottom. But it's pretty good. You could buy a whole-house filter for $7,000 that's really good, but most people don't have seven grand to drop on a whole-house filter. I would recommend the Berkey's.

Ian: I got one on the shower head too.

Ty B: Yeah, because you'll absorb more through your skin in the shower than you'll ever drink. That's a good idea.

Ian: My research on this has shown that the safest thing is to start with R. O. water, which is like distilled. It kills everything in it. Because there are so many pharmaceuticals and other things in there it's unbelievable. And then I have the shower head too. I don't know if it gets all the fluoride, but I know it gets all the chlorine and everything else out. So, water is very important, clean food is very important. What are your thoughts on Dr. Ryke Geerd Hamer and the "German New Medicine"? How most cancers are connected to an emotional tragedy or some similar experience? For example, in the one case, Eric: his wife died due to Big Pharma because she was on Coumadin I think, the blood thinner. She died. Then his daughter got leukemia about a year later which I hear is a textbook case. What do your years of experience say about this?

Ty B: You know, several years ago I didn't see any relationship, or I was ignorant of it. I had not studied it. But over the last couple of years, I've been at that more closely and I think there is often times a very close link between tragedies, traumas, emotional stress and the inception and progression of cancer. As a matter of fact, many practitioners will deal with the emotional aspect as well as a physical aspect at the same time. And they feel like you can't get a long-term control of the cancer, as long as the emotional aspect is still there. So, they'll try and free them up emotionally as well as physically. So, I think there's something to that. I'm not by any means an expert on that. That's really, probably relatively new to me, over the last 16 to 18 months. But I definitely see a connection.

Ian: Right. In your opinion do you think that alkalinity is pretty much key? Have you ever known anybody to cure cancer that didn't end up with a PH of 7.2 to 7.4? If you have a blood cancer your PH may be too high, if you have a tumor it may be too low. Isn't it true that through diet and whatever else you get your PH to be balanced to 7.2 – 7.4?

Ty B: Yes, drop processed foods, genetically modified foods and you go to an organic raw diet, by definition you've just gone to an alkaline diet. Not only are you going to raise your body's PH level, but then at the same time you're going to also be providing your body with the nutrition that it needs to heal itself naturally. So, I think that the organic raw-type diets and the alkaline environment go hand-in-hand. And so, by doing one you're going to necessarily do the other. And that's going to give your body the internal terrain that it needs in order to heal itself.

Because of all that a good diet for cancer treatment does, it doesn't cure cancer, it puts your body into the state where it takes care of the cancer the way that it's supposed to. Before you get started getting bombarded with all of these toxins, these pesticides, these genetically modified organisms (GMOs), the chemtrails; all the different toxicities that you're being hit with that we were not intended to ingest. And it puts your body back into the natural state that it heals itself.

Ian: Exactly. And now this is what I would tell people when they ask me about what Angelina Jolie did by getting her breasts removed "in case she gets breast cancer someday" – because of that stupid test that she did. I actually called my scientist buddy Michael McDonnough, from the Camelot Cancer Center and asked him, he said, . . . well, first of all, that test is bogus, it's pseudo-science at best. So, I ask him, "Can't you just keep your pH at 7.2—7.4? And he's like, "Yeah." So basically she could have looked at her pH and if it was 7.2 cool, and if five years down the line the test was true and she was going to get breast cancer, she could just up her pH and then forget it.

Ty B: But see, Mike Adams has written a really good article, about that and the connection with Myriad Genetics. Because if you remember Myriad Genetics was the company that tried to patent that gene. And shortly after all this happened Congress came back and I'm thankful that we finally had one good ruling and they said you can't patent that gene. You can't patent life, for lack of a better term. And so that kind of fell by the wayside. But it was just interesting the way that all of this double mastectomy, all this hoo-hah about Angelina Jolie and the BRCA gene, however you want to say it, and then the Myriad Genetics trying to patent life; it all happened at the same time. I think they were looking at the venues that could have been generated by manipulating women into getting a double mastectomy.

Think of all of the money that could have been made by the testing for that gene, and then by the surgeries, and then by the reconstructive surgeries, man, you're talking about a lot of cash! And when you compare that to the fact that when we look at Epigenetics, the things that you can do to suppress that to which you might be genetically inclined toward.

Now, I'm not going to admit that that gene, the Brack gene, the BRCA gene has anything to do with cancer, because Mike did a pretty good job of dismantling that. But, let's just say that it does. There are a myriad of things you can do to stop that gene from activating. There are all kinds of lifestyle choice that you can affect the outcome and so that's what modern cancer treatments don't address. They don't even say what you can do to eat, your exercise, the type of water that you drink; all kinds of different things that can affect that gene and cause it to remain dormant and never to act out.

Ian: Yeah. Yeah. I still to this day am wondering if she did it on purpose and was being compensated, or if she's really that dense. (Ty laughs) I mean, you can go to a Yoga class and learn about PH levels. So, I don't understand why she wouldn't know. And like you said, this is what I said when I made a video about it, "If that test is real and accurate who cares? Wait till your PH drops down to 5 then think about cutting it out, but hey why not try an alkaline diet?" Do you know what I mean?

Ty B: Yes. You know what is interesting, Mike Adams and Robert Scot Bell, they did a video about that a couple of days after the story broke, they did a video talking about Myriad Genetics factor and where they tried to patent life, and the fact that the BRCA gene has anything to do with cancer. And they were also questioning whether she ever actually had a double mastectomy or whether it was all just a big story to influence people to do this. They posted this video out on YouTube and it was censored and taken down within hours!

Ian: Really!?!

Ty B: Yeah! Yeah. So, YouTube censored that video. So, it's interesting that if you get censored, you must be pretty close to the truth, right?! I mean, they're not going to censor false things. So, when you're out there and you're getting censored like that, then maybe they're on to something (i.e., Mike Adams and Robert Scot Bell).

Ian: Yeah. You look at the fact that even though Camelot Cancer Center closed, that's actually a "first prize". You guys win first prize. They're closed because they were curing cancer!

Ty B: Yep, yep.

Ian: Horrible, horrible. What do you think is ever going to happen, man, because, I ask all my intelligent friends from both sides of the fence, whether they're sheep or not. Do you think there is going to be a financial collapse? I'm curious. Do you really think that's coming?

Ty B: Yeah. I mean the way that our monetary system is structured with the Federal Reserve notes, there has to be a collapse. Because what we're doing is, we're printing money from nothing. And so, for someone who doesn't understand the financial system, the Federal Reserve system was set up in 1913 is a misnomer. It's an oxymoron because it's neither "federal" nor are there any "reserves"! It's a consortium of private bankers and there are no reserves. They print money out of nothing. It's like monopoly money. And so, what happens is to 1970-something our money was on the gold standard. Then it was taken off the gold standard and since that time the printing presses have been running 24/7! And so, what happens when people think of inflation; the prices of good going up. That's not actually what's happening. The price of goods has remained the same.

What's happened over the past 30—40 years is that the value of the dollar has gone down, because the printing presses have been running full speed. Let's say that there are 100 dollars out there in the money supply, and the Federal Reserve says we've got to print more money, so they put another 100 dollars out in the money supply. So now, instead of having 100 dollars in the money supply, there are 200 collective dollars. Well what they just did is they just devalued each dollar that was out there previously by 50%. And so, they've been doing this for the last 40 years. So, what we really have is not inflation of goods, what we have is a devaluation of the dollar. And as they continue to print more and more money to cover our debts, trillions and trillions of dollars of printing, then the value of the dollar is eventually going to go down close to nothing.

And so, I think that the financial collapse of the dollar is inevitable. Now, what will follow that in the United States? I don't know. But I don't think it's going to be a pretty scenario. I don't have a lot of money anyway, but if I had a lot of money it wouldn't be sitting in the bank! Because eventually one of these days it could a hyper-inflationary scenario, which is really the collapse of the dollar, and all your money in the bank is not worth anything.

If you are familiar with history and the Weimar Republic, pre-world war 2 Germany, their money was worth nothing and they would take wheel barrels full of money to the bread store, in order to buy a loaf of bread. As a matter of fact, if I remember correctly, they would pay workers twice a day because if they waited until afternoon to pay the workers, the money that they would have earned the first half of the day would have devalued to such an extent that they couldn't buy anything if they went the store; because their money was devaluing at such a quick rate. Could that happen here? It could. I mean I don't know, I'm not a financial expert but it certainly could. The "writing is definitely on the wall" for our financial system, especially with the Federal Reserve notes that we call dollars.

Ian: Yeah, I'm always the optimist so I'm just hoping and praying: the Pleiadian's will come down and save this earth or something, or, we'll do what Iceland did. Let's just we the people stand up and get rid of the politicians, get rid of the bankers, let's start over.

Ty B: That's a solution. (smile)

Ian: We all know at this date . . . I mean I don't know what else to do, but again, I don't know if it's the fluoride or what…and I'm not an evil guy so as much as I get angry and I love to say that I'd go shoot them all, I just can't take another person's life. That's not my job.

Ty B: Not mine either. But it'll be interesting to see what happens because you've seen what's happened
recently did the "haircuts" on savings? I'm trying to think if that was Greece. Anyway, just across the board, the government confiscated everything above 40% of their savings. There are several European countries that are collapsing.

Ian: Wow!

Ty B: I'm trying to remember . . . it wasn't Greece . . . it's alluding me – the name of the country. This was within the last six months that this happened. The government basically came in and took people money!

I got an email forwarded to me – uh, I think it was Robert Scot Bell had an email from somebody that lived in that country – and I wish I could remember that country – that said about his mother: she said, "I went to bed a wealthy woman, I had saved for the university for my grandkids and for my retirement and I woke up a pauper." The government had taken all of her cash.

Just think what would happen in the United States if a similar scenario occurred where people had worked their whole lives for their retirements, their 401Ks – whatever, and they go to bed one night with X-number of dollars in the bank and the next morning they wake up and it's gone; because the government "confiscated" it for "the greater good." I mean, it's not going to be a pretty scenario if that happens.

Ian: No, I know. They'll get a revolution then I'm afraid. People out there, you've got to be your own best advocate. You can't expect your leaders to do anything for you, unfortunately. In the last couple minutes here, let's just bring up anything else that you want to offer to those out there with cancer. You wrote a book about it. You've been for at it a long time. For the person out there who has just found out for the first time and is freaking out because they've been told they have cancer, what would you say?

Ty B: By the way, the country was Cypress where that happened about six months ago. What I would tell people that have been diagnosed with cancer is don't freak out. Because my whole message is that there is always hope; that the cancer doesn't need to be a death sentence. In spite of what your oncologist tells you. You see they've been trained that cancer is not curable, that you can only use drugs to prolong your time here, but you're eventually going to die from it. Most cancer diagnoses are a death sentence according to conventional wisdom. That's kind of an oxymoron . . . because that's wisdom that conventional oncologists don't have! (Laughter!) But according to conventional oncologists, it is going to be a death sentence. Don't believe them! Because, as we talked about it earlier, a good portion of your cancer diagnosis and your cancer treatment, your remedy for cancer is your emotional state. And so, if you go into a cancer diagnosis and the first thing that you hear from day one is, "You're dead in six months" you're going to believe it, and you're not going to do well with your treatments. So, don't believe your oncologist.

Cancer doesn't need to be a death sentence. There are a lot of natural treatments that you can do to put your body back into the state it needs to be in to fight the cancer on its own. So, my message is, "Don't believe them!" Don't listen to them. Read my book and read other books that have been written, do your research. Empower yourself with knowledge so that you can fight that diagnosis when it comes. Because according to the WHO in 2010, 41% of the people alive today will face a cancer diagnosis. That's a lot of us. 41%. So, empower yourself with knowledge for when that diagnosis comes. You'll actually know what your options are, and you're not ramrodded into a choice of "chemo, radiation or surgery, and there's nothing else we can do for you." Those aren't good choices. There are more choices. But if you don't know about them, you're not going to fare well when you face that diagnosis.

Ian: Yeah, that's why I put this show out, and make movies. But to finish a point that I started earlier: the one Tijuana place that I keep bringing up the American Holistic Care, they do chemo, radiation, and surgery, but only if they have to. They do all holistic first. But they change the order of it. Instead of just scooping it out and then bombarding it with chemo and radiation like they do in America, they give a low dose circle around the tumor of cobalt radiation, low dose chemo in the blood so any rogue cells get out as they're cutting gets killed and sterilized, so the cancer cannot spread. And they've now incorporated the best holistic stuff. They know everything about holistic. I grilled them and they're on it. Then if they have-to-do IPT or low dose chemo they can.

Ty: Yeah. Sure.

Ian: I'm glad I was able to get that out. Just letting you know folks. So, folks, if you're going to do chemo, radiation and surgery go to Tijuana where the AMA and the FDA can't mess with you because they can do it in the correct order. But I would always do holistic first.

Ty B: Sure. There are some good clinics that do integrative medicine. They'll do both. And so, I'm not opposed to that if that's what somebody chooses to do. But I think what our mission to do is to empower people with knowledge, and to fight against the tyranny, so that people have an option, because if we live in America, the "Land of the Free and the Home of the Brave" supposedly, shouldn't we have a choice in our own healthcare?

And if somebody wants to go traditional, chemo, radiation and surgery, that's fine, that your choice. Somebody wants to go completely natural, that's their choice. If you want to go integrated, that's your choice. The thing that I am opposed to and that you're opposed to Ian, is a heavy-handed Federal government breathing down people's necks and saying, "you have to do this to treat your disease." That shouldn't be. So, it's all about the freedom to choose what you want to do and the knowledge to know what you should do.

Ian: Yeah. It's like we're living in the Nazi state again. It's unbelievable. . . . . Well, I really appreciate your being on the show. You're one of my heroes. I've always followed what you've done and it's an honor. So, thank you very much, man!

Ty B: Ah, back at you my friend. You're one of my heroes too. So, we'll keep up the good fight together.

Ian: Well right on. Ladies and Gentlemen thanks for tuning in for another I Cure Cancer on ZenLive.TV. Everybody have a good night. Be safe. Peace.

[See Pic 22.1]

CHAPTER 23:

INTERVIEW WITH DR. KELLY RABER

Ian: Hi Dr. Kelly. How are you today?

Dr. Kelly Raber: I'm doing well. I'm doing great. So, the website is, www.tumorx.com and there you can read different articles that I've put together for research, clinical studies and such, that demonstrate how the different materials work, what their mechanism of action is. It's some generally good information that I think most people will easily be able to understand and wrap their arms around.

Ian: Okay. Great. Your father was in my film ICureCancer.com. At the very beginning of the film there's a very powerful moment, he comes in and says there are three kinds of people that be cured of cancer: 1) their time is up. God's calling them. There's nothing you can do about it. 2) Folks that benefit from their disease. That's the scary one. Some people like the attention they get when they're sick, and unfortunately, they'll take that over living and end up dying just for that reason.

Dr. Kelly Raber: Well . . . some people are just too far gone that there's nothing that will work. Other people who should be too far gone but they turn around. So, this is arguable, you have to put a little destiny in. There are just some people no matter what you do they're going to die. There's just nothing that can be done. There are other people who benefit from the disease for whatever reason and then there are some people who want to reinvent the wheel every time they turn around. So, they just don't listen well. They become their own experiment, their own guinea pig.

Ian: Yeah, that's the one I was missing (3). They don't know how to follow instructions. And the key is following instructions folks because you're not just on a Jenny Craig diet where you're just going to remain fat. You're probably going to die if you don't get that alkaline level correct. You've either got to either bring your PH down because you may have a blood cancer or bring it up because it's too low because of a tumor … it's 5 and you want to get to 7.2 to 7.4. This is very key.

For a change, I actually have a list of prewritten questions for you. I hardly ever do this, but I have a friend called me with them, so I'm just going to go through this list of questions. Tell us about yourself Dr. Raber, your education, your career, in a nutshell just so people know that we're talking to a very smart man.

Dr. Kelly Raber: My background is biochemistry. I've been working on these types of say that formulation is really my niche. That's really what I do quite well; at least I hope I do. And in the process, I have made everything from dietary supplements to creams, lotions, you pretty much name it. And I've done lectures inside the U.S. and I've also done lectures outside the U.S. The main one where I've done a lot of them is in the Philippines, for the Filipino College for the Advancement of Medicine Foundation. It's a pretty decent organization that has been spearheading using natural products over there and teaching the doctors how to use natural products incorporated into their practices. I've done about six lectures over there for the Department of Health and for the Filipino College of Medicine.

Ian: Isn't it amazing. . . any thoughts on how it is that a country like that would be interested in these kinds of things, and your work and that nobody in America seems to be?

Dr. Kelly Raber: Well, the thing with the Philippines what I would suggest is that there are a lot of traditional healers over there. I think it would be fair to say that it's not the richest country on the planet. So, what they're looking for, and what the government is looking for is economical ways that people can extend their life and reverse these diseases. People all over the world get sick. Right? From the richest country to the poorest country – we all have the same fundamental problems. We age, we start having health breakdown, we start having issues. Over there, what they're attempting to do is open it up for everybody to have an opportunity to have the highest and longest quality of life possible. I'm probably going to get the exact date wrong, but about eight years ago they passed a law over there that the allopathic medicine, that is the MDs over there had to learn about alternative health. One of the first lectures I did over there, was for that particular conference at the old air force base – I forget the name. The point is that they really are dedicated to trying to find different ways, alternative ways of bringing down the costs of their treatments so that more people can have a higher quality of life.

Ian: Wow! What a concept! I didn't even know countries did that, while our country is trying to kill us!

Dr. Kelly Raber: No, one of their things is "medical tourism." They do everything from stem cell research to you-name-it over there. A lot of people have a misconception that the only place that there is technology is the U.S. I would suggest that there are probably more skyscrapers being built in Manilla than Atlanta. It's a small world is what I'm saying. Just because it's the Philippines doesn't mean it's always a horrible place. There are a lot of nice places over there. But the thing is the government officials that I have met have been dedicated to trying to get their people healthier. And they're looking at nutrition, they're looking at other ways of doing it to bring down the cost so that everybody can afford to do it.

Ian: Well that's amazing and very valiant and the way America should be and will be again soon if I have anything to do with it. Now, in a nutshell: people say, "Ian how did you get into cancer? Did you have cancer?" and I like to say "No, but a girlfriend of mine did. J Cynthia Brooks who co-hosts my I Cure Cancer, show. What is your story? How did you even learn to care about cancer, just out of curiosity?

Dr. Kelly Raber: Well, it's kind of an interesting story, hopefully not too long. I'll try and put it in a nutshell. The first time that I was actually exposed to it (cancer) was when I was quite cynical. The person had a method of killing cancer, basically a formulation of paste that you'd apply topically. It was an old family recipe that this family—he told me about. He said that if you applied this topical ointment it would kill the cancer cells. I was quite frankly cynical about it. I was thinking, "Well if this is true, then everybody should know about it, and since by trade you're a crop duster, why do you know?" And he told me it was his old family recipe.

He and my dad were friends, and they asked me to put it together for them. So, we put it together and made about a kilo of it. Then my dad tried it out on about a dozen of his friends. Twelve out of twelve were cancer free in less than a month! THAT'S what got my attention. Because at that point I had to realize one of two things: the government already knows about this, or, they know about it and are suppressing the information.

Years later, after we had done a fair amount of research and looked at it, we documented some of the methods on how it works and tried to get a better understanding of the herb. I found a book in England called Chemo Surgery Gangrene And, Infections by Frederic Mose of the University of Wisconsin, where he did a 12,000 human, clinical study. Imagine it. 12,000-person clinical study! He had a 97.7% success rate of curing topical cancers. (This is the exact opposite of the success rate of Chemotherapy, which has 2.1% success rate!!!) So, a lot of the work we were attempting to validate I found that in fact it had already been done in 1956. That's what also grabbed my attention even more. Because then it starts looking like even more of a conspiracy. Here you have Frederic Mose of the University of Wisconsin – I think we can all agree that that's a good university. Right? We're not going to say that's a second-rate university. That's a good university; Frederic Mose – well-respected oncologist! He does a 12,000-person study and the work is not seriously looked at even though it has a 97.7% success rate. I don't know of anyone, of any treatment today that would even come close to those types of numbers (excluding natural healers). And this is 1956.

Ian: WOW!

Dr. Kelly Raber: So, this is what started grabbing my attention. And then, later on, another one of my dad's friends was Dr. William Donald Kelly. Dr. Kelly cured himself in the 1970s using megadose levels of pancreatic enzymes. As he would take these enzymes the cancer would die. The thing we have to understand about pancreatic cancer is that it is one of the worst cancers out there. The chances of surviving it – you almost have a better chance of getting hit by lightning twice than surviving pancreatic cancer. So, the fact that he overcame it was astounding.

Dr. Kelly was credited with saving over 100,000 (a hundred thousand) lives using his mechanisms, using his technology of enzymes. One of the things that really gave me an insight was because he was friends with my dad, and I got to spend a lot of time with him. We got to discuss how the enzymes worked, what their mechanisms were when they failed, why they failed, or why he believed they failed. Sometimes he believed that the enzymes themselves were adulterated. They weren't just as pure as they should have been. This is one of the reason when I do formulations, I keep Dr. Kelly's thoughts in mind. I never formulate with fillers and additives. He believed that the reason that a lot of his people passed away, not because the enzymes weren't capable of killing the cancer, not that the person wasn't sincerely wanting to kill their cancer, but because the fillers and the additives—the chemical garbage that they put in there to make them flow a little bit easier, to get better production—was actually poisoning the patient.

So, with that thought in mind when I do my formulations I do not add fillers or flowing agents or any of those synthetic chemicals. This is one of the reasons because of what I learned from Dr. Kelly. So, he was a brilliant guy. The other thing that got me interested … for the big picture: When we look at his collective work, over 100,000 people cured. We have to also ask ourselves, "Why not more people?" Why did it sometimes fail? This is where I came into this…I had seen how well the paste worked, and the active ingredient was bloodroot. And all the literature I had read on bloodroot basically suggested that if a person takes greater than a gram that they'll have projectile vomiting, possibly hallucinate, and all kinds of fantasy things they wrote about it. But basically, it's a "poisonous herb." I found this to be completely untrue. I've seen people take large doses of it, and I've seen people who have taken Bloodroot orally and their cancer died. Now the research that's been done on that I think is interesting. The active ingredient is Sanguinary Kilorythrian down-regulates survivin, induce apoptosis (death of cancer cells) and allows the cancer cells to naturally express its death. That is kind of interesting? That's how I got involved; was knowing other people that had great successes and they needed to take it a step further.

Ian: Wow! I'm blown away. I forgot, or maybe it just went over my head . . . but I was not aware that you and your father were actually personal friends with Dr. Kelly. Are you kiddin' me? That's huge! No wonder you're learning what you're learning. So, you obviously just went with it. You ran with it. Explain what you call your protocols? How do they work? People listening have different types of cancer, are their side-effects? Do you want to just give us a brief explanation of what you have for people that have cancer?

Dr. Kelly Raber: Well, what I put together are: Different Mechanisms. So, depending on the type, the aggressiveness, what I would suggest is that I give you an example. If somebody has "garden-variety" skin cancer. What I have found is if people take Bloodroot – apoptosis protocol – package number one. If they take package one, typically their cancer will start to fade and disappear within from five to twenty days. I would suggest that if we do not see that action, it's one of two things: either we're not taking enough of it, that is incorrect, or we have a bigger problem than we are really aware of. So "package one" for picayune little skin cancers.

"Package two" is for people who just want to do an enzyme therapy. They want to basically follow Dr. Kelly's work. Where my "package two" is different from Dr. Kelly's is that I add another enzyme – to make the nausea go away – following Dr. Beard's work. That way they feel good through the whole thing. Why not? Who wants to suffer? But then on the other hand if you need to do it on a budget then you can consider using mainly just pancreatic enzymes and doing coffee enemas. "Package two" contains the combination of enzymes more closely related to Beard's research than Kelly's; to help detoxify the body as you're doing an enzyme therapy.

"Package three" is for someone who wants to do an aggressive package. They want to use the herb Bloodroot, sanguinary kilorythrian being the active ingredient, and they want to use enzymes together because the combination is phenomenal. There's a protein that is produced by cancer cells that are called survivin. Survivin is the protein that is at work when a lot of oncologists come to their patients and say, "your cancer has mutated." That is, it has changed and thus the drug they are using is no longer working. would suggest there is no mutation. What there was instead is a survivin production increase. As survivin production increased, the capability of the cancer cells to spread, to metastasize, also increased. And mitosis or cell division took place. Why I'm bringing this in is because sanguinarine down-regulates survivin. So, apoptosis can take place – that is cell death or cell suicide. So that particular package combines the two to make the enzymes, or allow the enzymes to work more efficiently. And then there's another protocol that I put together called package No. four. Package Four – is typically used for people who are suffering from starvation. The thing to keep in mind is . . . besides keeping PH in balance . . . that cancer secretes lactic acid or lactate. Lactic acid through the 'quarry' cycle can be converted back into glucose. Because it is converted back into glucose, what happens if a person doesn't consume enough food, the body goes into conservation. So, their body literally begins to cannibalize itself. The body literally starts to eat itself because of the acidic environment. In this acidic environment – what Warren points out – cancer cells have a tendency to replicate quicker, and become more aggressive. So, you can convert the lactate back into glucose using ATP, or "adenosine triphosphate." That nucleonic will convert the metabolic waste of the cancer into a relatively harmless substance, glucose or sugar.

Now, a lot of people at this point tend to freak out and say, "Aren't we trying to stop all glucose?" Right. But keep in mind that if we're eating fruits and vegetables, all those carbohydrates are sugar. And if we don't have enough nutrition, remember the body through glycogen through the liver will break it down fat and protein with ketones left over and produce its own sugar. There is no effective way of stopping sugar production in the human body. Does that make sense?

Ian: Yeah.

Dr. Kelly Raber: So more of the mechanisms that I've looked at are not necessarily trying to prevent all sugar. They're to convert the harmful waste by-products of the cancer cells into a relatively harmless by-product, taking the burden off the person. By doing this we're able to reverse starvation. Now, a lot of people say that there are other mechanisms out there that do that. I have not really seen it successfully done with other mechanisms other than an ATP.

Now, what I want to really stress here so as not to be misunderstood: if a person is suffering from starvation, eat more food and starvation stops. If a person has cachexia, this is completely different. With cachexia, the body is literally digesting itself. The person typically doesn't even feel hungry any more. At this point, their body through glycogen is breaking down the fat and the protein and glucose are being produced.

Remember, part of the trophoblast theory, Beard's research, is that cancer cells were like fetuses or embryos. His point was that the cancer gets fed before the person does! So, it is the first in the food chain. The person, the host, is the second. If Beard is right, and I believe he is based on all the research that I've seen over the years, Beard and Warren were ahead of their time. They were brilliant, brilliant men.

What they figured out were some fundamental truths. If we look at their fundamental truths and then apply them to what we know we can start seeing why cancer cells require us to have proper nutrition, not starvation. There are hundreds of foods out there that contain flavonoids, sanguinary chelerythrine, anthocyanins, that in fact will kill cancer cells. So, by using these mechanisms and methods we can kill the cancer. But it's not through necessarily changing the PH - and here again, I don't want to be misunderstood – if a person is eating junk food, they're basically giving jet fuel to their cancer. So, don't misunderstand me. I'm not suggesting junk food here.

What I am suggesting is that if a person eats a good quality diet that contains foods, for example, carrots. Let's assume they're juicing carrots. I would suggest that carrots are incredibly sweet. It's basically a ton of fructose, right. And most of the time you'd argue that this has no beneficial value to a cancer patient because of all the sugar. But it has also been shown that carrots also contain flavonoids that have anti-cancer properties. So why not consume them? So, I don't think it's always about changing the PH of the urine. I think it's more about targeting different foods.

Here's another good example: Mushrooms. Cordyceps or Shitake or Rishi. The beta glucans. They have a really good method, and those sugars – that's, really what beta glucans are – go into the cancer cell and give the cancer cell a little death package, it allows those phytochemicals to kill the cancer. So, I think what we need to consider is that it's not just one or two mechanisms that you want to use for killing the cancer. I think you want to use your diet; I think you want to be to get your proper nutrition; not that you want to have a body index of 40. I'm not suggesting that. You want to have a proper ratio because obesity is a triggering mechanism for example, for women who have breast cancer.

The thing to keep in mind is, because the extra estrogen that is being
produced, is jet fuel for the cancer. It's just like eating too much sugar. So, you want to use the nutrition that you have, as well as the understanding of your particular cancer to help have a strategy that will effectively allow the cancer cells to die. By integrating non-traditional foods like Bloodroot, that has in fact been used since the 1600s in the U.S the means of killing the cancer is speeded up. Dr. Hucksy was another brilliant person who used non-traditional foods who opened a clinic in Mexico. That was one of the ingredients he had in one of his formulae also. I wish we could claim that we're the smart ones on the planet and only we figured it out, however, that's just a fantasy. The reality is we all stand on the shoulders of giants. And I've been fortunate enough in life to know a lot of great people, read a lot of fantastic research, and hopefully be able to step back and look at it and put it in perspective where other people can also benefit from these great people.

Ian: Yeah. Absolutely. About the PH thing, I just wanted to clarify for the folks, because my mentor is Dr. Bernardo, and he cured more people than anyone I've ever met. He was also one of the first ones I ever met, who, like yourself, had a really lot of success, and was "alternative" you know. He was saying the PH thing is to get it to 7.2, 7.4, most cancers are typical – like breast cancer – are going to make your PH around 5 and you need to get your PH up to about 7.2. As far as measuring your PH the way he said to do it, was to measure the saliva, so it wasn't urine, although you could do both. The most important one was under the tongue to get your intercellular PH. Do you recommend that as well?

Dr. Kelly Raber: I have nothing against it. But the thing we have to keep in mind … is that we have different PH values in our body. Our saliva is more neutral as he pointed out. Our stomach PH is about 1.3 to 1.5, then we go into the small and large intestine and you're basically going to argue that it's neutral again. What happens is that the pancreas secretes the bicarbonate. This is why I don't make a big issue about it. I would partly agree with Bernardo because lactate has a rough PH of about 3 - 3.5 if I remember correctly. So, obviously, that's going to change the extra sale(?) of fluid. But, remember that's going to be the localized area. That's the point. As the lactate moves to the liver to do glycogen then you're going to be able to detect it in the blood. But keep in mind if the PH of the blood drops more than say 0.3 – 0.4 % the person is going to go into shock and die. So, if you have a really good PH meter, you could draw some blood and pick that up. But if you don't, litmus paper is a waste of time. There's no way to check that with litmus paper. How I've looked at litmus paper is just to make sure that you don't destroy your PH meter as you're setting things up. So, it not that I necessarily disagree, because I honestly don't know enough about his technique to be fair. What I suggest is simply this: if you type in the average PH of a fruit or vegetable you'll find that most of them have a PH below 7. And if it's anything below 7 we could fairly argue that it's acidic, right?

Ian: Yeah.

Dr. Kelly Raber: Well if anything below 7 is acidic and we're eating these acidic vegetables and they're going to alkalize us then it's not the rough PH that matters. Let me suggest that because the stomach is acidic, that acid environment is going to pull the minerals from the food. And it's those alkalizing minerals like magnesium, potassium, calcium, that are going to help alkalize the body. So, we should be checking that we're eating enough (fresh raw) fruits and vegetables to make sure that you're pulling down your urine PH. Also, looking at it from an endocrinology standpoint, a lot of times saliva indicates what's going on with the adrenals.

Ian: I shouldn't have got on that tangent, because it's really . . . bottom line folks, it's eating right. Google "alkaline diet" and eat it. If you want to take a litmus strip and test your PH in the morning, everybody that I know that's ever done it, it does show if you've got an alkaline diet, it'll go from 5 to 7.4. And then they live cancer free. Then if they get off that diet, like one of my friends, and their PH got low again, they got cancer again and died. You've got to get your PH up there and keep it there. This is just street science that I've seen. Just out of curiosity what are these protocols looking at financially? Just some quick numbers about what people can expect to pay for the protocols 1, 2 and 3?

Dr. Kelly Raber: Well, (sigh) I'll give rough numbers, and also understand, that I don't actually sell anything. So, if you get it you have to buy it through the manufacturer. Roughly, if you buy it through the manufacturer: Package 1 will be around $200. Package 2 will be around $500. Package 3 will be about the same as package 2, maybe a little bit more. Bloodroot is not that expensive. Package 6 is probably one of the more popular packages, is for stage 3 and 4 Cancer will be around $1,200 to $1,400 a month.

Ian: And that includes the enzymes, right? And that's why?

Dr. Kelly Raber: Yes. That's what makes it so expensive. The herb itself is relatively inexpensive. You can a bottle of say, apoptosis easy to digest 90-count or even full strength for around $20.00 you can get a 540-count roughly for $100 or a little more. But then, that's 540 capsules too, so that's a fair amount of it. Understand that these herbs and mechanisms are all dose-size dependent. You want to get as much of the herb into the body as possible. So, we take a little bit of this and a little bit of that – and I wouldn't expect it to work well.

The key that Kelly brought us, is to get as many enzymes into the body as possible. E.g., If you go to cancer.gov where we see that the federal government actually agrees, that you can kill cancer naturally – type in "enzyme Gonzales" go to Gonzales PDG health professional, click on overview and you'll see that the Gonzales regimen used was about 150 capsules of pancreatic enzymes per day. This kind of gives you the idea of how many it really takes to work. But he took the survival of about 20% success rate the first year, they also brought it up to an 83% success rate the same first year. So, he went from dismal failure (although that is an incredible success compared to Chemo, radiation, and surgery which has a success rate of 2.1%) to really not so bad (83%). And these were late-stage pancreatic cancer patients. As I said, pancreatic cancer is like getting hit twice by lightning. It's very uncommon.

Ian: Yeah. It's unreal. And Dr. Gonzales also was good friends and learned a lot from Dr. Kelly. But somebody told me that they looked into the research and although Kelly may have had a 95% success rate in curing pancreatic cancer that Gonzales doesn't and nobody else has come as close to that success rate. Is that true? Do you know what's going on there?

Dr. Kelly R: I don't know what Gonzales's number are. I don't have a clue. I know Kelly's main point was like mine, mega-dose. I believe that's also where Gonzales is coming from, from the little bit that I've read about his stuff.

Ian: Yes.

Dr. Kelly Raber: But I would say, as a general rule of thumb, we also have to look at what the people are doing. It's not just about eating enzymes. It's not just about adjusting PH. It's about correcting the diet and correcting how we think. Because a person who has a "woe is me" attitude probably is not going to turn their cancer around!

Ian: Exactly!

Dr. Kelly Raber: All of this is connected. It's not just one mechanism being used. You can't just look at a small section of a human or of a body and say if I correct this the whole body will get under control. As I said, I don't know what his success rates are, what I have seen is that people who follow the protocols properly, and really get aggressive with it, have a high success rate. And the ones who decide to do it their way, they don't. But I have seen that people who use pancreatic enzymes that it helps detoxify their body, it helps with the millions of cells dying, it helps change their PH. It helps with all of that. And it also removes HCG.

Ian: Right. I didn't want to pick on Gonzales or you or anybody. Everybody brags about Kelly's success rate, but I don't know anybody today that has that. Of course, people are kind of scared to talk about their success rates period. Do you have one? Do you want to talk about that?

Dr. Kelly Raber: Well the thing is . . . let me explain this properly. If we look at people who have skin cancers, their cancer is going to disappear in about 5 to 20 days. If we use them in the statistics, oh yeah, 99% whatever. It just depends on how many skin cancers you're dealing with.

Ian: Right, well thanks for being really honest...And this is a perfect segue way to this, the moment I found out about this I've been screaming it ever since: This Bloodroot we're speaking about folks, as far as I know, anybody that has put it on skin cancer it worked 100% of the time. Put it on the skin cancer and it ripped the skin cancer right out. It hurt like childbirth, but it worked. So, when I'm asked, I say "what I hear is that it works on skin cancer, and, also internally, it is not painful. But skin cancer is very painful. So, let's speak about that.

Dr. Kelly Raber: Well, I'd say you're relatively close. That's more like Mose's research which is at 97.7% success rate. The more people that apply this the better or worse the numbers get depending upon the percentages of all they break out. But in the 12,000-person human clinical study, dealing with early stage 1 cancer, 97.7% success rate. That was Frederic Mohs. When it was stage 4, late-stage cancer (remember there is no stage 5; stage 4 is late stage cancer) then he hit about a 45 – 50% success rate. That's why you want to combine other mechanisms to go along with it to have much higher success.

Ian: Gerson therapy itself which is internal in which you basically juice for six weeks or whatever, they have 100% success rate I heard with skin cancer, but they're only allowed to say 50%. At least it's better than 3% big pharma gets And that's totally different than putting something on your skin. Gerson is inside out treatment. So, personally, I'd do something like changing my diet and apply the bloodroot. And I've also been told "don't be shy to use morphine, or whatever it takes to be able to bear the pain when the cancer is ripped off. Does it feel like childbirth does it not?

Dr. Kelly Raber: Oh absolutely, it hurts like hell. However, for most individuals, they really don't need to use the paste. E.g., Let's assume you're a lady and you have breast cancer and you go to your oncologist and he says, "you know what? The cancer is too large. You're not operable. Go home and die. We're not going to do surgery, we're not going to do anything. The tumor is too large." If that patient applied the paste to the tumor in all likely hood it's going to kill it. She might remove a section of her breast the size of a fist . . . truth is her breast may be the size of a fist and she loses the whole breast.

Ian: Right.

Dr. Kelly Raber: And these are all possibilities. So, for that person, I think it's really worth it because at the end of the day the oncologist just gave her a death sentence. "Go home and die." So, I think for that person I think using the paste and doing anything she had to do would be reasonable. On the other hand, let's assume that you have skin cancer. Now, you could use the paste, but I would ask "why go through all that pain for no reason?" Take the capsules, five to twenty days later it disappears.

Ian: So you're saying that you could have the skin cancer and just do it internally and it'll heal the same way as if you'd used the paste on your skin, and saved yourself all that pain and misery?

Dr. Kelly Raber: I'm actually saying, taking it internally, would do a better job because there's no pain, there's no scarring, no discomfort, all it is, is eat a bunch of pills and watch it fade and disappear!

Ian: Okay Good!

Dr. Kelly Raber: And I think at the end of the day that's a far better method than hellish pain on the skin.

Ian: (laughter!) I know some women that have given birth and they say it doesn't feel all that great man! (major understatement) You just saved a lot of people a lot of pain man! And me too, because I would have taken bloodroot on the skin if I wasn't able to get Cannabis/hemp oil. That's the other thing, Cannabis/hemp oil works on the skin too from what I've been seeing. And it doesn't hurt. We'll just forget about the bloodroot and skin cancer for now. It's good to know that it works internally. Do any of your protocols recommend bloodroot for prevention, or is it strictly medicinal for once you're sick?

Dr. Kelly Raber: No, it's a supplement. You can take it anytime you want. It's just that if you take a little bit, it works as a supplement. If you take a lot, it works as a therapy against cancer. It's a dose-dependent action. So, if you have a few cells, take a little bit. If you have a lot of cells that need to die, take a lot of it. It's a dietary supplement at the end of the day. It's a mechanism that the body produces about 10,000 cells a second through the process of apoptosis kills about 10,000 cells a second. So, the body is constantly regenerating and killing cells. That's no big deal. All that Bloodroot is doing is allowing the natural process of the body to take place. It's the malignant cell that's defective. What the University of Wisconsin showed — about 12 years ago — how the mechanism on how it induced apoptosis. And what they showed was a DE laddering of DNA. So, all it's really doing is allowing the natural process of the cell to take place. Nothing more. Nothing less. It's just allowing the body to repair itself.

Ian: Do you have the numbers of the people who have used your protocol successfully? And if there are any examples that jump out in your memory, we'd like to hear about them.

Dr. Kelly Raber: What do you mean by "numbers"?

Ian: Yeah. How many have you treated successfully?

Dr. Kelly Raber: Again, it depends on the stage of the person. It's going to depend on their health. It's going to depend on how wealth they're listed. I'm hesitant. We can all say 90%. It depends on how you look at it. What I would suggest for everybody is that's it's 100%. They have 100% failure, or 100% success.

Ian: (laughter) I love it. That's great. (more laughter)

Dr. Kelly Raber: But either way, they're going to experience 100%. And this is why a person really needs to be proactive about their health. This is why a person really needs to be their own best advocate. What I'm suggesting is that foods contain compounds that kill cancer cells. I'm saying that there's nothing abnormal in our food. I'm saying it's part of the natural process, just like taking foods with natural antioxidants in them. There are enough foods out there, I think we can fairly argue, that the mechanism of the cancer dying is just as normal and is just as healthy. Does that make sense?

Ian: Yeah, yeah.

Dr. Kelly Raber: When you look at most of these mechanisms, they're dose-dependent. The analogy I've always used is if you're taking enough product to kill five million cells a day and your body is producing ten million, you're going to lose. There's no way that you're going to overcome your cancer. On the other hand, if you're killing ten million cancer cells a day and your body is only producing five million, how can you lose? The math is on your side. It's not "how does my body respond to it," or, "how does your body respond to it," but how does that individual's body respond to nutrition? And I think this is also where they need to do proper testing. We don't want to be in hopes, dreams and wishes and wishful thinking. If the lab report shows that you're getting healthy, well, you're getting healthy.

If lab reports show that you're getting worse, believe the lab reports. You're not getting better. You need to fundamentally re-look at your diet, and what you're doing. But hopefully you have enough understanding, or, you're working with a Naturopath, or somebody else. For example, if you're watching your PH, one of the reasons that our PH is going to bottom out, it's going to go down is because of lysis, right? So, as we kill millions of cells, we can expect the PH of the urine to drop. But that's actually a sign of success. So, you have to put it all into perspective and understand what you're doing, and the mechanism. In the example of skin cancer, if you can't see the cancer fading then you have to use lab work.

One of the tests that I like is done at American Metabolic Laboratories in Hollywood, Florida. They look at things like HCG. Simply, HCG is a symptom that you're pregnant. And Ian, let me suggest that if you come up with high levels of HCG, I don't think you're pregnant. (smile) It may be not from a lack of trying . . . (laughter) but it ain't going to happen. (laughter from Ian) So, you're not pregnant. What you have is a cancer cell. I think that's a good way of looking at it. If that's true, then you can do some simple blood work to determine if, in fact, you have cancer. You can also see how your numbers are changing if you are improving.

The difference between this and the Navaro test (done in the Philippines) is that in the Navaro test numbers tend to be static for two or three months. At least that's what I've noticed. The advantage of Navaro's test is that it's only about $50 - $55! This is affordable for anyone. So, it's a great test but it's only a one-panel marker. Whereas the American Metabolic Laboratories gives a five-panel marker.

Ian: I don't want to say anything bad about the Navaro test, but it didn't work for my friend's child who had leukemia. It was saying that she was fine, and then, all of a sudden she wasn't. So, FYI, I know it does work for a lot of people, and it sounds like this place in Florida is even better. Who is the doctor?

Dr. Kelly Raber: Dr. Shandel.

Ian: Yeah. Dr. Shandel. I interviewed him for my film too. Yeah. So, he has the best test around?

Dr. Kelly Raber: It's hard to say, "the best" because there are a lot of great tests out there. He has a very good laboratory and he does excellent work. But I'd also say that about Navarro Test too. The thing to keep in mind is that when you're using tests, there is no perfect test. The more tests you do the better likelihood you see toward the truth. (The more accurate the reflection of the truth.) I have seen people who had normal HCG and their CEA numbers were high. So, it doesn't mean that the test was wrong, it just means that they didn't have any HCG that they could find. Does that make sense?

Ian: Yeah.

Dr. Kelly Raber: So, it's not necessarily the lab technician or the method it could just be that individual person's cancer. That's why I was warning earlier about "success rates." More people, more years, and the numbers change. How well does the person listen? Do they really take it seriously? One problem that I have seen over the years is that people tend to bounce from one treatment protocol to another. So, they'll do a month with this one, and a month with that one and a month with another one. Or they'll be halfway within the middle of—one, and change their mind and do something else. They're all over the place like a bunch of rabbits jumping from one thing to another. These people typically don't get well. Then you have the other group that doesn't want to do lab tests. They don't want to invest the money to see what's happening. They have a conspiracy theory that the lab is somehow making oodles of money and so, they don't want to spend the money on it. What I would suggest is asking, "How do you know that you're getting better unless you test?"

Ian: Is there a number of tests that you can name for our audience right now so that they can make a list?

Dr. Kelly Raber: I think Dr. Navaro's test is a great test especially if you're on a budget. I think American Metabolic Laboratories' test is a great test. And I think if you have early-stage cancers, the AMS test done by Onco Labs in Boston, Massachusetts, is a really good test. However, when you read their study on it, it's only for early-stage cancers. They have, if my memory serves me correctly, they have 7% false positive and a 5% false negative error results. But their claim is that they can detect cancer five years before any other testing method can. So, let's assume you get a good clean bill of health from any of the testing facilities, then what I would use after that would be Onco Labs.

Ian: Is that AMS?

Dr. Kelly Raber: Yes, the AMS test was done by Onco Labs in Boston, Mass.

Ian: Okay. This is great stuff man. Thank you!

Dr. Kelly Raber: To check it out, you go to http://www.oncolabinc.com

Ian: Good. Now, what I did folks . . . especially since when I was younger I partied hard, smoked, drank, did everything you can think of, etc., and all of a sudden at age 45 earlier this year, I had a PH of 4 - 5 for about six months. I knew that if anyone came to me with a PH of 5 for 6 months, I'd say, "you've probably got cancer and I would assume that I did if I had that, or that I would have within 5 or 10 years. If you keep a PH of 5, you're very acidic. You're probably going to die, I assume. So, I just got my PH back up to 7.2 – 7.4, nipped it in the bud, and my prostate markers were high, and they're back down to normal. So, to be honest I think I may have just saved myself probably a lot of money, a lot of pain and suffering, and possibly even death just because I knew to take that PH strip in the mornings and see where my PH was. I now am healthy again. So, I would highly recommend that for everybody else. Would you not do that?

Dr. Kelly Raber: I definitely don't see, how it could do harm. And if you PSA went back to normal, fantastic. I think you know the red flag is above 4 – is the belief. From my perspective, anything above one (1) would be horrible. So, the lower you keep your PSA, I think, the better. And that's just good advice for any man.

Ian: Yeah. You don't want to lose that prostate man! 'Cause, you know, there's no more hanky-panky and I just found out you actually have to wear diapers! Holy smokes! Yeah. Get your PH up, get alkaline and stay healthy.

What I also wanted to ask you was, could you talk about the cachexia? Someone specifically asked: What causes cachexia? And how can you reverse that? Isn't ATP useful for that? How much ATP can one consume? Is there a limit to what is safe? You've already touched base on that, but did you totally kill that question already, or is there more you can add to that?

Dr. Kelly Raber: We can go into a little bit more. 1) What causes it that the body goes into conservation mode from not eating enough nutrition, or, there is so much metabolic waste getting dumped into the system that the high levels of lactate are what triggered it. I've found, along with clinical studies, that ATP works effectively. As a rule of thumb, from 12 to 16 capsules per day will generally reverse it.

2) The other thing to keep in mind is that because the body is in conservation mode, the body doesn't produce enough stomach acid. When the stomach doesn't produce sufficient stomach acid you don't break down your food properly. If you don't break down your food properly you don't alkalize. So, if you want an alkaline body, you have to have an acidic stomach. So, one part of it is, if their body is not producing enough stomach acid they need to take something like stomach advance. It's a pretty good formulation I've put together. What it contains is Betaine-hydrochloride, pepsin and stomach extract. The reason for the stomach extract is for the intrinsic factor so that you can get the B-12 and such into the body.

3) The other thing is that the best way to reverse it is to eat high-quality nutritious foods, making sure that you have enough enzymes to break it down. Then obviously, converting the lactic acid back to glucose; because as long as the body is too acidic, the body will be in conservation mode and digest itself. Therefore, what you're having is that the highly acid ketones are left over. Ketones are like super fuel to cancer. It's like jet fuel. So, the more starvation that the person experiences, typically, the faster the cancer grows. What produces more lactate, the more acidic the adjacent cells become. Make sense?

Ian: Yeah.

Dr. Kelly Raber: So, to reverse it change the environment, changing the PH, get great nutrition in and then convert that lactic acid back into glucose. So, the whole chain is broken and get healthy cells functioning properly.

Ian: That's right. This is beautiful man. It's kind of a catch-22 or bitter-sweet, but recently one of my friends died named Ronnie Smith. He was a big advocate for the cannabis-hemp oil movement. It's sad that he passed on, but it kind of made me jump into a couple of his groups and I'm trying to pass the information to some of them that may not have realized yet that there's definitely a lot more to cancer healing than just cannabis. That's a great little thing, medicinal approach, but you must balance your PH, you must boost your immune system, detox and all that as well. Am I correct Doctor?

Dr. Kelly Raber: Absolutely. I think the people who use a one-prong approach they may get lucky and it may work for them, but I would say more mechanisms and the more methods they use for killing the cancer, and then verifying that it is working; these are the people who typically conquer cancer. The ones who don't understand how they can do all this, they need to get with somebody who they can work with, whether it's a naturopath, an alternative doctor, someone like that who really understands and knows what they're doing.

Ian: And you are one of those people, and I have to give you props. Ladies and Gentlemen, this man has been helping people for over twenty years, and he will spend time on the phone with you. I'm all excited to tell my friends about him. And they already know. They go, "Oh, yeah, Dr. Raber. . . I talk to him all," I go, "Oh, okay. Cool." (laughter) They say he's a great guy to talk to.
Is there anything else you want to add before we end this talk?

Dr. Kelly Raber: Well, the main thing is that all these mechanisms that we've been speaking about are dose-dependent. The more you take in, the better it works. If you decide to use my formulations or use similar herbs, keep in mind that the good rule of Dr. Kelly is, "Make sure it doesn't have any fillers or additives." I really do think that those materials hinder the body's ability to repair. The reason I've done a lot of different work and that I prefer using special laboratories methods, is that they test everything three times, they make sure it is exactly what they say it is, they do micro-tests and they do chemical identification on everything twice before it is ever dealt with. So, when you get stuff from them you get exactly what your body requires, and this is why I like them. They don't cut corners. They make high-quality products.

That's one of the main reasons I like them. So, there are a lot of places getting herbs, and if you know that the bloodroot you're getting is good, fantastic. Just remember that the formulation I put together is buffered in the stomach, so you don't puke your guts out. So, the herb is wonderful, but it does have some difficulties. And, this is what has been really difficult for people over the years; taking enough of it to be beneficial. Right now, I've been able to get people up to 45 capsules three times a day! And I've seen some people report a 65% tumor reduction within the first 30-40 days.

Ian: Wow. That is really good news and again amazing news that you can take this internally and don't have to suffer through the pain of the physical-topical application of it on the skin. What a great show. I'm not sure what else to say, except TumorX.com. I think that's it, unless you have one more thing there, brother.

Dr. Kelly Raber: No. That's it. If I can help anybody, just let me know. If you read the website, go to the cancer's page. There's a lot of information. The other thing I did do for the entertainment of the government, that I have the government site that shows that cancer can be healed – cancer cells die "apoptosis" siting clinical studies that have already been done demonstrating that bloodroot does, in fact, kill cancer cells. So, educate yourself as much as humanly possible. Whatever you do, verify it using tests, and hopefully, you'll be cancer free. As you know my dad had esophagus cancer, he was stage four, two-and-a-half months later he was 100% cancer free.

Ian: Unfortunately, he passed due to a car accident.

Dr. Kelly Raber: Yeah. It was a logging truck.

Ian: To the public audience, give us a call. As far as I'm concerned, cancer is not a death sentence. It's just a wake-up call.

Dr. Kelly Raber: Absolutely, absolutely. It's just time for you to get serious and get under control

.

Ian: Right. Right on. Well, I can't tell you what a pleasure it is Dr. Kelly Raber. I hope to speak to you again. And, we'll definitely stay in touch, okay?

Dr. Kelly Raber: Okay. Sounds good.

CHAPTER 24:

RICHARD GORDON ON QUANTUM TOUCH

I just happened to be at my friend Bobby Williams and Mariel Hemingway's ranch one day on a visit when Richard Gordon stopped by and I just had to get my camera out of the car and shoot this guy. I was just learning about energy healing so it was good timing to meet this master. www.quantumtouch.com

Richard: I'm Richard Gordon and I've been doing energy healing for 36 years. I founded a business called Quantum Touch which is in over 50 countries.   And what we found is a very clear direct way to teach people how to move the energy through their body, to raise the life force energy, to allow their body to heal itself naturally, to accelerate the healing process.   And that's a really exciting process; but only in the last two years did I discover a new way of doing it that completely astounds me. You'd think after all these years I'd start to get a little jaded or tired of what I was doing, but this opened the doors to a wide range of possibilities using the advanced form of what we call quantum touch we're able to move the awareness in such a way where you don't even have to touch a person to see dramatic results.

We can actually just send the energy, and you can even see the bones spontaneously move back into correct alignment just without even touching them within seconds and it isn't just like a some of the time sort of phenomena, this thing happens like all the time. It's virtually 100 percent phenomena. Well out of the last couple thousand times I've been trying this on people I don't remember it not working one time. And one of the really cool things we're doing is, we're aligning this sphenoid bone with the occipital reds these are some bones inside the head and when they get aligned they phenomena is that the hips immediately align themselves front and back and the occipital ridge is aligned as well and what makes this so unusual is it tends to keep the alignment over a long period of time.

Now the reason I get so excited and talk way too much about alignment isn't because the work focuses on alignment, we work on the organs and glands and systems of the body, we work on the structural issues, we work pretty much on whatever it is, on pain relief, bringing down inflammation, but I can't show those things in real time. If somebody said, "Well let me see what your work does!" I can't show how we're affecting the mitochondria in the cells or we're affecting these sorts of things. I can show, however, how we're affecting structure because if the structure shifts in a few seconds then we have a really clear picture that I was able to do something.

And the other really exciting thing about this is that perhaps for the first time we've got a clear visible teachable way of showing that consciousness affects matter, and this could be the biggest story since Galileo. Four hundred years ago Galileo was showing off his telescope that the earth was actually going around the sun and that it wasn't the other way around. Well, now we can show that our love and our consciousness actually affect matter and changes the very structure of life. This would be the biggest shift of consciousness that we've seen, and it just seems so important that the word gets out that human beings can do this.

Ian: Like are you telling me that you basically can do what a chiropractor does with your mind?

Richard: Not only what a chiropractor does, but we can do things that a chiropractor can't do. For instance, the chiropractor couldn't work on getting... well if they are very bright they could figure out how to align this sphenoid bone and the occipital ridge so that the hips don't go out. But very few of them know how to do that because people need to keep coming back week after week to see the chiropractor cause, they'd be coming out of alignment, we're actually, able to get it to where it stays, but we can also work on things chiropractors can't touch.

For example, say somebody's sprains their ankle and as an athlete, you've experienced that. Well, typically people put ice on the ankle. I worked with the men's basketball team at UCSC demonstrating how the healing worked to accelerate the healing process. And what we saw was that an average ten-minute session reduced their pain by 50 percent. And that was like 12 years ago I did the study. And now we're even better than we were then.

But you could bring down the inflammation on a sprained ankle very quickly you can accelerate the speed that it heals. So, we're able to do things that touch on many different fields, including chiropractic. And to do things that people really, generally, don't know how to do, like how do you take the pain out of a burn? Recently, a few days ago, I interviewed someone who had worked on herself and she had severe rheumatoid arthritis to the point where she couldn't comfortably walk, she couldn't stand and do the cooking for the family and her doctor, one of her doctors told her that in a year she'd be in a wheelchair and that she'd be blind. And she said, she took in the information and just said, "No thank you", to him and then immediately met someone who was doing quantum touch and learn how to do it herself, was working on herself a lot had some sessions from people and her symptoms completely reversed, that's way beyond chiropractic.

Then just this week in one of my classes one of my students who was doing sessions and not only did the woman's scoliosis shift that she worked on, but she says she doesn't think she needs the knee replacement operation anymore as the doctor said. She's going to get the diagnosis soon, we'll find out. But she also said that her compulsive eating shifted where she did feel the need to eat, over the entire weekend she only ate two meals and didn't feel like she was missing anything. She just felt really grateful inside. So, we're seeing a wide range of phenomena that this healing work affects.

Ian: Is there any way you can explain to the layman what quantum physics is, how this works, cause the average person is just going to say you're full of it, there's no way you can use your brain to do this?

Richard: Well you know people should believe that this is crap. Because if they haven't experienced it or they haven't seen research on it then I would fully go along with that point of view. There's a lot of stuff out there that's basically crap.

But the general principle of quantum touch is that what we're doing is we're learning to use breathing and body awareness to raise our own vibration in ourselves and we lift what's called the life force energy of our bodies, now the Chinese call it Chi and the Japanese call it Qi and the Yogi's call it prana and many cultures around the world have acknowledged this life energy. And by using various breathing and body awareness exercises we can lift our vibration, really high; to a high place. Then through a process of resonance and entrainment, the other person's energy matches yours and then their body intelligence does the healing.

So, we like to say that the definition of a healer was someone who was sick and got well. And a great healer was someone very sick who got well quickly because we don't actually heal anybody else. What we're doing is creating a frequency of vibration. Now that frequency of vibration could be done with the hands and for 33 years of my work I was using my hands as the way of moving the energy. But then I just got the idea that, Wow we could do it directly without even the hands and it's faster and it's easier and it's more fun than it's ever been before. And now I can work much more quickly and more profoundly. But anybody who says that energy healing is the answer to our problems is exaggerating. It's an answer. It's a great answer. It's an important answer. But on a deeper level are the emotional causes of why we generated the problem.

Now about 85-90 percent of the time you can create a really nice shift to symptoms with the energy work. And sometimes that's all the person needs, in fact, often, that's all they need. But when it doesn't work, that's when I really like to go find the emotional causation of what they were experiencing emotionally that wasn't completed that they're now expressing through the conditions in their body.

Oh yeah, there's a lot of stuff that goes in there, especially with your hip that's been out for so long and the injuries and the discomfort that it causes, there are expressions, emotional expressions.
Now I like the idea that I could give you analgesic help which we did a little while ago and that's great. But if that's not enough, if you haven't healed those emotional issues in your life then we could actually work to find emotional causation and what's so exciting is not only do the symptoms disappear, but people will even feel really grateful for having had the condition because it showed them how they'd stopped loving.

The body had the ability to be sick not as a dysfunction but as a communication from your own higher consciousness to show you how you could be well. And using my system I'd be able to figure it out probably we could figure it out in ten or twenty minutes, and know exactly what the particular issue was not as a generalization but as a very specific emotional set of circumstances that you could then process and release on your own time.

Here's the deal, the body heals itself. And we've got a few thousand practitioners around the world in over 50 countries and they're working on pretty much everything and we don't know the limits of this work, but to say that it's going to fix A, B or C decondition is not true because the body heals itself and when things are aligned, yeah, we see tremendous affects. But again, the healer was the one who was sick and got well and we cannot predict the outcome. It's neither something we know how to do nor something that's even legal. We can't do that.

But what we can do is provide the energy and we often see wonderful things happening.
So, for instance, there's an oncologist who writes wonderful things about quantum touch. He says how it reduces their fear, it reduces their pain, it reduces scar tissue, it heals the scar tissue faster, it gives them greater mobility, it raises their spirits. He mentions a ton of things. He might get into trouble if he said, it was actually healing them.

And we know that if somethings raising their spirits and it's accelerating the healing of wounds then the body's healing itself faster so whatever capacity the body has to heal itself would be enhanced and that's about as far as I can go because that's what we do, we enhance healing. We don't heal anything particularly, we enhance the bodies capacity for self-healing. Because think about it, there is no drug that heals people, there's no surgery that heals people. It's the cells that have to heal themselves that are doing the healing.

So, what we're doing essentially is creating an environment where the body can do that stuff for itself.

Okay one story that was just outlandish and it blew my mind was when I first met my teacher and he was working on my girlfriend and she's standing in front of the room and we're staring at her back and I realize, "Wow, look at that she really has significant scoliosis and he said, "Well this all moves," and he touches her and the bones move back to alignment and this moves here and within about ten minutes she was like halfway straightened out. I was shocked.

Then shortly after that, after I learned how to move the energy myself. I... this is really funny, this friend brought a rabbit to my house and the rabbit was hopping all around the house. I thought it was really cute until I realized there were these pellets all over the floor. So, I had to put the rabbit back in a box. So, it takes me a while to corner the rabbit and I have the rabbit underneath my hands and it's trembling, figuring, in rabbit language that is was going to be dinner. So, I started running the energy into the rabbit and the rabbit relaxed, stopped trembling and a couple of seconds later the rabbit stretched its front paws forward and its back paws back as far as it could. And then I continued running the energy, my friend is watching, like this and the rabbit flips itself over on its back and lays there all stretched out on its back like it was sunning itself on the beach in Hawaii.

Ian: And you were giving it love, were you?

Richard: I was just giving it love. Yeah. And of course, I really believe now that the reason that happened is that the rabbit was so scared. Had the rabbit been relaxed it would have just not really noticed much of a difference from its normal state to a slightly more relaxed state. But when you take it from terror to total relaxation and he just continues going, "Okay I can be totally relaxed now."
And I just met a woman who had the same experience with a rabbit. She had a scared rabbit, ran the energy and it flipped over on its back. At first, when it was flipping I thought it was going to try to run away. And then when it flipped over on its back [chuckling], oh my God my hands were on its belly and it's just all stretched out.

Ian: Wow, you just validated something for me. A little dog, like one of these little ones.
Richard: Yeah.
Ian: Got hit by a car in front of our house one time.
Richard: Yeah.

Ian: like crazy all the neighbors are coming out just going...

Richard: Yeah.

Ian: I went out, swear to God... cause, I learned this through the Essene meditation that I was studying, and I didn't even believe in it and I thought my girlfriend was whacked but I went because I liked this girl. But I did it, just for shits and giggles, I put my hand on the dog and I pictured light from God come in my one hand.

Richard: Yeah. Sure.

Ian: and into my body and in that dog through my other hand and it chilled out right then and there.

Richard: Yeah.

Ian: I freaked myself out. And then I just blew it off as coincidence.

Richard: Well here's the deal. Virtually any technique you come up with whether you make it up or you hear it from somebody else is going to work for energy healing.

Now there are techniques that can raise your energy, really profoundly. Just lifting your spirits as you did. You know to ask and then to be there, that'll work, that's a technique, there are thousands of them. What we like about the quantum touch work that makes it quite unique, as far as I know, is that by using breathing and body awareness to lift our own field of energy, what we're doing is we're creating an extremely high frequency of vibration, and so we never get tired or drained from doing the work. But many people are using their own energy, or they don't know how to raise their spirit sufficiently, so they don't entrain or match the vibration of the person they're working on which is what causes them to get tired or drained. We just walk people right through from the beginning, right through, so that by the end of a weekend workshop, everybody's doing some pretty awesome work.

Ian: Just, you don't have to tell me right now, but am I in the right ballpark, do you like envision suns filling you full of light, that kind of stuff?

Richard: No. No. I'll tell you what we do. We use body awareness exercises where we're feeling awareness moving through our body. We're just feeling ourselves essentially. And we're learning how to move it in certain patterns and then we link it with certain breathing patterns.

So, we're moving body awareness and linking it with breathing. Now if somebody wants to pray or if somebody wants to connect to source or whatever it is, great, go do those things, cause that's what you, that's what works for you. Somebody can just think of how much they love their cat and that works too. But what we're wanting to do is get you feeling connected with yourself. And in that connected space, as you're using the breathing, as you're using the body awareness and you're linking them together, then we get this awesome effect.

That's why I would say that everybody is able to move bones back into alignment before lunch day on the first day of a workshop or their money back because it works. That's using your hands. The level II work that I just come up with recently is where we do it with consciousness directly.

And that's what gets so exciting for the scientists and the physicists is they can pass off the energy work to placebo or some other psychological mechanism and say, "Oh, yeah", but when something works on infants and animals and people under general anesthesia, plants fluids minerals and be able to adjust people at a distance when they don't believe it or when they're hostile against you, that's when it gets really interesting, because, that's paradigm changing information.

I was at a consciousness conference in Tucson not too long ago. And I had a big sign on the wall and the sign said, "Consciousness affects matter, free demo!" And the scientist is like, "Come on." I say, "Okay, what you got here?" I said, "Well let me measure your hips." "Oh wow, they're really off about as far off as you usually ever see them, about like that." And I said, "Well I'm going to attempt to put them back into alignment without touching you. And he goes, "Well that's impossible!" I said, "Great. Hold that thought!" So, I wanted to make it a little harder.

And then I said, "In fact, while we're at it, why don't you kind of lock your hips and just kind of make it so they can't move." So, he, alright, so he's kind of like that and ten seconds later I measure him. "Oh, look they're completely level." He said, "Well yeah, I used reverse psychology on me." And I said, "Well that's an interesting hypothesis. So, do you consider yourself a faith-based scientist?" He said, "Well of course not I'm empirical." I said, "Oh, wonderful. Well as an empirical scientist why don't you watch me do this, eight or ten more times and see if I'm using reverse psychology?" And he said, "If I let myself believe this just happened, everything I know about science would fall like a house of cards." And I said, "Well, as an empirical scientist, don't you want to let the cards fall where they will?" And he said, "Not today!"

Because it's too big a shift for most people to go from a completely mechanical viewpoint of the reality to more of a quantum perspective where it's all energy and it's all consciousness and energy and consciousness responds to itself and to each other quite clearly and quite easily.

If they would visit www.quantumtouch.com that'd be a great place for them to start and they could learn about the basic workshop, the advanced workshops, we've got the advanced workshops in Europe, Australia, Japan, what's left of it, Hawaii, most of the United States, Canada.

So, we've got them out there and the beginning workshops they're everywhere. And people can also watch the video as a DVD and soon we're going to have them online where you can watch them on demand.

[See Pic 24.1]

www.quantumtouch.com

CHAPTER 25:

MARIEL HEMINGWAY & BOBBY WILLIAMS

Ian: Alternative Medicine is not really even heard of much back then so what...

Mariel: Right.

Ian: Why are you different and why didn't you go with the flow of Western?

Mariel: Okay. I'm Mariel Hemingway. And the reason why, I guess my interest in, I guess nobody is really interested in cancer [chuckling] but my sort of understanding and delving into what is behind cancer and how to prevent it came because my mother had cancer when I was growing up and I was her primary caregiver when I was about, she got it when I was ten years old and I took care of her for years. I used to... sleep in the same bed and when she went through chemotherapy and radiation, you know, I held her hand when she threw up bad, you know, I held her head when she threw up, you know. It made her really, really, sick and I think that, I really think that the cure for cancer is what killed her.

Now granted this was... 30 years ago, you know, something crazy or even more thirty.... never mind [chuckling]... it's a lot of years ago. So, you know their so-called technology has changed and they say that they are more directed and all that stuff. But then cut to my ex-husband... 11 years ago contracted stage 4 melanoma on the top of his head. And you know, basically, they write you off. Stage 4 is, as you know like it's bad. And melanoma is bad. Usually, chemotherapy and radiation don't respond well to, you know melanoma, melanoma doesn't respond well to chemotherapy and radiation.

Yet it didn't matter, they still wanted to do it. And I just said to him, "Look, I was around cancer my whole childhood. It destroys a person. The cure for it destroys a person. I really think that we can address this in a different way." I remember reading something about a Buddhist Monk saying that it was really one of the great gifts that a person can get is cancer. Because it's a way to learn about yourself and is a real way if you get the message. It's a real way to understand who you are, change your lifestyle, become more aware... self-aware on a physical, mental and spiritual basis.

I started to look at what it was that was the cause of cancer and I know spiritually or emotionally it has a lot to do with resentment, resentment, anger, the things that are, you know, bottled up inside. Not that a lot of diseases don't have that but that seems to be one of the underlying core factors of people that get cancer they have sort of, whatever it is, some pent-up thing that deals with this resentment. Thinking back at my mother, she was definitely a resentful, angry, unhappy person who hadn't dealt with things from her childhood and that kind of thing. So, there was that level of looking at it. But then there was food. I mean, just think about food itself.

My ex-husband was a sugar addict. He was an "A" type personality. I mean he'd just go, go, go all the time, worked all the time. And the more he worked, you know, he felt that he was better, and you know, high-stress level, massively high-stress level, drank, ate badly. You know, all these different things in combinations. I started to say, okay, let's... number one, let's look at your food. Let's not feed the cancer. What do cancer cells eat? What do all cells eat? But what do cancer cells grow on? Sugar. Let's get sugar out of your diet. Sugar, carbohydrates... and people say, "Oh, sugar, you know, that's the ice cream and cookies." Well, it's actually, ice cream, cookies, white flour, you know, bagels, pasta, bread... whatever it is that is processed and not pure and whole.

We tried to give him a diet that was a whole food based diet. So, he had a whole food based diet, no sugar, no carbohydrates, except for berries because they are great antioxidants and doing a supplement program, food-based supplements that were high antioxidants and you know, helping with this whole, you know, fighting the cancer. We did a lot of research and a friend of ours mentioned a thing called bloodroot, which is an American Indian, you know, cure for cancer. It actually attacks cancer only. Which is just bizarre, but it's ancient. So, these are all alternative holistic ways to go about attacking cancer.

So, he started doing that, and what's really interesting because I said, "I want to try it." Cause I want to know if it... and it just gave me a stomach ache and didn't do anything. But for him, he could feel it in his system working, working away. He did acupuncture, he did Chinese herbs and he learned to meditate. I mean he changed his life spiritually and he... you know, he brought his stress level down.

So, all these things are powerful tools, to actually heal. But when people get cancer, so often they say, "I got cancer." And they give all their power over to a doctor, you know, whatever huge doctor, you know, huge system medical center blah blah blah that's known for their cancer research and they give all their participation in the disease away. Because I've had people, friends of mine who have gotten cancer and have said, you know, and I've said to them, "Look, you know, my husband is still alive. He's 11 years into remission." That's HUGE. I mean that doesn't happen very often and he did it through food and exercise and life style because that's how... it really can be done. It doesn't mean that all of these systems will work. But like we did ozone for him. We looked into ozone therapy. Well in this country, "Oh, that's poison and it's against the law." Well, I'm sorry, it's used in Europe all over the place. We don't use it in this country. But there are so many modalities to heal cancer. To heal cancer. Where you don't get cancer again.

Most people that go through them, you know, the traditional medicine, they get cancer, they do chemotherapy and radiation, they might go into remission, but it usually recurs.

So, it really is about... look... it's about knowledge, you gotta have the knowledge and what I love that you're doing is you're getting information out there. I would never tell anyone not to do what they believed in. But you should know that you are part of the healing process. You know, what people eat, how they think, how they live their lives, what exercise they do. You know, whether they take some silence. It's all these different things, it's gonna heal them. You have to be part of the... you have to be your own doctor. You really have to participate in your own coming to health.

You know what, I think when the Buddhist was saying that, it's like, you've become self-responsible. When you get a disease or something it's a wake-up call to self-awareness. Who am I? What do I need to do? Why did this happen? Oh, it's not some horrible thing... it doesn't have to be a horrible thing. It can be your opportunity to really understand yourself in a deeper way. But you need to... the person with the cancer needs to take responsibility that they are part of the process, part of the healing. And not allow, you know, western medicine to just take them down. And just... you know... because I see people that will eat whatever they want. It's like, "Oh I feel bad, so I'm gonna eat more sugar because poor me I've got this horrible thing called cancer."

And the truth is when you're doing that food is medicine. You take an Advil and 20 minutes later you don't have a headache, you don't think your food does the same thing to you? It does. It has the same effect on us. Everything we ingest in our bodies has... it has a chemical and you know physical effect on us.

It reminds me... so my husband has this cancer. He has this melanoma. So, Bobby, my partner, who's gonna... I'm gonna bring him in here in a second. He has a friend who contracted the same cancer, the exact same... only stage 1, not even stage II, far less severe than my husband's and we desperately tried to convince him, please, you know, look... my, you know my girlfriend... Bobby was saying this to his friend Matt, my girlfriend's husband had the same cancer and they cured it holistically. Please give us two weeks, give us a month, give us something and see if we can turn this around.   And he was already, you know, they already had the chemotherapy, radiation, surgery all that lined up. And Bobby's gonna come in and read a letter from him that it is just heartbreaking.

Bobby: Yeah.

Mariel: So this is Bobby.

Bobby: And another thing is Mariel's husband did have a tumor removed at the hospital and he was gonna stay in and go the conventional way. And when he came out of surgery, Mariel, tell them what food they brought him or what looked like food.

Mariel: Oh yeah, yeah, yeah. Oh, I forgot that.

Bobby: So here you go to the hospital and you assume that everybody... that they have a knowledge about nutrition. So, his first meal that he was given after surgery... and he's there and he's got his head wrapped up. Cause they did do surgery to remove the tumor out of his... you know, near his brain.   And he is like swollen, he feels like crap, but he's kind of hungry, whatever... So, this is his first meal. They bring it out on a tray and I undo the thing... you know, I take the plastic over the top of the food. And it's a boiled chicken breast. It's some green Jell-O. A cup of coffee...And a piece of chocolate cake.

Mariel: And a piece of chocolate cake. Processed chocolate cake. And... and, and a thing of pasteurized milk.

Bobby: Yeah.

Mariel: And I'm like... I was infuriated. I was so MAD.

Bobby: She was like is this real food? Is this...

Mariel: Is this what you would give someone who just got out of surgery?

Bobby: Really, who just got out of surgery? And the doctor said, he goes, "Oh, it's fine."

Mariel: What's the matter?

Bobby: She goes, "This isn't even food." She goes, "This is the reason why he has the cancer."

Mariel: Yeah.

Bobby: And he was like, he was like, "Oh no. Don't worry it's fine." Same oncologist as Farrah Fawcett. The BEST. The BEST.

Mariel: And he's not a bad person, but......

Bobby: They don't, they don't have an

Mariel: their knowledge of nutrition and all that stuff...

Bobby: understanding... and health…

Mariel: was so crazy. And he was like, "You can do that acupuncture, that stuff, you know, oh, that'll help..."

Bobby: And when you ask them...

Mariel: "it'll help you feel good and peaceful."

Bobby: When you ask the doctors, you say, "How much time have you spent on nutrition in your six, eight, ten-year internship?" Most of them look away. And I'm like, "It's okay, I know you've only spent two weeks and you have no idea about that part of the stuff, you're emergency care and that kind of stuff... broken bones, best on the planet, you guys are fantastic, couldn't be in better hands." Preventative? That's something that we're gonna have to take care of ourselves.

Mariel: There's just not... yeah, exactly.

Bobby: So this is what I get from Matt. Identical cancer to Mariel's ex. I haven't heard from him in months and I wanted him to come over here and do ozone with us. By the way, statistics, Mariel's statistics with the ozone, 7,000 practitioners in Europe using ozone. Seven thousand. My grandmother said that she had it when she was a kid and it went away in the 40s and it went away when pharmaceutical companies came in. Because it's inexpensive...

Mariel: Doesn't make them money and...

Bobby: So there's that... and, and, and... then she also talked about the percentage of cancer coming back or not being put into remission or being put into remission and coming back. It's 97 percent change for it to come back once it's been in remission or if it got put into remission, 97 percent chance that the cancer's coming back even after this painful type of thing.

So, this is Matt's email to me and you know Matt, we know him from 20 years ago. Military guy. Okay. Green beret. Matt leaves a message saying "I would have called you to give you an update Bobby, but the side effects of the head radiation continue to impede my ability to speak. I don't think I'll be able to talk for another week or so." Now he sat down with a team of five people said that they were gonna localize the radiation. It's very small up here, no problem. Listen to this,

"Unfortunately, my recovery is going very, very slowly much slower than expected. I keep hoping for some significant improvement, but improvement is almost indiscernible. My treatments ended a month ago, my esophagus and mouth feel like they've been burned with a propane torch. My weight is down to 168 pounds and a lot of my hair is all gone." He was 225 pounds. Matt continues "I know it sounds irrational, but I'm actually growing a bit more scared. I'm experiencing a strange form of claustrophobia. I feel like I'm trapped inside my own body. I wake up ten times a night. I wake up ten times a night and taking a shower hurts and I still eat through a tube in my stomach." I was like... WHAT? This stage I that was gonna be localized. The doctors tell me, Eventually, you'll get your life back, but it'll be a different kind of life. I don't know what that means, but I just want to feel normal again. I'm tired of this whole thing and I'm feeling a little defeated. My next PET scans are scheduled for April and at that point, I'll learn if the chemo, radiation was effective, and my cancer is in remission. Thanks for checking up on me Bobby, you're a good friend. Matt."

Bobby: I mean, dude, come oooonnnnnnn.......
Mariel: How heartbreaking is that. It makes me cry every time. It's sooooo sad.

Bobby: I couldn't read it for the first ten times. I read it now and then I get angry while I'm reading it so I don't cry. Cause I couldn't... I would have Mariel read it when we first started reading it to people when we were talking in public. You know, come on. This is a green beret who... who can endure some of the greatest pains and all and these doctors sat there .... and I wonder.... are they into, some kind of oath... they're telling them this. Well if it's so.... you know, not that bad for you. Then why don't they do it themselves and show us how it's not that bad for you.

Mariel: I know.

Bobby: You know, and we know many people that wouldn't even go to the doctors. Doctors themselves wouldn't go to the doctors that get cured for cancer. Who are we kidding here? You know, is it a business? I don't know. I'd like to think that people aren't that evil, you know.

Mariel: And it makes us think, you know.... and we get, we get things, you know there are these wonderful causes out there, you know, walk for the cure or marathon for the cure or whatever it is... **let's cure breast cancer or something like that. And we always ask the question...**

Bobby: We ask the celebrities.

Mariel: Yeah.

Bobby: We've asked the celebrities, "Where's the money going?|"

Mariel: And they're not... they have a good heart and it's a good intention. "Where's the money going?" "Cancer Research."

Bobby: What does that mean?

Mariel: Really? What does that mean?

Bobby: I don't know.

Mariel: I don't know.

Bobby: So you're raising 2 million dollars to give to somebody that you don't know, and you don't know what's going on? And you just assume it's gonna be this? It's the same thing, over and over again. It never stops. It's like... it's like... you know, Jerry's kids, he's been doing telethons for 40 years, the same kids come out on stage. When are they gonna be healed? How much money does it take?

And it always... we always go back to the same thing. It starts with you. We have to start with ourselves. We have to start asking the questions and looking into this ourselves. And if we do that... well then, we'll figure it out.

Mariel: Yeah. Cause it's not about pointing fingers and saying somebody's bad or doctors are bad. It's just about saying, "Look, take responsibility. That was the thing."

Bobby: These things aren't working.

Mariel: It's not working. And quit telling us that it is working because it really isn't.

Bobby: And when you...

Mariel: I mean there are a few small cases where it goes in remission. In cases where cancer is not that strong, or it's not a really severe version. Maybe... maybe then. But I'm telling you for the most part... it doesn't work. That whole system doesn't work. There's a holistic way to go about it. And it's not woo woo, it's not crap. These are... it's centuries long.

Bobby: You know that... that was a big... that was a big word you're using... holistic! It's not alternative... what they are doing is alternative.

Mariel: is alternative.

Bobby: We were told that we live an alternative lifestyle for the longest time [laughing Mariel] my dad called me up like a month ago and he said, "Bob," he's like, "it's us that's, we're living the alternative lifestyle. We eat chemicals. We eat processed food. We eat this alternative stuff."

Mariel: We eat synthetic food that's not even real.

Bobby: He said, "You guys are eating simple." Milk straight from a cow that's healthy and taken care of. You know, chickens that are really free-range and biodynamic. Real fruit. Fruit and vegetables and stuff from the farm and you know where it comes from.

Mariel: They have to be radiated, you know, and there are no pesticides.

Bobby: And he's like, so you're...

Mariel: Natural.

Bobby: So we're simplifying our lives and saying, "Hey, nature has the answers. Let's look there and see how nature is. You know, instead of trying to speed everything up, package things, shelf life, money, money, money. It's all driven by the same thing.

Mariel: And then people will say to us, like, "Yeah, but you know, that's a great idea." I mean even in regard to cancer, "but it's so expensive to eat that way and do all these things." I'm like, "Go to a hospital, get cancer and see what those bills are like."

Bobby: Right.

Mariel: That's … I mean talk about taking your life down. Most people at the end of their life.

Bobby: Far more expensive to get sick. It's far more expensive to get sick than it is to spend a few hundred dollars extra a week on organic food. You won't have to go see a doctor.

Mariel: To just save your life. It will save your life.

Bobby: And by the way, Mariel and I are two hundred years old today.

Mariel: [Laughing] Yes.

Bobby: We don't look at it, but we're feeling good.

Mariel: [chuckling]

Bobby: Go that route.

Mariel: Laughing...

Ian: That's awesome man. You're the best. Wow.

Mariel: Laughing.

Ian: I mean, I got tears coming out of my eyes knowing the good this interview will do. So many look up to you guys. Any thoughts on what... if you two had a child and you wanted to treat that child, you couldn't until it's 18 you have to get that child chemotherapy and radiation or they'll take them away, they'll get you on endangerment. Can you speak about that?

Mariel: If somebody tried to tell me that I had to put my child on chemotherapy and radiation... I would leave the country so fast. I'm sorry. Not my kid. I'm not going to put my kid in the hands of somebody who's going to kill them.

Bobby: No, we'd be smart about it. We'd be, "Sure we'll see you next week. Next week will be a great time." And then you'd never hear from us again.

Mariel: Laughing. Disappeared ooooooo.

Bobby: Where'd they go? Ahh, show up a year later. "Oh, he doesn't have cancer. Guess he doesn't have to go. Misdiagnosis.

Mariel: Yup. Oh, they must have made it up. You know, right.

Bobby: Again, we're not saying that doctors don't have the knowledge to fix things and work on things and do emergency care, and these things but certain things aren't working. Well if the same thing is happening, over and over again, that's the definition of insanity, right. Einstein said it, "Why keep doing the same thing?"

Mariel: If it's not... yeah.

Bobby: You're getting the same results.

Mariel: You're getting the same results. And it's not working.

Bobby: Everyone is dying it's not working. But hey, wait a minute, James Hopson? liver cancer, cured, Mariel's husband cured. Several people at the Venice Raw Store are cured. Several people that I know in my life cured, cured, cured. Hodgkin's disease cured. Dave Schultz? Cured. Oh, he's never gonna have kids. You know, he's got Hodgkin's, he's not gonna... he had two boys after.

Mariel: (Pointing to Ian) Your ex-girlfriend.

Bobby: Your ex-girlfriend. Cynthia.

Mariel: J Cynthia Brooks whom I saw in your movie... And she took... and what I love is she took.... she was self-responsible. She said, "This is my life. I'm gonna do something about it." And that's what a person has to do when they get cancer. They have to go, "Okay, bummer." [Chuckling] "Not fun. I don't like it." But look at every aspect of your life. If I were to give anybody advice like... pull your life apart. Look at yourself, emotionally, spiritually, mentally, physically... all these different things and say, "What can I do", which is everything.

Bobby: And we talk about the emotional body. The emotional body is just as huge as the physical.

Mariel: It's everything.

Bobby: But people don't pay attention to it. There's … there's a bunch of different types of bodies that we don't look at that doctors don't look at. They're... they're starting to know. And they're starting to say, "Hey, stress is a big part of all these diseases." Well, wow, let's take-a-look at that. So, it's starting to happen there as well and there's a lot of doctors that are saying, "Wait a minute, there's something with this food thing." And there's quite a few you know sort of going Eastern/Western both philosophies.

Mariel: Which is beautiful.

Bobby: That's fantastic combining the two.

Mariel: Yeah.

Bobby: And that's where we want to go. That's why we aren't gonna say, "Doctor's don't know anything."

Mariel: Cause that's not true.

Bobby: We get a little angry about the cancer part because look at the suffering that is going on. When they go in, they go in healthy. They come out, they're what?

Mariel: I mean, they are like Matt C.? It's not right. You know, it hurts.

Bobby: Something obviously doesn't work. It's become a little bit barbaric. You know, and if Matt were to come to us and we said just give us two months. You've been waiting this much time and your chemo doesn't start until December. So, October, November. We give you ozone. You do infrared saunas. We change your diet. We teach you how to meditate. We get rid of the sugar. We teach you to exercise. And this is what I wrote to him, Ian. You're gonna become bigger, faster, stronger and happier with us. And then go to the hospital and see if the tumor is gone. If not, choose your route. Okay.

Mariel: It's up to you.

Bobby: I want to guaranty you that the tumor will shrink in two months. Couldn't get him to do it. And that was the result. He thought that he was gonna be fine. I mean, eating out of a tube in his stomach. This is Matt the mailman who used to deliver. What's he delivering now? You know. And I feel BAD for him

Mariel: Yup.

Bobby: This is the way it is.

Ian: Yeah.

Bobby: So let's fight back man. Let's take a look at ourselves and figure all this stuff out. Get the information.

Ian: I mean, we are teaching by example.

Mariel: Absolutely.

Ian: So is there anything else we can do besides teaching by example?

Mariel: Well... my thing is... is like how you raise kids. If you want kids to do something, you have-to-do it yourself. So, if you want somebody to not eat sugar and live a healthier lifestyle you have to live a healthier lifestyle yourself. You have to cut those things out that you don't want another person to do.

That's the biggest teacher that anybody can do. Is, you know, we're just... we share who we are and how we live and there's no question that how we live is reflected in our life, in our energy, in our vitality, in our joy, in our happiness. So, if you can show up as an example (I tried to be an example and save those people with cancer from causes they haven't thought about because they are so focused on food … again, I feel what those autistic babies are feeling, and many parents do not know, and those babies are in toxic environments breathing those ubiquitous toxins. Even those who think they are doing well, for instance, Seventh Generation is full of pesticide. And what are they washing those babies clothes in, and who is holding those babies, that second hand "toxicants" causing those babies the inability to breath and intense internal burning they can't vocalize and seizures from grand mom's favorite "fragrance" or because Aunt Sue thought she was doing a good thing by using hand sanitizer before holding that "sick" baby? You can show up as an example that's the best thing you can do. Cause telling people what to do doesn't really work.

Bobby: Yup.

Ian: Politically, is there anything we can do?

Mariel: ehhhh

Bobby: Politically turns into an example, again. We feel like we are being more political than people that are into politics by changing ourselves as individuals and inspiring people to change themselves.

Mariel: To ask questions.

Bobby: And ask questions. One of the things in politics is you're supposed to question the government, nobody does. They say, "Well the government wouldn't do that. Or this wouldn't be this way, or the FDA wouldn't be set up like this? It's just not like that. They sit there and say, that, "Everything is fine." So, we stopped asking questions a long time ago and started following.

Mariel: Yeah.

Bobby: Just because a million people are following doesn't make it right. I think you need to step back from the crowd and ask the questions of why? How does this work? What's going on?

Mariel: And get involved...and tell your congressman that, you know, you're upset that you didn't know that your food can be tampered with every single day.

Mariel: They can change the regulations on organic and give you 35 chemicals in it! You know the FDA can change things. So, it's about knowing that we are the power. It's like... so when we say, you're your own guide, you're also your own politician, your own... it's taking responsibility. When you take responsibility, you start asking questions of your government, of your community, of all these different things because it's our responsibility to do that. We need to do that. If you want to close your eyes. Look the other direction then let everybody else take care of you, but don't be upset when you're sick or when things don't work out the way that you want them to.

Bobby: Or how about the government for that matter and how it's set up? They work for us. We pay their salaries with our taxes. They work for us. We are supposed to ask them questions about how this stuff works. We just stopped taking responsibility that's all it is. So, Mariel and I are trying to teach everybody to take responsibility for themselves first. And then for their families and then for their community. And that's what this place was supposed to be based on.

Mariel: Yup.

Bobby: That kind of thing. I mean the bartering system of food went on when I grew up. We had farms all around. You know, my family grew, you know, corn and tomatoes and had chickens and we'd trade with somebody who had the milk and you know, the wheat and... and, you know, the peppers and the broccoli. You know, we'd barter. We'd be like, "Okay, I'll trade you this for that, this for that, this for that. And everything was sort of equal. All the people are really well but, they didn't have to grow everything. So, if there were ten farms around and each farm grew ten things, you know, that's a hundred things and everybody got to have those things and you lived that way. We've gotten so far away from that.

Mariel: Yeah, and we just encourage people cause not everybody is gonna have a farm or even a garden, but you know, go to local farmers markets. Support your local community because your local community can be your... you know, your power base. And that can also be your health base. You can find health within your local community. A local farmer's market is unique... in its ability to give you something that enriches your life. So... you can change energetically on sooo many different levels just by what you ingest.

Bobby: and you want to be happy immensely go out and play again.
Mariel: Yeah exactly.
Bobby: I say to all these corporate people that we sit and talk in front of. I ask them a question. I say, "When is the last time you went out and played?" And they're like, "What are you talking about?"

Mariel: I got to the gym.
Bobby: What do you do for fun? They say, "I go to the gym." And I said, "But what do you do for fun?" "I go to the gym."

Bobby: I'm like, "That sounds like torture."
Mariel: Laughing.

Bobby: When is the last time you went out and played basketball? Or played with your kids? We look at them and watch them play, yet we stopped playing as adults for some reason. I mean, I don't. But, you know, mostly everybody else does. I have Mariel playing with me all the time, we go out and play all the time. And it raises your emotional body and it changes your energies in your body to be able to go out and play.

Mariel: And that's another healing tool. People have no idea how much laughter heals you. Laughter, fun it heals you. It makes you younger and if you're not well, it will make you well.

Bobby: Here's a great...
Mariel: It's one of the tools.
Bobby: Here's a great analogy we use as well. This is fantastic, and everybody relates to this. That, you know, has gone to school.
Mariel: Yeah.

Bobby: Do you remember how long the summers were when you were in elementary school or junior high school. You'd get out of school, you know, at the end of June, you're like, we don't have to go back to school until next year. And the summers were forever. It was for 12 weeks. If I told an adult today, that in 12 weeks...

Mariel: You have 12 weeks...
Bobby: to deliver such and such. They're like, "Oh, my God."
Mariel: I have no time.
Bobby: I have no time at all. But when we were kids.
Mariel: It was the world.

Bobby: We were so like in the moment that that was forever. And we lost touch with that. And Mariel and I are working our asses off trying to get back in touch with what it was like to be that. To be in the moment the whole time and to live in the now. And it's really important!

Mariel: Yeah.
Bobby: It's really important!

Mariel: Yup.

Bobby: And connect. Connect. Connect. The technology is really great but, to not connect like we're connecting not you're getting an original instant message from Mariel [chuckling]. We're all connected.

Mariel: The original …

Bobby: Yeah, it's fantastic. You nod your head, or smiling and stuff, you know.

Mariel: We know... yeah...

Bobby: What's going on. Instead of a text that, "Why did he say that?"

Mariel: Laughing.

Bobby: "What did he mean by that?" He left out a word or something or just the email, whatever. It's great to get in touch with, really quick. But to BE together and eat together... and that's Mariel's big thing... you know, communing.

Mariel: Ceremony and ritual involved in food. And all these things. All these different things, I mean getting back to cancer. All these different things are part of your healing modalities. Creating a sacred space in your home. You know, as simple as that, creating a space that you feel at peace. You feel calm. That's a healing environment. But it's also a living environment. You know.

Bobby: So that's it, that's all. What else do you need Ian?

Mariel: – Laughing.............

Ian here... FYI, Bobby and I were roommates and good friends in Hollywood back in the day. Starving actors, stuntmen, "Roxbury" VIP security for the stars and truth seekers from the get-go. He taught me raw, unpasteurized milk was healthy and pasteurized milk was poison in the early '90s. He was the first one I knew on the raw diet by Aajonus Vonderplanitz Way ahead of his time and a hell of a wrestler. [See Pic 25.1 and 25.2]

Mariel Hemingway_is Ernest Hemingway's granddaughter and the nicest movie star yours truly has ever met and I met 'em all as a VIP security guy in Tinsel Town. Mariel is an Oscar nominated actress and author of living/cooking right/raise your vibe, books. [See Pic 25.3] Love you Bobby and Mariel!

CHAPTER 26:

DR. WALLACH - DEAD DOCTORS DON'T LIE

(CLIP FROM ICURECANCER.COM)

My name is Dr. Joel Wallach. I'm 65 years old and I'm a physician.

I think the thing that makes my view different on health is that I'm a veterinarian as well as a physician. And in veterinarian medicine, we don't have insurance for animals like we do people. If we were to use a human health care type of system for livestock it'd be a sticker shock for ya. Your hamper? would cost you $275 a pound just to pay for the health care. We learned in the animal industry that we could keep the price of animal products down where the average person could afford to eat them every day simply by eliminating health care costs.

We do this with these little alfalfa pellets. Everybody's seen these little alfalfa pellets, mouse pellets, rat pellets, and hamster pellets and gerbil pellets. The reason why we put these animal feeds into the pelletized form is so that every mouth full is biochemically perfect. Every mouthful is perfect. Even the stupidest animal in the groups gets a perfect diet. And we have been so successful over the last 75 years we've eliminated 900 different diseases with this little program.

One of the things we learned in animals in 1912 was that the word nutrients could reduce the risk significantly of cancer. The original was selenium. In the Western world, this was actually in Germany and we learned that this trace mineral selenium could actually prevent and reduce the risk of certain cancers. Ten thousand years before that the Chinese realized that arsenic, a trace mineral, was a great treatment for certain types of blood cancers like leukemia and lymphomas and so the concept of nutrients being a preventative and treatment for cancer is not new.

We do know that antioxidants are just exceptional nutritional therapies for cancer and also preventative. For instance, you can reduce the risk of colon cancer with a single multiple, this was a nurse's health study from Harvard Medical School, they looked at 90,000 nurses over a 15 year period. They found that they can reduce the risk of colon cancer by 75 percent! That's right, 75 percent. There's no drug that would reduce the risk of colon cancer by 1 percent.

And then you take the antioxidants that are found in dark berries, such as blackberries and blueberries and black raspberries and black cherries and strawberries. These antioxidants that are found naturally in these dark berries can reduce the risk of colon cancer by 80 percent according to the University of Ohio.

And so there's an enormous amount of evidence to show that food substances and foods and trace minerals and vitamins can, in fact, reduce the risk of cancers. And some of them, like the trace mineral selenium, is an excellent choice for somebody who has prostate cancer, breast cancer. An enormous amount of evidence to show this.

If something would happen to somebody that I care about personally or if a patient would ask me, say, "Dr. Wallach, what would I do? I've been diagnosed with cancer; I want to know my options? What are all my options?

And personally, I would never recommend chemotherapy and radiation. There are times when surgery is important to remove large masses obstructing a blood vessel or maybe the digestive system and you have to do what's called de-bulking the system where you're removing a physician mass that's obstructing something. On occasion that's necessary. But there's more damage caused by chemotherapy and radiation than there is benefit. And you want to support the immune system which is the best friend of any cancer patient with all the known essential nutrients. People forget that the immune system needs nutrients to function just like everything else.

I would support their immune system with all the known essential nutrients. And then very specifically, I would throw in all of the antioxidants and I would err on the side of excess when it comes to the antioxidants. Doctors who treat cancer patients with chemotherapy and radiation, they get all concerned about people taking antioxidants when they're giving chemotherapy and radiation because they're afraid that the antioxidants will neutralize the damaging effects of the radiation and chemotherapy.

Well, I'd rather just leave out the radiation and chemotherapy and use only the vita-nutrients and the antioxidants.

Now personally I don't like to try to cure cancer because if you cure cancer you usually kill the patient. To kill cancer is very easy. But the side effect is the patient dies. So I'd rather talk about managing cancer. Where you support the immune system and you allow their immune system to defend them.

There are people who are told by their doctors, they had weeks or months or years to live and 30 years later they're still going. They still have their cancer, but their bodies have been given enough raw materials that the body's been able to learn to manage that cancer and keep it kind of walled off or keep it in the box as I say. So it doesn't kill the patient. So if you were to examine that patient they would still have the cancer. But it didn't kill 'em over a 30-year period when the doctor said they had six months to live!

Dr. Wallach's - Supplement's: Youngevity: http://iccessential.my90forlife.com/

CHAPTER 27:

EXTRAS

Here are some supplemental materials in the forms of links, videos, and so on, that you might find helpful:

Baking soda/maple syrup:

https://www.youtube.com/watch?v=gtT2dsAel9w

Cannabis oil making videos:

https://www.youtube.com/watch?v=Rm3o9IcsWfg

https://www.youtube.com/watch?v=qAyhQnBDE_I

https://www.youtube.com/watch?v=7m-l5PPDIhI

https://www.youtube.com/watch?v=0vmMR4RRA0k

I didn't have time to add another chapter right now but if I did it would be on **Jim Humble, Mark Grenon** and gang!   Their service to humanity by discovering and spreading the news about MMS Miracle Mineral Solution which kills pathogens better than any anti-biotic available.

http://genesis2church.is

Long story short, Jim Humble was in the jungle and his workers were dying of malaria. Someone said to try the stuff they use to purify our water systems.   Sodium chlorite is presently being promoted as a miracle mineral supplement or MMS with superior antimicrobial activity. You can appreciate its power from a statement by the discoverer of this remedy that all 75,000 individuals with malaria that have been treated were cured within a day, with 98% being cured within 4 hours. This obviously has great ramifications not only for self-healing but also for the drug industry and medicine. In the following I want to comment on these issues. (click that link for the article)
MMS is a unique chemical oxidizer that has the ability to enter the water, it kills pathogens that are causing diseases and touch absolutely nothing else.

Well, it worked for his workers' malaria then he went on to cure tribes of HIV with the Red Cross only to be chased out of the jungle by big pharma mafia. I highly recommend you research this man and his work.

Jim Humble:

https://www.youtube.com/watch?v=miJNgSOTLAQ&t=130s

Mark Grenon's - How to: MMS For Cancer.

https://www.youtube.com/watch?v=HgOC4ZwaAWs

MMS HIV:

https://www.youtube.com/watch?v=j9NbanNCAFQ

MMS Documentary:

https://www.youtube.com/watch?v=B6d0VZbDT1g&t=2897s

To Buy MMS:

https://g2sacraments.org

OTHER PRODUCTS I ENDORSE

Oceans Alive Sales Page Better Than EFA's!

http://www.activationproducts.com/jointventures?AFFID=61185

Panaseeda Oils: From makers of Ocean's Alive Phytoplankton. Top end oils like black seed oil, 5 oil blend, etc...

http://www.activationproducts.com/panaseeda?AFFID=6118

Ease Magnesium

http://activationaffiliates.com/?a=61185&c=21&p=r&s1=

Clar8ty Supplements for Health.

"To live as a "Master" does not mean to be "perfect." It means to be who you are as a Soul in a Body, and to express your Soul in alignment with Spirit, in everything that you experience and manifest on Earth." – Unknown

EPILOGUE

This book was to be released 3 years ago but apparently, the universe wasn't ready. I don't question Source. Now that it's finally transcribed and typed and corrected and re-corrected and added to and taken away, pictures lined up, up on Kindle, back to manuscript up again on Kindle, it's finally done! My truthful look at how folks have been curing themselves of cancer for decades. They do it holistically. Because you are not dying of cancer, you are just acidic and need to balance your alkalinity to a saliva pH of 7.2ish. That's it. No big deal. Follow Dr. Bernardo's protocol and I don't see how you can fail. I mean there is no silver bullet but there is a universal law of free will. Your free will, combined with non-toxic, noninvasive therapies will give you the best shot on the planet that I know of now. When I made the film, I realized my main job was accomplished to show you Western Medicine is not a choice. Just go holistic baby. Only way.

I'm happy the way Source worked through me to get this to you. It started with the documentary I Cure Cancer. This book although includes some of that, much of it is new material to back up the film. And of course, luckily, we salvaged a couple of versions of Dr. B's protocol to include.

I'll be making one more film on this subject called iCureCancer2.- Baby Killers. or something like that. Because sure I brought the world this documentary and book so you can now cure your cancer or have the best shot at it compared to the dismal and deprecating chemotherapy and radiation treatments Rockefeller medicine will give you. But you couldn't use it on your child. Can you believe that? In America, and the west in general, if you refuse chemotherapy and radiation on your children you get thrown in jail and they go to child services. I think everyone needs to know this.

Do you know what's funny? The reason I slowed up and never quite got I cure part 2 rolling was simply that YouTube came around and I just built the www.youtube.com/icurecancer2 channel. It's easier and quicker to just find the light or 411 and boom put it up for you there.

California decided to force vaccinate their children in 2015. So, I spent the summer fighting sb277 the law (YouTube series on this below) that says kids can't go to school if they don't take their shots. To make a long story short we lost and they now force vaccinate. Guess what's happened in their education budgeting? They need more special ed teachers because so many kids are getting Autism. Just like anyone with a brain knew would happen.

When I was a kid, there were 3 shots maybe. Now there is 70 plus before kindergarten. The reason is the Jesuits work with the Zionists and sacrifice our children to Lucifer. Only they got you doing it for them now. Do 2 hours of research on the ills of vaccine and you will understand the powers that be need you to suffer for the black magic demons they use to run the world. Don't believe me? Watch my series below and get the inside scoop from insiders like Sandi White, Janice Kirkpatrick, and Rosie Ferdin Cruz. (all front line sb 277'ers.) on how they have always known peanut oil in the vaccines cause SID's but Bush Sr. made a law stating they don't have to tell us what is in the vaccines instead of taking the peanut oil out. Or that the nagalase molecule injected into humans via vaccines ensures Cancer industry profits 'locked in'. It explains the aggressive vaccine push. Research that, if you don't believe me.

All diseases were dead thanks to nutrition, cleanliness, and plumbing. They did not stop Polio or Smallpox. The pharmaceutical companies just lay claim to the cure but it's not true. Just like the rest of our history. The Rothschild's have run the show from the get-go with the Masons and the Zionist's and Royals. Till we deal with these Mafia's we will be their slaves. So wake up!

157 Research Papers Supporting the Vaccine/Autism Link

https://www.scribd.com/doc/220807175/157-Research-Papers-Supporting-the-Vaccine-Autism-Link

Provaxxers debunk this. Her eyes, not the statistics.

https://www.youtube.com/watch?v=mMdObIbP8zs

Jury Nullification:

Everyone needs to know this. If you were a juror about to send a man to prison for 20 years because he grew medical marijuana that was curing people of cancer you could say you don't believe in the law and say not guilty! Or a parent doesn't want to inject unknown substances from big Pharma mafia into their kid's veins. Very important everyone knows this! So spread it around! The judges and lawyers won't tell you this!

http://law2.umkc.edu/faculty/projects/ftrials/zenger/nullification.html
http://silverunderground.com/2013/10/jury-nullification-ad-appears-in-subway-near-dc-superior-court

This graph [See Pic 28.1] is checkmate for any provaxers out there. Sorry, you have been duped. All diseases have gone thanks to cleanliness, nutrition, and plumbing. Sorry, Charlie. It's over.

Today I'm still making films. After I Cure2 I will be making "Space Cadet" next. A documentary on the stars.

On the side, because I can't say no to people in true desire for true medicine, I'm basically a cancer coach. And I teach kickboxing better than most, thanks to the trainers I've mentioned earlier. I work with my best friend Raul Rodriguez, who's a celebrity trainer for the stars and invented the R30 program. I used it to rehab after my recent full hip replacement and continue to do it daily with him today. We are starting a YouTube show called **Muscle Brain Fitness**. We have combined his pro trainer/rehab specialties with my kickboxing training and Holistic Health Coaching. This will be quality video content for those that can't make it to us in person. We plan to have plant-based cooking show's as well.

Dolphins – The Holistic Clinic

Another future project of mine is to make "Dolphins". A holistic health-and-wellness clinic in Costa Rica where the Dolphins hang out. Just swimming next to them is healing. Their frequency of the chirps and squeals they use for talking goes through us and heals us. That would be just one of the things to do while healing in the jungle/beach area I've got mapped out. Why not do Dr. Bernardo's protocol somewhere tropical? With waterfalls and dolphins to meditate with. It's going to be beautiful.

https://www.youtube.com/watch?v=qwEukGXnG5Y

Now that this book is done, I can get iCureCancer2 edited and out to the world as well. To show again that cancer is curable if you stay away from your oncologist but btw if your kid gets cancer you have no rights how they are treated. You have to give them chemo, radiation and surgery none of which would ever be my first choice for disease. You are not sick you are just out of balance. The government must rid us of the medical mafia once and for all or this world will continue to be in a pathetic state-of-affairs. One of suffering.

And if the Pleiadians don't come down in 2020 and just 86 the Rothschild's and all their minions... ahem... spiritually speaking of course... then we need to get 5000 people around each of their houses with pots and pans. Literally. Okay so I'm banking on the space brothers but whatever it takes. Are you with me? Godspeed then!

Watch this Expert Weapon YouTube series of mine and spread the news. Notice there is no 50-year-old Autistics? Cuz the shots didn't go up till the late '80s. Expect the demand for Special Ed teachers to continue to rise.

Ian Jacklin was the Expert Weapon in Martial Art films in the '90s and now for "We the People" enlightening folks on how to cure cancer holistically and why saying no to Vaccines now could make a champion later.

All on my http://www.youtube.com/IanJacklin

Trailer: https://www.youtube.com/watch?v=mXtjqcNCM0M

Expert Weapon 2.0

Episode 1: https://www.youtube.com/watch?v=xQt2UxmwlH0

Episode 2: https://www.youtube.com/watch?v=D2804xqLWAQ

Episode 3: https://www.youtube.com/watch?v=NPaHOmd8ATU&spfreload=10

Episode 4:   https://www.youtube.com/watch?v=pqHCQ-b4i8I&t=1389s&spfreload=10

Episode 5: https://www.youtube.com/watch?v=Wq8vpLkRtVc&t=635s&spfreload=10

Episode 6: https://www.youtube.com/watch?v=aemFAVhBDFk&spfreload=10

Episode 7: https://www.youtube.com/watch?v=0u6N_Jjcna0

Episode 8: https://www.youtube.com/watch?v=3m0z9tqqKQ4&t=9s&spfreload=10

Peace,
Ian Jacklin
April 30, 2019

Last thoughts from Ian:

You will keep reincarnating in the flesh till you learn to not hate, envy or be greedy. So good luck. Heaven awaits. On earth and off. Balance your pH, balance your life. My undying love to you all. I hope this helped.

Studying Blavatsky, I learned your soul is a piece of Source or God. Hence, we are all truly... God. Together. We are one.

Peace,
Ian Jacklin

ABOUT THE AUTHOR

[SEE PICTURE 29.1]

Ian Jacklin is documentary filmmaker, concert promoter, actor and kickboxing champion and holistic health coach. With three films produced and one world kickboxing title shot under his black belt, he's a warrior who persists until the fight is won or the project is done.

Jacklin, is a graduate of Joanne Baron, method acting, school. His 20-year acting career in Hollywood includes starring roles in Death Match and Expert Weapon as well as lead roles in several other action movies. His television credits include appearances on Days of Our Lives and the sitcom Just Shoot Me. His acting years coincided with his 10-year professional fighting career.

In 1990, he was chosen to be the light heavyweight in the camp of heavyweight boxing champ Lennox Lewis. A black belt in Kenpo karate, Jacklin went on to become the Canadian International Sport Karate Association's and the World Kickboxing and Karate Association's North American champion. He was ranked number two in the world by WKA in 1992.

During the last 15 years, his focus has been producing documentaries and health videos as owner of Co-dependent Pictures, Inc. His first two films were Rockumentaries one in NYC and one in upstate NY. Jacklin's current film, icurecancer.com is about people who cured themselves of deadly diseases after their doctors were unable to help them using holistic medicine. A short of it called Dr. Bernardo Majalca won runner up in the Magic Lantern International Movie Festival 2007.

Countless people now have healed holistically due to the film and now book while Jacklin works on editing: iCureCancer Part 2 – The Baby Killer Documentary. If you force chemo or vaccinations on children, I and all that is holy will find you. Expect us.

For more information about Ian visit www.archangelstudios.org and www.icurecancer.com.

PHOTO GALLERY

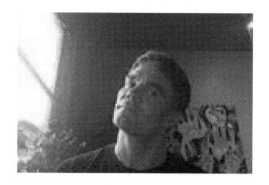

Ian Jacklin Dedication Picture

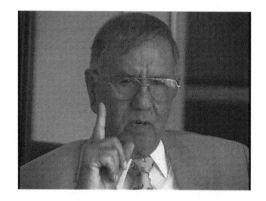

Dr Bernardo Majalca 2004

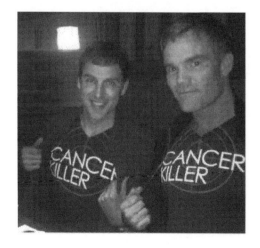

Chris Wark interview Picture 1.1

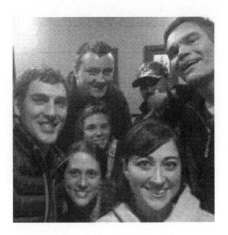

L.J. Devon and wife, Howard Hoffman, Chris Wark, Joni Abbott, Rachel Rene, Ian Jacklin,
Changing the world one seminar at a time. Picture 1.2

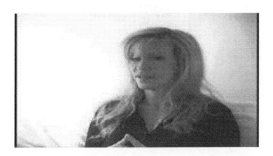

Cynthia Brooks Picture 2.1

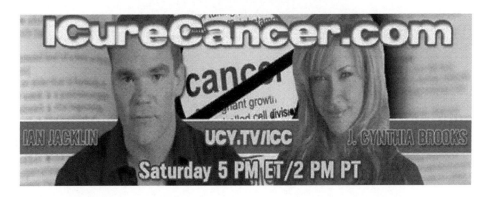

Radio show Cynthia and Ian did together. Picture 2.2

PHOTO GALLERY

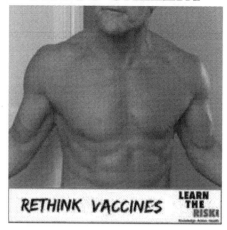

Rethink Vaccines Picture 2.3

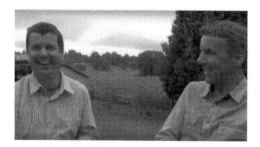

Ian Clark from Oceans Alive and Adrian Quinn organic farmer chat on holistic health Picture 5.1

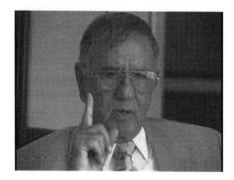

Dr. Bernardo Maljaca Picture 6.1

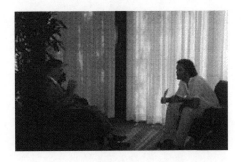

Ian and Dr. B at the 2004 Cancer Control Society– Picture 6.2

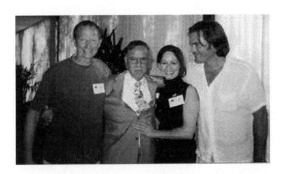

Jim Hawks, Dr. Bernardo, Jessica Biscardi, Ian Jacklin Picture 7.1

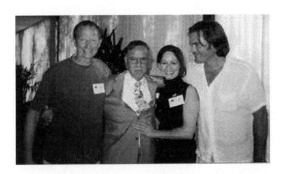

Sample Supplement Order Form Picture 7.2

PHOTO GALLERY

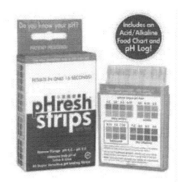

pH strips Image 7.3

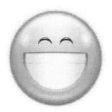

Attitude Makes a Big Difference Image 7.4

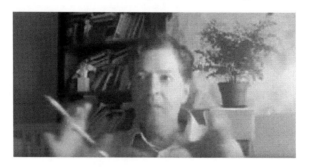

John Forrester Handed me this interview before he died knowing I would make sure it got to you. RIP.
Picture 8.1

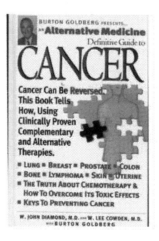

Burton Goldburg Picture 10.1

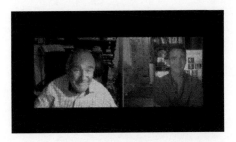

Burton and I on ZenLive.tv for one of our many interviews. Picture 10.2

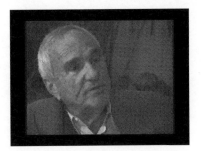

BurtonGoldberg.com @ CancerControlSociety.org – 2004 Picture 10.3

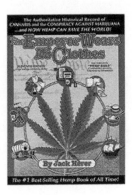

The Emperor Wear No Clothes By Jack Herer Picture 11.1

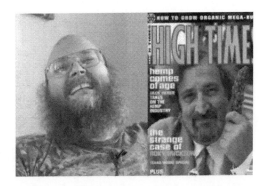

Ronnie Smith and High Times pic with Jack Herer on it Picture 11.2

PHOTO GALLERY

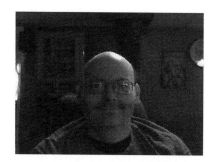

Ronnie Smith Picture 11.3

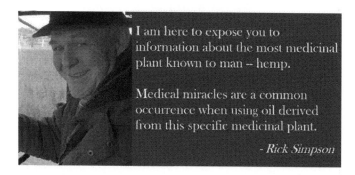

II Cure Cancer ZenLive.TV with Rick Simpson Picture 12.1

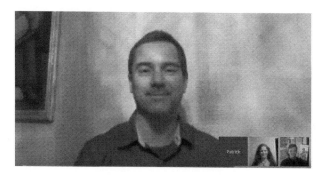

Dr. Vickers, Organic Lynette and Ian Jacklin on ZenLive.TV Picture 13.1

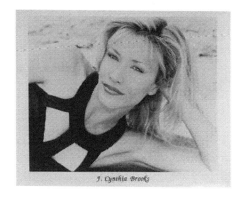

J. Cynthia Brooks Picture 14.1

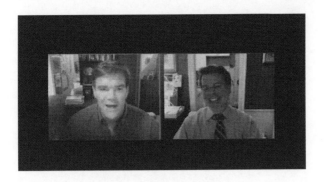

Nick Gonzales and I on ZenLive.tv Picture 15.1

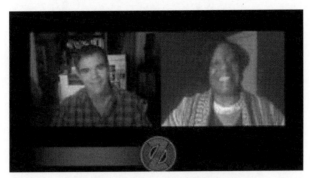

Ian Jacklin and Essene Rev. Lynne Deverges on ZenLive.TV Pic 16.1

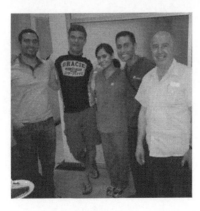

American Biodental Clinic TiJuanna Mexico Picture 18:1

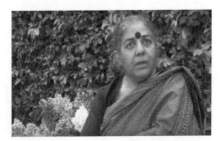

Vandanna Shiva at AXE Venice Beach Picture 19.1

PHOTO GALLERY

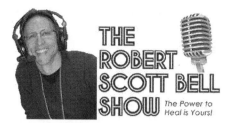

The Robert Scott Bell Show Picture 20.1

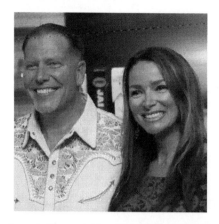

Real life superhero's Ty and Charlene Bollinger Picture 22.1

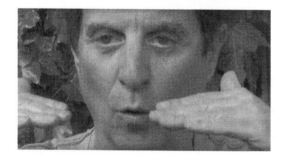

Richard Gordon - Quantumtouch.com. Picture 24.1

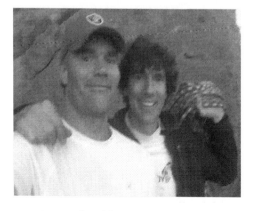

Ian and Bobby Picture 25.1

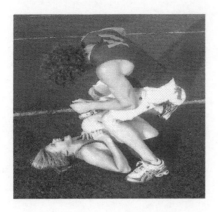

Bobby Williams and girlfriend, Mariel Hemingway. Pic 25.2

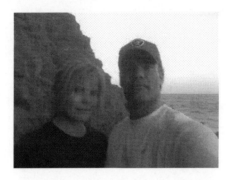

Mariel Hemingway and Ian Pic 25.3

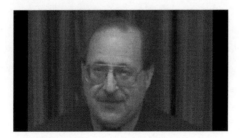

Dr. Joel Wallach – Author of Dead Doctors Don't Lie Picture 26.1

PHOTO GALLERY

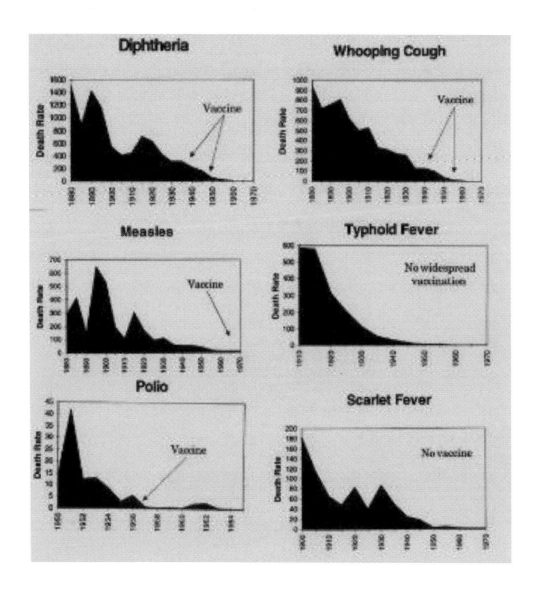

Vaccine/Disease Chart picture 28.1

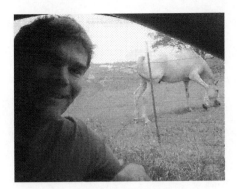

Ian Jacklin Picture 29.1

MORE PICTURES OF IAN JACKLIN

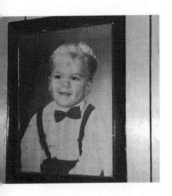

Born August 22, 1968

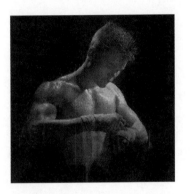

Became a Championship Fighter

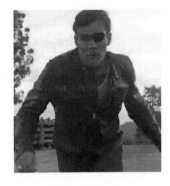

Became and Action Hero

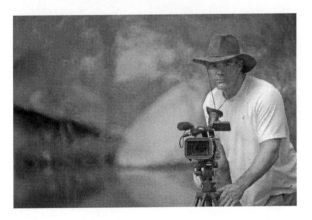

Became a Filmmaker

PHOTO GALLERY

My first dream was to fight for the world title. On the way to the title I had some really good fights like this one with Louis Neglia's fighter John Kenny at Madison Square Garden. I was on that night, he wasn't so I took a unanimous decision.

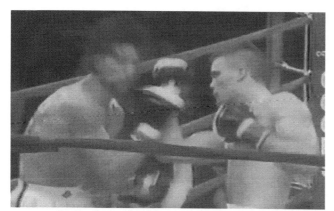
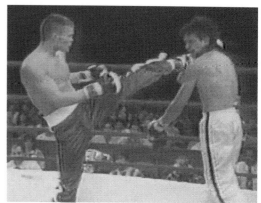

I also boxed with Lennox Lewis stable as the Light Heavy in 1989 after he won Gold

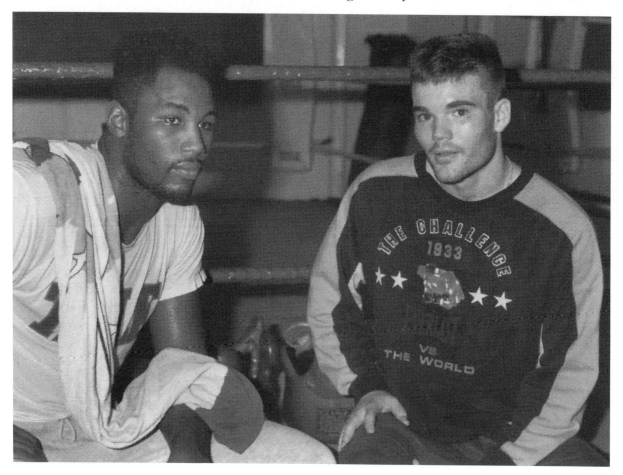

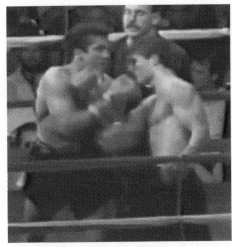

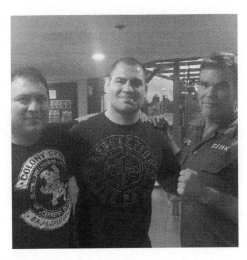

World Title – Javier Mendez Vs Ian Jacklin. Promoted by Scott Coker.   Javier, Cain, and Ian

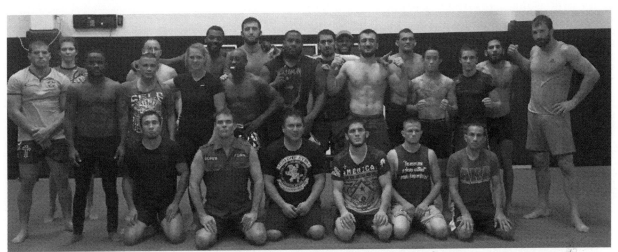

Luke Rockhold & Khabib Nurmagomedov and gang.

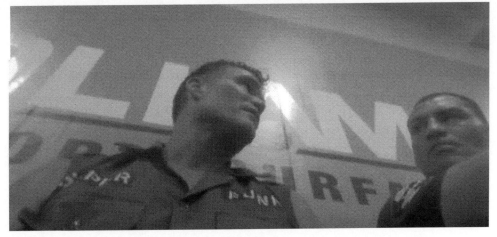

Cain Velasquez learns the ills of vaccines firsthand

PHOTO GALLERY

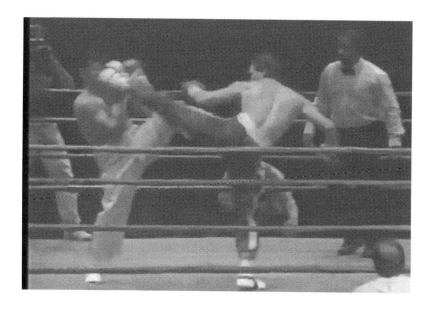

Javier thought it was a jab I was hitting him with he told me. He said my corner yelled no that's his foot. He's kicking you in the face! What a war that first fight was. Another fight of the night but back in those days there was little money. I got $2400 to fight him for the world title in 93.

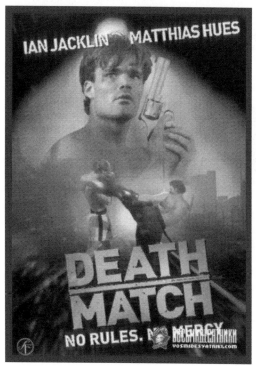

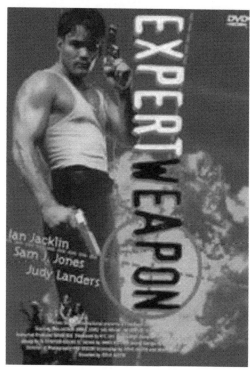

My other dream from childhood, other than fighting for title, was to star in a movie. And I And I got to do that too! So always dream. That's how you manifest things…!

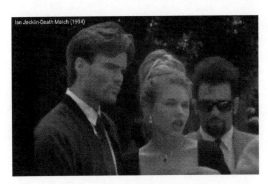

Ian Jacklin with co-star Rene Allman

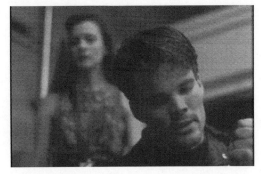

Ian Jacklin with co-star Julie Merril

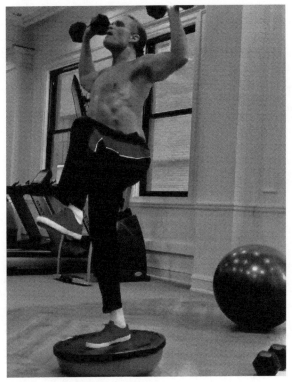

Still reaching for the Sky

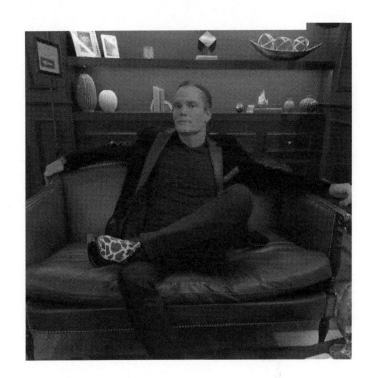

IanJacklin.com

Printed by Amazon Italia Logistica S.r.l.
Torrazza Piemonte (TO), Italy

15903092R10243